CONCISE GUIDE TO

The Psychiatric Interview of
Children and Adolescents

American Psychiatric Press
CONCISE GUIDES

Robert E. Hales, M.D.
Series Editor

CONCISE GUIDE TO

The Psychiatric Interview of Children and Adolescents

Claudio Cepeda, M.D.
Clinical Associate Professor
Department of Psychiatry
University of Texas Health Science Center at San Antonio
San Antonio, Texas

American
Psychiatric
Press, Inc.

Washington, DC
London, England

Note: The authors have worked to ensure that all information in this book concerning drug dosages, schedules, and routes of administration is accurate as of the time of publication and consistent with standards set by the U.S. Food and Drug Administration and the general medical community. As medical research and practice advance, however, therapeutic standards may change. For this reason and because human and mechanical errors sometimes occur, we recommend that readers follow the advice of a physician who is directly involved in their care or the care of a member of their family.

Copyright © 2000 American Psychiatric Press, Inc.
ALL RIGHTS RESERVED
Manufactured in the United States of America on acid-free paper

03 02 01 00   4 3 2 1

American Psychiatric Press, Inc.
1400 K Street, N.W.
Washington, DC   20005
www.appi.org

Library of Congress Cataloging-in-Publication Data
Cepeda, Claudio, 1942–
    Concise guide to the psychiatric interview of children and
adolescents / Claudio Cepeda.
        p.   cm. — (Concise guides / American Psychiatric Press)
    Includes bibliographical references and index.
    ISBN 0-88048-330-X
    1. Interviewing in child psychiatry Handbooks, manuals, etc.
2. Interviewing in adolescent psychiatry Handbooks, manuals, etc.
I. Title.   II. Title: Psychiatric interview of children and
adolescents.   III. Series: Concise guides (American Psychiatric
Press).
    [DNLM: 1. Interview, Psychological—methods—Adolescence
Handbooks.   2. Interview, Psychological—methods—Child Handbooks.
3. Interview, Psychological—methods—Child, Preschool Handbooks.
4. Psychiatry—methods—Adolescence Handbooks.   5. Psychiatry—
methods—Child Handbooks.   6. Psychiatry—methods—Child, Preschool
Handbooks.   WS 39 C399c 2000]
RJ503.6.C46   2000
618.92'89—dc21
DNLM/DLC
for Library of Congress   99-26053
                                                                                            CIP

British Library Cataloguing in Publication Data
A CIP record is available from the British Library.

This book is dedicated to my wife, Rosalba;
to my children, Rene, Adrian, and Joe;
and
to the memory of my niece Yvonne ("Bombis"), my
nephew Edgar Hernando, and my dear friend
Hector Tejada, M.D., all of whom passed away
while this book was being written.

CONTENTS

LIST OF TABLES

LIST OF CASE EXAMPLES[1]

[1] Patients' names and some biographic data have been changed to ensure confidentiality.

INTRODUCTION

to the American Psychiatric Press Concise Guides

The American Psychiatric Press Concise Guides Series provides, in an accessible format, practical information for psychiatrists, psychiatry residents, and medical students working in a variety of treatment settings, such as inpatient psychiatry units, outpatient clinics, consultation-liaison services, and private office settings. The Concise Guides are meant to complement the more detailed information to be found in lengthier psychiatry texts.

The Concise Guides address topics of special concern to psychiatrists in clinical practice. The books in this series contain a detailed table of contents, along with an index, tables, figures, and other charts for easy access. The books are designed to fit into a lab coat pocket or jacket pocket, which makes them a convenient source of information. References have been limited to those most relevant to the material presented.

Robert E. Hales, M.D., M.B.A.
Series Editor
American Psychiatric Press
  Concise Guides

INTRODUCTION

FOREWORD

I was delighted when I first read the manuscript for *Concise Guide to the Psychiatric Interview of Children and Adolescents* by Claudio Cepeda, M.D. Many issues came to mind that excited me. I have been a child and adolescent psychiatrist for more than 30 years and during most of that time have been involved in practice, teaching, and exploring the reaches and boundaries of child and adolescent development. My preoccupations never culminated in formal research, yet I was always asking and seeking answers to the big questions—"What?" and "Why?"—and, of course, exploring the issue of "How?"

As long ago as 1974, I postulated that the special medical discipline of child and adolescent psychiatry had become a science. I contended that the evolution of our training had followed the qualifying criteria to become a science and that our practices encompassed the following defining characteristics:

- Traditions/mystique
- Philosophy/belief
- Art
- Science
- Imitation
- Training
- Supervision
- Practice

Dr. Cepeda reminds us again that our discipline encompasses all of those components.

His thorough analysis and descriptions of each of the steps of the psychiatric interview brilliantly exhibit those elements that derive from philosophy, tradition, art, and science. His approach keeps our formulations and diagnoses in the most relevant realm and, therefore, our treatments most appropriate for the complete and accurate understanding of our patients.

Additionally, his skillful detailing of the psychiatric examination renews our commitment to the concept of mental illness as biopsychosocial. He keeps the several components in their particular places in our special field. Dr. Cepeda writes clearly and precisely about the psychiatric evaluation and does not go far beyond what we can and should learn from the accomplishment of a complete psychiatric examination. Nothing of value is overlooked, and no guesswork is endowed with truth.

The author's dedication to the completeness of the psychiatric examination of children and adolescents is the hallmark of this work. It is this quality that will interest, enthuse, and educate the student, while providing the veteran practitioner with refreshing reflections, remarkable reminders, and enlightening reassurances. True to the author's aim, the volume can also serve as an excellent resource for information and techniques for all other medical practitioners and mental health care providers. We have long needed such a volume. It's very good to have it at last.

I am delighted that Dr. Cepeda wrote this book, delighted that it is available for you to read and study, and finally, delighted to have this opportunity to endorse such a monumentally detailed and valuable achievement.

Lawrence A. Stone, M.D.
Past President, American Academy of Child and Adolescent Psychiatry
Clinical Professor of Psychiatry, University of Texas Health Science Center at San Antonio
Executive Medical Director, Laurel Ridge Hospital, San Antonio, Texas

INTRODUCTION

Contemporary interviewing is direct and syndromically oriented. The examiner specifically seeks clinical complexes that correspond to identifiable illnesses or disorders. Once a defined disorder has been identified, the examiner proceeds to uncover comorbid disorders or conditions most commonly associated with the primary disorder (see Note 1). At the same time, the examiner observes and pursues major characterological patterns of coping and problem solving and the relevant psychosocial stressors that activate or maintain the ongoing psychopathology. Contemporary assessment of children and adolescents demands, as an essential component of the diagnostic process, direct interviewing and formulation of the children under investigation. This component is considered a sine qua non element of the psychiatric evaluation. The systematic psychiatric examination of children created a real revolution in the field of child and adolescent psychiatry. The individual diagnostic assessment is being extended, now, to the earliest disturbances of infancy.

Performing mental status examinations on children and adolescents is a recent development in the field of child and adolescent psychiatry. Not long ago, child psychiatrists had a reserved attitude toward diagnosis and were wary about the nosological labeling of children. Child psychiatrists used to relegate the diagnostic data gathering to other mental health professionals and based their diagnostic inferences primarily on parental reports and play observations. This approach was partly the result of the limited credence given to the children's own accounts.

Direct interviewing and direct questioning of children regarding specific symptoms started 30 years ago. Systematic interviewing of children and adolescents is a more recent development. Many factors have promoted the need for a systematic and reliable interview process and for an accurate diagnosis: major advances in psychiatric nosology and epidemiology, the growing importance of longitudinal studies, the progressive influence of outcome studies, the unparalleled progress of psychopharmacology and other allied fields, and the revolution of managed care in the provision of heath services.

There is an increasing recognition that child psychiatric syndromes have equivalence to adult syndromes and that many adult disorders start in childhood. The continuity of a variety of childhood psychiatric disorders into adulthood has been demonstrated. This is particularly true of attention-deficit/hyperactivity disorder, mood and anxiety disorders, and other disorders.

The recognition of childhood depression as a syndrome dates back to no more than 25 years ago. Childhood depression was not officially recognized in the United States until the 1975 National Institute of Mental Health (NIMH) Conference on Depression in Childhood (1, p. 709).

Spitz's pioneering research in infants, in which he observed the effect of separating children from their mothers, advanced the concepts of hospitalism and anaclitic depression (2, 3). However, his far-reaching insights did not gain extension into the analogous disorders of childhood and adolescence. It took clinicians a long time to recognize that the depressive syndrome could be precipitated by a multiplicity of factors other than separation from the mother.

The importance of the child interview increased when child psychiatrists determined that there were a number of symptoms or subjective states for which only the children themselves could give a valid account. Parents may be completely unaware of their child's inappropriate guilt, obsessions, depressive mood, self-esteem problems, delusional beliefs, suicidal preoccupations, anxious worries, hallucinations, and other symptoms (4, p. 381). In contrast, parents can provide invaluable information in the evaluation of externalizing disorders. They are also better informants in areas of development and in the medical and family history.

Progress in the field of psychiatric diagnosis and the expansion of therapeutic options have created the need for diagnostic validity and reliability, which has increased the importance of the interviewing process. These changes have given impetus to the development of reliable methods for conducting and documenting the mental status examination in children and adolescents.

New concerns with cost-effectiveness make it imperative that diagnostic processes be sound and that relevant therapeutic recommendations be implemented. There is nothing more cost-effective than performing an accurate diagnosis and developing a relevant treatment plan.

There are growing concerns that the extraordinary progress in neurosciences (e.g., biochemistry, genetics, imaging), the progress in diagnostic assessment (neuropsychological evaluation, in particular), and other diagnostic procedures may mislead clinicians into thinking that the interview process is no longer of fundamental importance. We strongly argue in favor of the primacy and importance of the clinical interview. This stance parallels Akiskal and Akiskal's point of view: "The mental status examination represents the most important step in the clinical evaluation of individuals suffering from or suspected of having mental disorders" (5, p. 25).

Many psychiatrists delegate diagnostic questions to testing procedures: psychological, neuropsychological, and others. Although these procedures are of immense value, they are only aids to the diagnostic process. Tests are not a substitute for careful and comprehensive diagnostic evaluation. It is the clinician's responsibility to guide the testing and to specify the pertinent questions that need clarification; this effort should not be delegated. If clinicians were to take advantage of the richness and possibilities of the interview, two positive cost-effective results in the utilization of testing would ensue: 1) improvement of the clinical usefulness of tests by obtaining responses to more specific or sophisticated questions and 2) elimination of testing redundancy.

Some clinicians believe that the existence of structured protocols for a variety of psychiatric conditions makes open and semi-structured interviews dispensable. This is arguable. According to Akiskal and Akiskal, "Although a multitude of structured psychopathological interview schedules are now available for clinical research, the evaluation of mentally ill patients is still very much an art that depends on experience and clinical judgement" (5, p. 49).

In spite of the great contributions of the neurosciences to psychiatric diagnosis, the field still relies extensively on methodical and comprehensive history gathering and on observations and inferences obtained during the interview process. Armed with the latter, the examiner advances an understanding of the child's psychiatric conditions and of the child's internal and interpersonal worlds. There are no better alternatives to reach an understanding of the patient's presenting problems or their emotional lives. Sensitive questions become the real "probes" of the mind.

Even with specific disorders, such as depression, oppositional disorder, and attention-deficit/hyperactivity disorder, the unstructured section of the interview (see Chapter 1) gives the patient opportunities to express ongoing concerns or other active emotional conflicts that contribute to the complexities of the clinical picture or that may have a bearing on treatment.

It is of very limited value to conduct diagnostic inquiries with the limited purpose of establishing a DSM-IV diagnosis. The child psychiatric diagnostic interview transcends the narrow objective of arriving at a diagnosis according to DSM-IV. Data gathering needs to identify the psychological sources of distress, the detrimental developmental forces, and other noxious circumstances that contribute to the child's overall dysfunction.

The process of interviewing the child or adolescent alone decontextualizes the child from family factors and other systemic realities; these factors may play a fundamental role in the child's overall maladaptation. To stress the obvious, the interview of the child or adolescent alone provides only part of the information needed to develop a solid diagnosis and a comprehensive treatment plan. The examiner also needs to collect data related to the child's personnel and interpersonal contexts.

In the field of medicine, the quality of the data gathered during the patient examination depends on the quality and thoroughness of the examination and on the degree of rapport established between the patient and the doctor. This is even more important in the field of psychiatry, where relevant data deals with private feelings, inner thoughts, and subjective experiences.

Progress in biological psychiatry may lead us to believe that new pharmacological agents will provide solutions to our human problems. Contrary to excessive claims, biological agents are for the most part palliative (see Note 2). Psychotropic medications are more effective when combined with psychosocial interventions, and multidimensional treatments are better than isolated psychopharmacological or psychotherapeutic interventions.

Most psychiatric pathology does not follow an acute, infectious course but a chronic one. In most cases, the psychiatrist must formulate a comprehensive rehabilitation plan to deal with the long-term consequences of psychiatric disorders and associated comorbidities. For this reason, the child and adolescent psychiatrist's long-term relationship with the developing patient is imperative. A secure step is taken in this difficult enterprise when the examiner gains the child's and the family's trust, and when he or she stimulates their interest in participating in the diagnostic and treatment process.

Skillful interviewing should be a fundamental teaching objective in the training of general psychiatric and child and adolescent psychiatric residents and of other mental health professionals. For the novice interviewer, examining children is baffling and intimidating. It is hoped that this concise introduction will help the beginner to become more confident and better equipped in this fundamental clinical skill.

Professional maturation in the field is reflected in the manner and efficiency (i.e., the art and science) with which the examiner extracts diagnostic information, and in the manner with which the examiner entices the child and family into further diagnostic work. In contemporary competitive practice, diagnostic ability, formulation of cases, and provision of relevant consultation to other child and adolescent professionals are skills in great demand.

■ ABOUT THE BOOK

This book contains general guidelines that are addressed to child psychiatric and general psychiatric residents and medical students.

This book also has relevance to other mental health professionals who deal with children and adolescents and their families. It is hoped that the interviewing principles presented will be useful in learning or improving interviewing diagnostic skills and in making the art of interviewing more fascinating and productive.

The author has more than 25 years of experience in the evaluation and treatment of severely disturbed children and adolescents and has enjoyed a rewarding experience of teaching the interview process for many years to psychiatric residents and to child and adolescent fellows in the Department of Psychiatry at the University of Texas Health Science Center at San Antonio.

The case examples presented in this book were gathered in the multiethnic and rich cultural and historical background of south Texas, which has been enriched even further by many mixed marriages between American military personal and persons from Europe and from the Middle and Far East.

The book consists of 11 chapters. Because the ultimate objective of the diagnostic interview is the development of a DSM-IV–oriented diagnosis and the creation of a comprehensive diagnostic formulation, all the chapters converge to Chapter 8 (on comprehensive psychiatric formulation).

Chapter 1 deals with general aspects of interviewing, phases of the diagnostic interview, and strategies and considerations regarding different situations of the interview process. Chapter 2 is an introduction to nonverbal interviewing techniques. Chapter 3 deals with documentation of the mental status examination. Chapter 4 deals with the process of interviewing internalizing symptoms. Chapter 5 deals with the process of interviewing externalizing symptoms. Chapter 6 addresses the evaluation of some special symptoms. Chapter 7 is an introduction to the neuropsychiatric examination of children. Chapter 8 deals with theory and pragmatics of the formulation process and presents a model for a comprehensive psychiatric diagnostic formulation. Chapter 9 is a brief discussion of issues related to symptom formation and symptom maintenance. Chapter 10 deals with obstacles or resistances emerging during the diagnostic interviewing, and Chapter 11 deals with some issues related to countertransference responses surfacing during the diagnostic interview.

■ A WORD ABOUT CITATIONS

The vast majority of ideas in this book have been extracted from the body of knowledge existing in the field and from professional and teaching experience. It is impossible to give due credit to each of the concepts presented in this book. Standard sources, controversial areas, and recent contributions have been referenced. Some ideas may have not given a deserved credit to their respective creators. The author apologizes for this; the omission was not intended.

Thank you.

■ NOTES

1. The concept of comorbidity has been helpful in addressing the multiple dimensions of dysfunctional behavior implicated in any child's maladjustment. This concept has some potential for misuse, however. The increasing concern about polypharmacy in child psychiatry has comorbidity as one of its sources.

2. Long-term follow-up outcome data on bipolar disorders are rather sobering: "In spite of vigorous individualized prophylactic management, 37% [of the patients] had a recurrence episode of depression or mania within one year and 73% within five years. Of the patients who did not have discrete relapse episodes, 46% still had significant manic or depressive symptoms or both, and only 17% stayed euthymic or had minimal symptoms. Only 28% had good occupational outcomes. Relapses were more common in patients with more prior episodes or a history of psychotic symptoms and occurred sooner in patients with poorer occupational adjustment." (6, p. 4; 7).

■ REFERENCES

1. Weller EB, Weller RA: Bipolar disorders in children: misdiagnosis, underdiagnosis, and future directions. J Am Acad Child Adolesc Psychiatry 34:709–714, 1995

2. Spitz R: Hospitalism: An Inquiry Into the Genesis of Psychiatric Conditions in Early Childhood; The Psychoanalytic Study of the Child, Vol 1. New York, International Universities Press, 1945, pp 53–74

3. Spitz R: Anaclitic Depression: An Inquiry Into the Genesis of Psychiatric Conditions in Early Childhood; II: The Psychoanalytic Study of the Child, Vol 2. New York, International Universities Press, 1946, pp 313–342

4. Puig-Antich J, Gittelman R: Depression in childhood and adolescence, in Handbook of Affective Disorders. Edited by Paykel ES. New York, Guilford, 1982, pp 379–392

5. Akiskal HS, Akiskal K: Mental status examination; the art and science of the clinical interview, in Diagnostic Interviewing, 2nd Edition. Edited by Hersen M, Turner SM. New York, Plenum, 1994, pp 25–51

6. Yager I: Managing bipolar disorder. Journal Watch for Psychiatry 2:4, 1996

7. Gitlin MJ, Swendsen J, Heller TL, et al: Relapse and impairment in bipolar disorder. Am J Psychiatry 152:1635–1640, 1995

ACKNOWLEDGMENTS

I want to express appreciation and gratitude to the many individuals who contributed to the success of this project.

I extend special gratitude to my great teachers at the University of Michigan: Humberto Nagera, M.D., Jose Carreras, M.D., Mary Kemme, Ph.D., and Morton Chethik, M.S.W. They have been a source of ongoing inspiration. Gratitude is also extended to Carl Pfeifer, M.D., my former boss, who for many years supported my ideas and encouraged my writing.

I am especially grateful to Robert Leon, M.D., former chairman of the Department of Psychiatry at the University of Texas Health Science Center at San Antonio (UTHSCSA), and to Kenneth Matthews, M.D., residency training director in the Department of Psychiatry at UTHSCSA, who gave ongoing counsel and encouragement throughout this project. Graham Rogeness, M.D., medical director of the Southwest Mental Health Center, supported the writing of this book by allowing me to take time off from the busy clinical group practice. He also read Chapter 8 and offered useful suggestions. Clark Terrell, M.D., director of the Psychotherapy Training Program in the Department of Psychiatry at UTHSCSA, and Geoff Gentry, Ph.D., director of psychological assessment at the Southwest Mental Health Center, also read Chapter 8 and offered valuable ideas regarding emphasis and clarity.

I am indebted to David Fuller, M.D., who created the AMSIT, for allowing the use of its format in Chapter 3.

Many thanks are presented to Robert E. Hales, M.D., editor of the American Psychiatric Press Concise Guides Series, for his multiple suggestions in making the text more didactic and focused; to Pamela Harley, managing editor of the American Psychiatric Press book division, for her help in bringing this book to print; and to the American Psychiatric Press editorial and production staff for the multiple suggestions and modifications of the manuscript that made the text more clear and coherent.

Particular gratitude is extended to Larry Stone, M.D., former president of the American Academy of Child and Adolescent Psychiatry, for his interest in and support of this book and for his willingness to write its foreword.

I am deeply indebted to many people for improving the organization and readability of the text. James Smith, M.A., former director of the adolescent program at San Antonio State Hospital, read a preliminary draft and offered many corrections and helpful suggestions. Marie Beyer, M.A., L.P.C., lent her time and support on multiple occasions and read and corrected preliminary drafts. She also read and corrected the book proofs. Her support and assistance in the completion of this book have been immense. Kay Pergrem, M.A., L.C.P., L.C.D.C., offered valuable suggestions on organizing the draft. Her interest and support are highly appreciated. Linda Rasmussen, M.Ed., went over the whole manuscript with a fine-tooth comb and meticulously reviewed the text's grammar and syntax. Her contribution to this project is especially recognized.

Many psychiatric residents and fellows in child and adolescent psychiatry assisted me in a variety of ways and on many occasions volunteered to conduct bibliographic searches. Angie Montoya, M.D., read the manuscript and offered suggestions to improve its clarity. Juan Campos, M.D., helped in gathering the references for Chapter 8.

I am particularly grateful to the secretarial support provided by Joyce Jones and Sandra Smythe at the Psychotherapy Training Program in the Department of Psychiatry at UTHSCSA and by Marcy Barrera, Sherri Moczygemba, and Susan Barger at the Southwest Mental Health Center. Marcy aided in so many ways that it's difficult to give enough credit to her help; Sherri printed and reprinted multiple drafts and helped to format the original manuscript. Susan provided immense assistance in the final formatting and presentation of the original manuscript.

Special recognition is given to Sharon Stanush, former president of the Southwest Mental Health Center, for making the Center's resources available to me.

Last but not least, I thank my wife for her unending support with this project and for her patience and understanding during the many hours this effort took away from our marital and family life.

GENERAL PRINCIPLES OF INTERVIEWING

Diagnostic interviewing is a collaborative process that involves the psychiatric examiner, the identified patient, and the patient's family. Its purpose is to reach a comprehensive diagnostic formulation (see Chapter 8) that will form the foundation of a comprehensive treatment plan.

■ INTERVIEW SETTING

The diagnostic interview is usually conducted in a professional setting, ideally in an appropriately arranged office space; however, it may take place in other locations. For example, productive interviews can occur in a classroom, in a hospital at the child's bedside, or in a playground. The setting is determined by the spirit, purpose, and objectives of the interview rather than by the nature of the space or the environmental features surrounding the patient and the examiner. The most important element of the interview setting is the climate of receptivity, warmth, and cooperative interest that the examiner creates. No matter where the interview is carried out, the child and the child's family need to feel welcome, respected, and understood. An attitude of hope and helpfulness should permeate all transactions with the child and the family.

Safety—the child's and the examiner's—is a basic consideration for all evaluations. In professional settings, any objects found in the examiner's office (e.g., items used to decorate the office) may be used during play with the child, but the child could also use such objects as weapons in a moment of dyscontrol. The examiner should keep this risk in mind when making decisions regarding the examination space and the office decor. Similarly, children (especially preschoolers) should not be left in the reception area without adult supervision while the parents are interviewed; this is especially true if the child has a history of impulsive or destructive behavior.

■ PREPARATION FOR THE PSYCHIATRIC EXAMINATION

Ideally, children and adolescents should be prepared for the psychiatric examination. Parents need to receive guidance on what to tell the child regarding the examination. The type of guidance needed depends greatly on the relationship between the parents and the child. If open hostility exists between the two, the child may not be amenable to adequate preparation.

In general, parents need to address the distressing symptoms that disturb the child or the problematic behaviors that put the child in conflict with others. If the child feels depressed, for instance, parents will tell the child that he or she will be taken to a child psychiatrist in order to find out why he or she feels that way and to get help. In some cases, parents will want to tell the child that the psychiatrist will help the child discover why he or she is getting into trouble at school or at home.

Parents are often not forthright with a child regarding the need for psychiatric evaluation. When parents feel intimidated or when they fear the child's response, they are likely to be less than candid. In these circumstances, parents often cajole or deceive the child by saying that he or she will be taken to a medical doctor, a counselor, a special school, or somewhere else. In crisis or emergency situations, the preparatory aspects of the interview are usually dispensed with.

Children rarely express explicit concerns about their symptoms, but this does not mean they are happy with their problems. Children with psychiatric symptoms are unhappy to a greater or lesser extent but prefer to save face rather than acknowledge responsibility for maladaptive behaviors; however, they may be willing to change when the right person and the right circumstances present themselves. If the child is given this opportunity, the chances for involving him or her in the examination and in the treatment process may increase.

For some children the interview may become a turning point in their lives and may have a long-lasting, positive effect. The interview needs to be considered in a wide perspective rather than with narrow and immediate objectives. If the examiner is unsuccessful, or, worse, if he or she becomes critical, aversive, or psychologically negative to the child, the end result may be detrimental for future evaluations or psychiatric interventions.

■ INTERVIEW PROCESS

Before a face-to-face interview with the parents and the child, the examiner needs to clarify the nature of the problem(s) that prompted the evaluation. Contact with the referral agent (e.g., school or other agencies) helps the examiner sort out issues that need to be addressed during the assessment. The referral agent may be able to provide additional information or clarify the questions at hand. This preliminary review of the situation will stimulate the broad hypotheses that give the psychiatric examination its initial organization.

It is important to ascertain who or what has prompted the need for the assessment. Does it come from within the family or from external sources? It makes a big difference if the concerns come from within the immediate family rather than from external sources (e.g., school, court). For the most part, when the evaluation is initiated by someone outside the family, it is fraught from the very beginning with greater difficulties and overt obstacles (in the form of open resistances) (see Chapter 10).

Conducting the Family Assessment

It is good practice to begin the evaluation by meeting with the child and the parents together. This enables the examiner to observe the child interacting with other members of the family and allows the examiner to observe important aspects of family dynamics and parenting behavior. The assessment of parenting—particularly of the quality of parenting—is an important part of every child psychiatric evaluation (1, p. 272). Although family interviews offer the psychiatrist several benefits, child psychiatric evaluations often do not begin with them. Beginning the evaluation with the whole family gives the psychiatrist the only opportunity he or she will have to "observe pure family interactions, untainted by biases that can result from alliances created with family members later in the process" (2, p. 449). The psychiatrist can observe problems as they unfold and "the resulting anguish that has driven the family to seek help. The family interview also may give the psychiatrist an initial understanding of unconscious motivations and defenses that maintain the symptom structure within the family" (2, p. 449).

In the initial family meeting, a number of observations may be made: Who is the family's spokesperson? Does the family exhibit concern, love or affection, or indifference and distance? Who sets the rules and structure? What are the dominant subsystems within the family? What is the family's emotional atmosphere? How strong is the parental subsystem? Is there any evidence of enmeshment? What are the intergenerational boundaries? Is there any evidence of affection or tenderness? These observations will aid in the parental and family dynamics assessment (see Chapter 8).

Frequently the examiner will observe psychopathology in individuals other than the identified patient. At times it may seem as though the identified patient is not the person in need of the evaluation, because other family members obviously have greater need for psychiatric assessment. For example, in cases of affective disorders, other family members commonly have mood disorders. This is equally true of other psychiatric conditions (e.g., anxiety disorders, substance abuse, psychotic disorders, and conduct disorders).

In the following two case examples, observations of family interactions revealed evidence of psychopathology in individuals other than the identified patient:

Luis, a very small, 10-year-old Hispanic boy, was evaluated for suicidal behavior. The child was profoundly melancholic and had tried many times to kill himself. Approximately 18 months earlier, his 12-year old sister had died of a fulminating pneumonia. Luis felt responsible for his sister's death because he blamed himself for "coughing on her face." He missed his sister a great deal because she had been like a second mother to him. Luis very much wanted to be with her.

The family interview revealed that Luis's mother had recently been admitted to a psychiatric hospital after a suicide attempt. His mother was still mourning the loss of Luis's sister, whom she called her "best friend." She also expressed a desire to end her marriage. She said she was tired of her drug-abusing and alcoholic husband. Luis's father was also very depressed and had attempted twice before to kill himself. He was under psychiatric treatment at the time of Luis's psychiatric examination. The father was also in the process of claiming disability compensation for back pain. Luis had two remaining siblings: a 12-year-old brother, who was overtly depressed and reported having suicidal thoughts, and a 6-year-old brother, who stayed by his mother's side throughout the interview.

During the family meeting, the examiner observed the following sequence of behaviors: first Luis stood by his mother and gave her a gentle backrub; then he helped his younger brother to trace a picture from a book, guiding and holding his hand; and finally he moved closer to his older brother, engaged him in a verbal exchange, and made him laugh. The examiner realized, then, that Luis had taken over his dead sister's role, caring for the whole family.

The preceding case example illustrates two common findings in severe child psychopathology: first, severe psychopathology (in this case, affective disorder) is likely to be observed in the parents or in other members of the immediate family, and second, other risk factors (e.g., marital discord, parental dysfunction) that complicate treatment and prognosis may be present within the family. The next case example highlights important family dynamics issues that may become apparent during the diagnostic interview:

Rose, a 12-year-old Caucasian girl, was evaluated for aggressive behavior toward her mother. Her abusive behavior had escalated during the previous 2 months. Rose called her mother names such as "bitch" and "fat cow" (the mother was heavy); she also pushed, shoved, hit, and kicked her mother and pulled her hair. On one occasion Rose pulled her mother's hair while she was driving. Another time, again when her mother was driving, Rose kicked her mother's seat from behind, putting everyone in the car at risk. Rose had threatened to kill her mother many times. On one occasion Rose told her mother that she wanted to cut her to pieces. Rose also vented anger against her environment. Rose kicked through a door in fit of rage the night before the psychiatric examination. At the peak of Rose's dyscontrol, she would either threaten suicide or become self-abusive by scratching her arms or legs.

Rose's threats and intimidation toward her mother reached such intensity that her mother became afraid of her. Before the evaluation, Rose's mother could no longer sleep in peace; she feared for her life. The family learned that Rose took knives to bed in order to protect herself "if father were to come in at night and attempt to harm me." She also slept in her clothes.

Rose was a very bright student and had been enrolled in a gifted and talented program at school, although her grades had dropped during the previous semester. She complained that she couldn't concentrate and that her mind kept wandering. The family had noticed that Rose was very moody, was extremely irritable, and had problems sleeping. She frequently woke up at night and had trouble going back to sleep. In the mornings she felt tired and nonrefreshed.

Rose had felt depressed since she was 8 years old. She had felt suicidal for the previous couple of years. On one occasion she attempted to overdose with over-the-counter medications. She had tried to control her suicidal feelings by staying busy most of the time. Her parents also reported that Rose was a worrier: she worried about the environment, pollution, the poor, the homeless, and so on.

Rose's developmental history revealed that she had been a difficult child between ages 1 and 2 years. She had also displayed pica. Her mother reported that she regretted having been harsh with Rose during that time. Between ages 6 and 7 years,

Rose had been electively mute at school. She was also intermittently enuretic; she last wet the bed 4 months prior to the evaluation. No relevant medical, surgical, or traumatic history was revealed. She had no history of seizures or head trauma. Rose had no psychiatric history and had never received psychotherapy.

Rose's mental status examination revealed an attractive and articulate female adolescent with mild childish demeanor. She exhibited signs of depression, and her posture indicated tiredness and a lack of interest, if not regressive behavior. She appeared sad, angry, and tense, and she looked very anxious. Her affect was constricted but appropriate; she acknowledged suicidal ideation but endorsed no suicide plans. She admitted to feeling like killing her mother from time to time. There were no perceptual disturbances; her thought processes were intact. Sensorium, intelligence, and language were unremarkable. Judgment was fair, and insight was considered limited. Rose denied she was depressed and denied needing psychiatric help.

During the family session, Rose sat closer to her father than her mother and demonstrated clear hostility toward her mother. As soon as her mother said something, Rose would verbally attack her. Rose's father could say the same things without being attacked. Upon being attacked verbally, Rose's mother would start crying, exhibiting confusion, desperation, and helplessness. This made Rose angrier and more hostile toward her mother. Rose would tell her mother that she thought her mother was weak and that she never wanted to be like her. Upon hearing this, her mother's crying and sense of confusion and helplessness increased. At no point did Rose express negative feelings toward her father. Because Rose's mother appeared very vulnerable, she was evaluated separately.

The individual interview with Rose's mother revealed that the family had relocated to the area 18 months earlier. Her husband was on active duty with the military. She was a music teacher but had difficulty finding a job. She experienced depression 1 year earlier and reported that her "world crumbled to pieces" 5 months before the evaluation, when her husband failed to gain a military promotion. When Rose began to have problems, her mother got a further sense that "the world was falling apart." She wondered if she needed treatment and whether she was the cause of the problem. She also felt extremely guilty that she had been harsh toward Rose as a child and obsessed about being the reason for her daughter's problems. During the session, Rose's mother regressed, becoming quite helpless, crying easily, and seeming to need ongoing support. In a desperate manner, she asked the examiner in an insistent tone to tell her what to do and how to behave toward her daughter. She was pathetically ambivalent toward Rose.

The examiner made Rose's mother aware of her ambivalence and anger toward her daughter and of how guilty she felt for being so angry and for her perceived parental behavior when Rose was younger. The examiner also made her aware of her fear of harming Rose and of how her guilt and her fear interfered with effective parenting. The examiner told her that these emotions were blocking her capacity to set firm controls on Rose's abusive behavior toward her. When her anger toward her daughter was legitimized, she began to regain her composure and controls and began to smile. She was able to verbalize that she was afraid of harming Rose and that she was scared of her daughter. She said that she didn't want to be around Rose for a while. The examiner also became aware that the mother was depressed and that she would need a full psychiatric assessment at a later time.

Rose qualified for the diagnoses of mood and anxiety disorders and for a severe oppositional defiant disorder. Sexual abuse was suspected but was not substantiated.

Rose's history revealed some developmental delays, which are common in children who have severe psychopathology. The session with Rose's family and the individual session with her mother were revealing: they uncovered significant family and parental dysfunction and clear psychopathology in one of the parents. (Chapter 9 examines other family issues related to the formation and maintenance of symptoms.)

The examiner's recommendations for treatment had to take into account the mother's emotional state and her ineffective parenting. Without the family evaluation and the individual assessment of the mother, the treatment recommendations for Rose and her family would have been incomplete. A comprehensive treatment plan for Rose needed to include recommendations for treatment of the family dysfunction and other developmental interferences present in the household.

Maintaining Dependency Ties During the Interview

Many evaluations are marred from the very beginning because the examiner inadvertently or prematurely threatens to sever strong dependency ties between the child and the parents. This risk is greater during the examination of adolescents when the examiner assumes more individuation and autonomy than the child has achieved or more independence than the parents have allowed. The following case example illustrates this point:

Nick, a 17-year-old Caucasian boy, had just been withdrawn, by his mother, from an acute psychiatric hospital, where he had been admitted 48 hours earlier for an acute psychotic episode. The mother alleged that the former psychiatrist "had been insensitive" and that the doctor "had rushed into judgment regarding the diagnosis" (she was told her son had schizophrenia and that he needed acute psychiatric hospitalization). She complained that the psychiatrist had spoken to Nick "alone for only 10 minutes." She objected to having been separated from her son and was upset that she couldn't be around him for comfort. She said that she was going to start a national campaign "to ensure that parents of hospitalized adolescents can stay in the hospital with them." According to the former psychiatrist, Nick arrived at the hospital in a state of incoherence and, when evaluated, was floridly psychotic. His mother claimed that prior to the referral to the psychiatric hospital, she had taken him to a local emergency room where, "he had an episode of respiratory arrest." The acute psychotic break coincided with Nick's father's recent departure for a consulting job in another state.

Nick, valedictorian of his high school class, had been markedly driven to excel, had been an honor student, and was seeking entrance into an Ivy League college. He got up at 4:30 A.M. to study on a regular basis and was involved in multiple extracurricular activities. According to Nick's mother, most of the family members, including Nick's father, were shy. His father had a serious stuttering disorder. His wife used to speak for him in social situations. There was a strong history of bipolar disorder in the mother's extended family.

Nick was born a few weeks premature and at birth weighed

about 5 pounds. He was born with respiratory distress syndrome. His parents were told to make funeral arrangements for him. Nick survived; however, he required an incubator and oxygen for his first 3 months of life. At age 3 months, he had spinal meningitis but never had seizures. His development was delayed: he first sat at age 11 months and walked at 18 months. Nick's mother could not tell if there had been any delay in Nick's speech production. Nick had always been of smaller stature than his peers, and this had been a source a difficulty with his classmates. His superior intelligence was recognized when he entered school.

During the diagnostic evaluation, Nick's mother responded when the examiner asked Nick questions. She was very anxious and intrusive. She minimized the nature of the recent psychotic episode and did not lose any opportunity to extol the virtues and accomplishments of her "special child." The examiner recognized and accepted the dependent relationship of this adolescent with his mother and made no attempt to disrupt the symbiotic bond.

Nick was guarded and suspicious and maintained limited eye contact. He was thin and small and had a frail appearance. He was mildly depressed and very constricted in the affective sphere. He had problems developing rapport with the examiner. He was coherent, but his speech was moderately pressured and uninterrupted (he did not punctuate his sentences). His associations were loose and tended to be very circumstantial. Nick was overtly paranoid. A number of times he asked his mother to bring a lawyer when he feared the examiner might "tamper" with his mind. His mother appropriately reassured him at those times. Nick denied he was experiencing auditory or visual hallucinations but acknowledged that he had experienced them recently. He denied any suicidal or homicidal ideation. He also denied there was anything wrong with him. He wanted to go back home, right away, "to catch up with my studies and to continue the college search."

Nick's mother was told that Nick still needed intense psychiatric monitoring in an acute psychiatric hospital. She persuaded Nick to follow the examiner's recommendation. Nick recovered promptly and completely from the psychotic episode. Shortly afterward, his mother informed the examiner that Nick had been awarded the president's scholarship at a prominent university in New England. Despite multiple risk factors, Nick demonstrated an exceptional cognitive and academic outcome. His mother's fears for his life and Nick's behavioral inhibition had contributed to his strong dependency needs. Nick's psychiatric outcome was uncertain.

The preceding case illustrates the importance of beginning the evaluation with a family interview and alerts the examiner to the risks of prematurely separating the child from the family for the individual interview.

Conducting the Individual Interview

Once the family assessment has been completed, the child is interviewed alone. An important goal for the examiner during the individual interview is to facilitate the child's verbalization of his or her problems so that the child may put into his or her own words the nature of the difficulties or the manner in which he or she perceives them. Without this understanding, the quality of diagnostic data will be compromised. The child's verbalizations also help in building a diagnostic and therapeutic alliance.[1]

---

[1] The importance of the therapeutic alliance is in a state of transition. Striving to gain and to maintain an optimal therapeutic alliance was a major priority before the managed-care revolution. More recently, psychiatrists have been assigned preferentially the roles of diagnosticians and consultants. Because the psychiatrist no longer has the exclusive burden of clinical responsibility and the physician's involvement in psychotherapy has been discouraged, building a therapeutic alliance is no longer the top clinical priority. However, even with a limited or circumscribed psychiatric role, attention to the therapeutic alliance is still quite relevant. The patient and his or her family would most likely follow the doctor's recommendations if good rapport and a working alliance have been established. Obviously the therapeutic alliance remains an essential objective when the child psychiatrist assumes a psychotherapist role.

Creating Rapport and Engagement

The examiner needs to create a sensitive and empathic environment for the child and his or her family. The interview environment needs to be inviting and to communicate genuine warmth and receptivity. The child needs to feel respected and understood at all times. Except with preschoolers, with whom there is a universal tendency to use baby talk, the examiner should use his or her natural voice and intonation. Children sense when they are patronized or manipulated by adults or when they are addressed in an artificial manner.

Rapport refers to the emotional climate between the child and the examiner that evolves throughout the interview. *Engagement* relates to the quality of relatedness and the technical measures used by the examiner to facilitate the child's participation during the interview. In other words, engagement relates to the means by which the examiner increases rapport.

Engagement entails warmth, acceptance, playfulness, humor, compassion, helpfulness, and empathic attunement on the part of the examiner. Furthermore, the examiner must have an accepting and tolerant attitude and must be sensitive to and aware of the child's developmental, cognitive, and emotional levels. In order to engage families, the examiner must be equitable, compassionate, and tolerant of human frailty. Broad personal experience is also necessary.

The process of engaging the child and the family is facilitated by the examiner's equidistant relationship to them. Traditionally, the child psychiatrist has been cast in the role of the child's advocate. This special role should not be maintained at the expense of alienating the family or at the risk of being unduly partial to the child.

Experienced clinicians display an automatic behavioral repertoire and make instantaneous adjustments when they interview children. For example, they change body posture, vocabulary, tone of voice, and even their affective display. These adjustments of verbal and nonverbal communication put the clinician in immediate contact with the child's developmental level. The following case example illustrates the process of engagement in an impaired and defensive early adolescent:

George, a 12-year-old boy, was a very defensive and uncooperative child: he was clever and liked to outsmart adults and his peers. He had a history of chronic affective psychosis and had an extensive psychiatric history, including prolonged hospitalizations for suicidal and aggressive behaviors. He was intelligent but had a history of chronic school problems, including aggression toward his teachers. To control psychotic symptoms, George had received neuroleptic medications for many years and had developed a severe case of tardive dyskinesia. As a result, all antipsychotic medication had to be stopped.

When George was interviewed for the first time, he was in the hospital. He sat in a chair and fidgeted a great deal; at times he rocked the chair, tilting it in such a way that the examiner feared for George's safety. The examiner said to George, "That makes me uneasy." George reassured the examiner that he would not get hurt and continued tilting the chair back and forth. When he was asked what had brought him to the hospital, he said, "Drugs." The examiner asked, "Which ones?" George answered, "Marijuana." He said that he had used it for a long time, adding that his parents did not know anything about it. To this the examiner replied, "It takes a lot of cleverness to hide this from the family." George responded with an enthusiastic "Yes!" George then proceeded to talk about the buzz he got from gasoline: it made him feel like he was floating, as if he could fly. The examiner then asked George whether he had ever attempted to fly. George said that from time to time he felt like Superman and had tried to fly from the roof of his home. On one occasion he fell on his "belly and it hurt pretty bad." He denied he had broken any bones.

Later in the interview, when the examiner and George discussed his suicidal behavior and prior suicidal attempts, George said he had a secret plan to kill himself and stressed that he was not going to share the plan with anybody. He stated that he frequently daydreamed about flying over a highway bridge and being killed by a car. He said he believed he would go straight to heaven, adding that he was not meant to be in this life because he "can't make it in life." George then described how bad he felt about himself. For example, when he looked at himself in the mirror, he used to see a monster with horns. This monster talked to him and told him to do bad things. On one occasion the monster told him to hurt somebody, but George shouted "No!"

The preceding case example illustrates successful engagement of a resistant child. By joining the child's grandiosity, the examiner facilitated the development of rapport: the child provided meaningful information after the examiner achieved an emotional connection with him.

Using Nonverbal Engagement

Although verbal engagement is the most desirable technique, nonverbal engagement becomes a stepping-stone in the process of building trust and developing a diagnostic and therapeutic alliance. The following case example illustrates this point:

Pedro, a 5 ½-year-old Hispanic boy, was referred for a psychiatric evaluation for aggressive behavior. He was also unruly and oppositional. He had been in the care of his maternal grandmother since he was 2 years old. Pedro's mother was conspicuously neglectful and abusive; she would leave her children unattended for prolonged periods of time. Pedro's grandmother and other relatives would find the children unkempt, soiled, and malnourished on a regular basis. A number of times, his grandmother picked up the children from the streets, where Pedro's mother had irresponsibly left them.

The examiner suspected that during the first 2 years of Pedro's life, he had endured frequent maltreatment and neglect. A 7-year-old sister had decided not to stay with the mother any longer, because she "got tired of acting like a mom." The mother frequently put her daughter in charge of her two younger siblings. The grandmother was the legal custodian of the two older children and also had cared for the two younger ones. Although tired and emotionally exhausted, she couldn't bear the thought of leaving the younger ones in the care of her daughter.

Pedro was small for his age. He looked a bit scraggly and was very inhibited and submissive. During the individual interview, he was completely silent and remained distant, apprehensive, and reserved. Because he did not respond to simple questions such as "What is your name?" and "How old are you?" the examiner made an effort to engage him in play. Pedro was offered a set of animals, a group of dinosaurs, and a group of dolls. He did not show any interest in the toys. In an attempt to engage Pedro, the examiner began to place the animals in a circle, hoping Pedro would join him in the play; that did not happen. After a while, the examiner left the animals alone and began to play with the dolls; Pedro did not join in this play either. The examiner then attempted to engage Pedro in the squiggle technique[2]: he picked up a sheet of paper; put a pencil on the table, closer to Pedro; and invited Pedro to draw something with him. After Pedro refused a number of invitations, the examiner collected all the items from the table.

The examiner had a tennis ball on top of the desk. He picked it up and rolled it to Pedro. Pedro picked up the ball and rolled it back to the examiner. The examiner rolled the ball again, and Pedro rolled it back in return. The ball was rolled back and forth may times. At one point, the distant, unanimated child began to smile. Shortly thereafter, he began to throw the ball progressively more forcefully and somewhat aggressively: on two occasions he hit the examiner in the chest, and Pedro began to get more emotionally involved in the game. After throwing the ball back and forth a number of times, the interview was concluded.

---

[2]The *squiggle technique* is an engaging projective drawing technique in which the examiner stimulates a child to draw something from simple ambiguous tracings made by the examiner. What the child draws has important psychodynamic meanings. This technique was created by Winnicott (3).

Pedro was told, "Next time we will play some more."

This engagement attempt lasted for about 45 minutes; at no point during the interview did Pedro utter a word. Significant anxiety, language disorders, and cognitive limitations may have contributed to the child's elective mutism.

The preceding case example illustrates nonverbal engagement after unsuccessful attempts to involve the child in verbal interactions. Recognizing the child's mistrust, the examiner made plans to take the child to the courtyard for the next diagnostic appointment—"to play in the playground," he told Pedro. The novelty and intimacy of the office and the private nature of the examination (i.e., having to stay alone with the examiner behind closed doors) may have been too threatening for the child. A history of anxiety disorders, abuse, developmental language disorders, or cognitive limitations are common in children like Pedro and may contribute to difficulty responding verbally in an interview.

The quality of data gathered during the examination depends on the quality of the rapport and engagement. The better the trust and the more positive the quality of the engagement, the better will be the quality and consistency of the data the child and the family provide. If the child or the family feel apprehensive or, worse, defensive, the data will be partial, selective, or even inconsistent.

■ QUALITIES OF THE PSYCHIATRIC EXAMINATION

The quality of the relationship between the examiner and the child and his or her family has an important bearing on the accuracy of the diagnosis and on the patient's compliance with treatment recommendations. A good interview achieves its objectives when the examiner promotes optimal participation from the child and his or her family. This is achieved when defensiveness and self-consciousness are kept to a minimum. The interview process is, by its very nature, a stressful event for all involved, including the examiner. The art of interviewing rests on the examiner's ability to minimize discomfort and to foster natural interaction. If the interview is done in a tactful and sensitive way, the child's and the family's apprehension of being "in the hot seat" will be minimized.

First and foremost, the examiner should use language appropriate for the child's developmental level. Special attention is required to avoid the use of sophisticated or professional language. Furthermore, the examiner should understand that when the child or the family uses common words such as "depression," the meaning given to such words is not necessarily the same that the examiner gives to them (see "Communication Issues" section later in this chapter).

The examiner must ascertain whether the child understands the initial verbal transactions; if the child does not understand, an auditory sensory defect, delirium, or a receptive language disorder are most likely present (see "Interviewing Children Who Have Learning Disabilities or Other Neuropsychiatric Deficits" in Chapter 7). With children who have receptive language difficulties, the examiner will need to modify the communication approach used. He or she will need to speak slowly and in a deliberate manner to make contact with the child, striving toward attentive eye contact and face-to-face communication. The examiner could also use alternative media (e.g., play, drawing) to communicate with the child. If delirium is suspected, a detailed examination of the sensorium is mandatory. If the child does not seem to respond to the examiner's utterances, the examiner should determine whether the child's auditory functions are intact or whether autistic features are present.

The diagnostic interview should exhibit the following qualities:

Sensitivity. *Sensitivity* relates to the examiner's ability to empathize with the child and to adjust his or her approach to the child's developmental level. It also implies that the examiner is attentive to the child's level of anxiety and attempts to carry out the evaluation process with the least amount of stress possible. An optimal level of engagement and empathic attunement to the child's emotions and anxiety level are good markers of sensitivity.

Fluidity. The examiner strives to maintain a natural and smooth flow in the child's verbal and nonverbal communication. A sense of *fluidity* is created by facilitating smooth transitions from one topic to the next. By following closely the thread of the child's communications and abreacted affect (emotional expression), the examiner promotes a sense of cohesion and fluidity.

Depth. The examiner clarifies and explores the main issues at hand, including their ramifications and meanings, before moving on to other areas. He or she gives special attention to the child's verbal and nonverbal manifestations of affect. Every time an emotional abreaction (emergence of affect) occurs, the examiner asks the child to verbalize what made him or her feel that particular way. In the same vein, when the child is narrating events that are by their nature filled with emotion and the child does not display the corresponding affect, the examiner makes the child aware of the discrepancy. The examiner attempts to draw out the child's suppressed emotions. This approach gives the interview a sense of *depth*.

Coherence. As the examiner strives to connect and to integrate the information gathered during the interview, he or she gives to the process a sense of connection or *coherence*. Inexperienced examiners give the interview process a quality of discontinuity or fragmentation. An observer is left with the impression that the communication is unclear or disjointed, that certain areas were not explored adequately, or that certain topics were missed altogether. When coherence is not achieved, the patient feels irritated and misunderstood.

Specificity. *Specificity* of the psychiatric interview refers to the understanding and identification of the presenting complaints and to the clarification of the context in which the symptoms appear. A complementary idea is the concept of functional assessment. Because psychopathology and problems of adaptation do not go hand and hand, the examiner needs to clarify how psychopathology interferes with the patient's adaptive capacity.

Comprehensiveness. The examiner strives to be thorough. *Comprehensiveness* is achieved by exploring all the possible ramifications of a given problem in the context of the child's developmental history and his or her current family and school circumstances. For example, the examiner will take into account the child's relevant medical and psychiatric history.

Meaningfulness. The interview should make overall integrative sense. This speaks to the quality of *meaningfulness*. By following through with a topic and sticking to it until full understanding is achieved, the examiner gains depth and breadth of meaning.

Versatility. *Versatility* relates to the examiner's skill in meeting and engaging diverse presentations of child and family dysfunctions. The diagnostic interview needs to be tailored to the child's and the family's needs. In order to build a bridge of trust and to create an atmosphere of understanding, the examiner needs to address the specific issues related to the child's and family's presenting problem. A monotonous or ritualistic survey of symptoms will not fulfill this need.

Efficiency. The examiner needs to keep up a diligent pace in the process of diagnostic data-gathering. He or she must be efficient with time. In order to achieve *efficiency,* the examiner needs to have a flexible but clear plan in mind. The goals of the interview need to be pursued even in the presence of intrinsic or extrinsic pressures. The experienced examiner knows how to differentiate the essential from the unimportant. He or she learns to obtain the fundamental data in the least possible time and to use the obstacles he or she finds in data gathering as vehicles to increase his or her understanding of the child and the child's circumstances.

An efficient and experienced examiner is able to complete a comprehensive assessment of a child and family in 1.5–2 hours. Although a solid diagnostic interview may be accomplished in one sitting, circumstances may dictate additional diagnostic sessions.

■ PHASES OF THE PSYCHIATRIC EXAMINATION

Table 1–1 lists the phases of the psychiatric examination.

Beginning the Interview (Engagement)

The beginning, or engagement, phase pertains to the initial contact between the examiner and the child (and his or her family). Leon's comments regarding the first meeting between the adult patient and the doctor is applicable to child psychiatry. In the following quotation, "physician" stands for child psychiatrist and "patient" stands for the child and his or her family:

> Although the physician may already have seen many patients that day, this is the first meeting of this patient and doctor. For the patient, it is important. The patient has been anticipating this meeting with a mixture of fear and hope. The patient's fear comes from many sources. What will the doctor be like? Will

TABLE 1–1. Phases of the psychiatric examination
1. Beginning the interview (engagement)
2. Elaborating the presenting problem
3. Extending the exploration
4. Completing the mental status examination
5. Closing the interview
6. Interpreting the results

the patient be judged adversely? What will be found? Will the doctor want to help? The hope is that the doctor can relieve the stress. (4, p. 15)

In a similar fashion, Katz's description of the adolescent's anxiety preceding the initial interview with the therapist could be aptly applied to the first meeting between the child and the psychiatrist:

> While the first few minutes of an [initial] interview are significant with all patients, they are particularly significant with adolescents, as many of them are struggling for independence, trying to establish an identity, and choosing their place in the world. They are particularly sensitive to any signals from the therapist [examiner] that their power of decision, their intelligence, and their perceptions will be ignored. (5, p. 70)

Depending on how the preliminary contact goes and the first impressions that are made, a warm-up stage or engagement phase takes precedence in the initial encounter. The goal here is to help the patient and the family to feel at ease and as comfortable as possible; this will promote cooperation and a decrease in anxiety and resistance. In general, this phase is more prolonged with preadolescents and with younger, immature, and regressed children. With adolescents, this engagement phase may not take long. The extent and duration of this phase also depend on the degree of psychopathology, the degree of dystonicity (discomfort) caused by the symptoms, and the patient's awareness of a need to change.

The engagement phase allows the examiner to determine the patient's and the family's openness and their likely degree of participation in the diagnostic process. It also provides an incipient sense of the patient's and the family's *relatedness* (i.e., the quality of object relations within the family and within the individual child). These preliminary perceptions will guide the examiner in judging the degree of overt psychopathology, the level of cooperation and rapport, and the amount of *direction* (i.e., structuring) that will be necessary to ensure success in the diagnostic process.

Once the family concerns are explored and the family members are given the opportunity to express their views on the problem(s), the family is asked to leave, and the child's examination begins or, to be more precise, continues.

At the beginning of the psychiatric examination of the child, the examiner should start with a warm greeting and introduce himself or herself if this is the first meeting with the child. The examiner may start by asking simple questions such as "What is your name?" "How old are you?" or "Where do you go to school?" The examiner may ask the child if he or she knows where they are and what kind of doctor the examiner is. The examiner may also ask the child why he or she is at the doctor's office now or why he or she needs to see a psychiatrist. This is the time to start the specific interview process.

Rapport is fostered when the examiner gives the child positive feedback for behaving adaptively or in a developmentally appropriate manner. For example, when evaluating a 5-year-old boy who has a prolonged history of hyperactivity and destructiveness, the examiner could praise the child when, at the end of the session and upon hearing that the interview has ended, the child puts away the toys he has been using. Engagement is also facilitated when the examiner supports the child's adaptive efforts. This point is illustrated in the following case example:

> Benny, a 16-year-old Caucasian boy, was brought by his paternal grandmother to a psychiatric evaluation for aggressive and oppositional behaviors at home and at school. Benny and his 12-year-old sister had been under their grandmother's custody for many years. The children's parents were drug addicts and had been unable to care for them. Benny had an extensive psychiatric history, including acute psychiatric hospitalizations and residential treatment for anger dyscontrol, conduct difficulties, unstable mood, and drug abuse. Benny had spent some time at a juvenile detention center and had received drug treatment at a residential drug program. At the time of the psychiatric examination, he was on probation.

Benny's grandmother had previously brought her granddaughter in for an evaluation secondary to aggressive and extremely oppositional behaviors. At that time, the examiner learned that both children hated their grandmother and that both were abusive to her.

From the moment the grandmother and Benny entered the examination room, an atmosphere of tension and hostility was present. Benny stated at the outset, "Either she leaves and I stay, or I go and she stays." When the examiner attempted to elicit information regarding the grandmother's concerns, Benny issued a new warning, "I am not going to stay in the same room with her." When the examiner asked a general question to both of them, Benny stood up and left the room. The examiner asked the grandmother a limited number of questions regarding her concerns about Benny. She was concerned about his aggressive and unruly behaviors, and she suspected that he was using drugs again. After spending about 5 minutes with the grandmother, the examiner came out and invited Benny to rejoin him alone.

Benny was a robust and rough-looking adolescent. His hair was shaved close to the scalp, and he had several scars on his face. He was dressed seasonally in a short-sleeve shirt. A ¾-inch round cigarette burn was conspicuous on his left forearm. Benny repeated defiantly and hostilely that he didn't need to be examined and that he came to interview only "to get my grandmother off my back." Benny displayed a defensive and reserved posture and conveyed through nonverbal behavior that he wanted the examination to be over with as soon as possible.

When the examiner asked Benny about school, he said, "My grades are getting better this semester." He said that he liked school and that he had not been skipping school during the current semester. When the examiner asked Benny about his drug use, he responded proudly, "I haven't touched the stuff for 50 days; today is the 50th day I've been without drugs. I've been going to PDAP [a juvenile drug abuse outpatient program] regularly." Upon hearing this, the examiner stood up, walked over to Benny, and shook his hand, congratulating him. The examiner praised Benny for his effort to stay away from drugs and said that he hoped Benny would remain abstinent.

Benny smiled with appreciation, and his demeanor toward

the examiner changed dramatically. He apologized for his previous rude behavior, saying, "I'm tired of psychiatrists and of taking medicines. They don't help."

Because Benny seemed more open to further exploration, the examiner proceeded to inquire about Benny's self-abusive behavior. The examiner invited Benny to discuss the cigarette burn on his arm. Benny said that he enjoyed pain and that he didn't see it as a problem. He denied suicidal ideation. He said he was looking forward to turning 17, because he expected to leave his grandmother's custody at that time. He said, "That would be a relief!"

The examiner asked Benny how he controlled his anger. Benny said that he tried to control it all the time. He mentioned a couple of fights at school, explaining that he had been provoked and that he would not allow "those punks to run over me." The examiner said that Benny seemed very angry with his grandmother. Benny said, "I can't stand her." The examiner asked Benny if he thought about killing her. Benny reported that he thought about it all the time. He attempted to reassure himself by saying, "I am not stupid. I know that if I were to kill her, I'd be the first suspect. If I knew a way, I would do it." He added, "I don't want to have a [legal] record because I'm planning to join the Marines." Benny confessed that when his anger became too intense he would burn himself because "it helps me to get back in control."

Benny was able to review other difficult and sensitive topics (e.g., his relationships with his parents and his sister). Benny said that he would like to have more contact with his father. He was very negative and critical of his mother. He was happy she was in trouble and intimated that she was going to jail: "She's responsible for what she's doing, and she should pay for it." He didn't care about her at all. Benny did not seem to like his sister, either; she was in a residential placement at the time of the interview.

To close the interview, the examiner asked Benny if there was any way a psychiatrist could help him. Benny said that he didn't need any help right now. The examiner gave Benny his business card and offered his services any time Benny felt in need of help. Benny shook the examiner's hand warmly and appeared appreciative when he departed.

In the preceding case, the patient arrived at the evaluation with a very angry and antagonistic demeanor. He came prepared to battle with the examiner; however, there was a clear, if not dramatic, change in his attitude toward the interview after the examiner praised him for his efforts to stay off drugs.

Sensitive comments to the child about signs of illness or injury (e.g., sniffles or a cast) help the examiner to build rapport and increase the diagnostic alliance with the patient. For example, the examiner can convey to the child that he or she has noticed that the child is sick or that the child has been injured in some way. Rapport is also fostered when the examiner initiates the examination by picking up on themes or preoccupations the child brings to the evaluation. Consider the following case example:

> Rudy, a 14-year-old Caucasian boy, was being evaluated for paranoia. He brought to the examination two large drawings of dragons. The examiner demonstrated interest in the two drawings, which showed dragons puffing fire and no other figures or beings present. The examiner asked Rudy what the dragons were doing. Rudy said, "The dragons are puffing fire." The examiner commented, "The dragons seem very lonely; there is nobody else around them." Rudy responded, "The dragons don't like to be around other people." He added, "Others don't like dragons because they are very angry." The examiner commented that the dragons puff a lot of fire, that they are very angry. To this, Rudy said, "Although one of the dragons puffs fire, the other puffs only smoke." The child added, "I don't need anybody. I don't need to be loved." The examiner responded, "Love is essential for life. Without it we cannot live." Rudy said, "I am trying very hard not to need love." After this exchange, Rudy began to talk about the problems he had with his parents, and the interview continued in a productive manner.

The preceding case example illustrates the spontaneous use of drawing in the psychiatric examination. For more details about the use of drawing during the diagnostic child psychiatric examination, see Chapter 2.

The child may open the interview by talking about sports, a

movie star, a television show, or some other issue that at first glance may seem banal or immaterial to the main concerns of the examination. By joining the child's prevailing fantasy or immediate interest, the examiner gains a number of benefits: 1) The examiner creates or increases the alliance with the child; 2) he or she learns about important aspects of the child's psychological world; and 3) by paying close attention to the content and the process of the child's communication, the examiner may gain significant insights into the child's cognitive capacities, language functions, manner of relating, reality testing, and other psychological and adaptive functions.

The engagement phase needs to be as unstructured as possible. During this phase, the child should be allowed to speak about anything he or she wants and to discuss whatever is uppermost in his or her mind. As the examiner listens, he or she develops a sense or understanding of the sources of the patient's anxieties. This approach parallels an open-ended exploration. The examiner pays particular attention to the child's emotional expression and to the manner in which he or she articulates difficulties. This allows the examiner to appreciate the child's prevailing mood, cognitive organization, and adaptive resources.

Observations made during the engagement phase stimulate a number of clinical hunches, or incipient hypotheses. These impressions may serve as bases for exploring further and for probing a number of diagnostic areas. Also, by listening attentively and by demonstrating interest and empathy, the examiner conveys to the child that the child's concerns are considered seriously. In this manner, the child perceives that the examiner is caring and sensitive and is interested in what he or she has to say.

It is useful to facilitate the child's and the family's participation in defining the problem and in finding ways to solve it. If everything proceeds well later during the interpretive phase of the evaluation (discussed later in this section), there will be a convergence of the child's, parents', and examiner's views regarding what the problems are and what needs to done about them.

Elaborating the Presenting Problem

The major goal during the elaboration phase is to explore the presenting problem as fully as possible. This phase parallels what Brown and Rutter call the systematic exploratory style of interviewing, which involves a fact-oriented style and feeling-oriented techniques (6, 7). Systematic questioning and specific probing have definite advantages in eliciting factual information. This approach seems to be more successful in eliciting the "*detailed,* relevant data needed for an adequate diagnostic formulation" (8, p. 289). "The structured and systematic exploratory styles are far superior in providing evidence on the definitive *absence* of problems. . . . The implication is clear: if psychiatrists are to obtain sufficient detail about family problems and child symptoms for them to make an adequate formulation on which to base treatment plans, systematic and detailed probing and questioning must occur" (9, pp. 31, 32).

The examiner's priority during this phase is to obtain a clear and detailed account of the presenting problem. The examiner attempts to learn the *what*'s, *how*'s, *when*'s, and *where*'s of the presenting complaint. These questions relate to facts, events, and circumstances. Questions regarding frequency, intensity, and other factors that bring on the problem are of major relevance. After this exploration is completed, the examination of some of the psychological factors that may be contributing to the problem (i.e., the *why*'s) may be in order. The *why* questions relate to psychological explanations, rationalizations, and beliefs.

If the presenting problem is, for instance, anger dyscontrol, the examiner needs to consider the following questions:

1. What does the patient do when he or she loses control? Does the patient become aggressive? How? Does the patient become destructive? Does the patient become self-abusive? In what way? Has the patient ever tried to hurt himself or herself or to hurt others? (Note that the examiner is conducting a mental status examination at the same time he or she is exploring the presenting problem.)

2. How often does the patient lose control?
3. Where does the patient lose control?
4. How long does it take the patient to regain control?
5. What factors make the patient lose control?
6. What happens after the patient loses control? Has the patient ever received any treatment? Has the patient complied with therapeutic or medical recommendations?
7. How does the patient see his or her loss of control? Does the patient see dyscontrol as a problem?

Note that the most introspective questions come last. The same format may be followed with other symptoms (e.g., depression, suicidal behavior, drug abuse, running away).

When the issue at hand is suicidality or homicidality, standard questions are, in the case of suicidality, "How close have you been to killing yourself?" and "Do you have a plan to kill yourself?" or, in the case of homicidality, "How close have you been to killing?" "Whom?" and "Do you have a plan to kill that person now?" The examiner must assess the patient's potential risk to harm others and must remember his or her duty to warn potential victims, a result of the *Tarasoff* decision (10, p. 1140).

It is not enough to simply explore whether the patient has suicidal ideation. The examiner must explore all the possible means the patient has in mind. This point is illustrated in the following case example:

Matthew, a 6-year-old Caucasian boy, was referred by a social worker therapist for a psychiatric evaluation because of concerns with the child's depressive state and possible suicidal behavior. One year earlier, Matthew had undergone a psychiatric evaluation for aggressive behaviors at home and at school. His disturbance seemed to have started 1 year before the previous evaluation, when his father moved out and his older brother was hospitalized. Shortly afterward, Matthew began to kill small animals, trip and hit his peers, and hit his teenage sister. Matthew threw things around and was quite angry with his mother. Matthew's preschool teacher described him as very disruptive and withdrawn; he also was said to be careless and destructive with his schoolwork. Matthew displayed a prominent fear of fires; this had started after a fire drill. Matthew had not been abused but witnessed his father's abusive behavior toward his mother. Matthew's developmental milestones and history prior to his father leaving home were unremarkable. Both parents had depression and anxiety; Matthew's older brother was diagnosed with oppositional defiant disorder and organic brain disorder, possibly secondary to marijuana exposure in utero.

At the time of the current evaluation, Matthew's mental status examination revealed a handsome, bright, and articulate child who appeared his stated age. He looked unhappy and depressed and exhibited marked retardation in psychomotor activity. His affect was constricted markedly, and he appeared anhedonic and hopeless. When questioned about suicidal ideation, Matthew confirmed it readily. When asked how he thought he would kill himself, he said he had thought of using a knife. The examiner asked Matthew if he had considered other means of hurting himself. Matthew said that he had wanted to jump from the roof of the house. He had also thought about using a gun, laying down in the road so that he could be run over by a car, or somehow crushing his brain. He said that he had stood on his head many times, hoping to "drown" his brain with blood.

Matthew missed his father a great deal and hated living with his mother. He was very unhappy with his mother's recent remarriage. Also, he hated school and had difficulties concentrating. No psychotic features were present. Matthew was given the diagnosis of a major depressive episode and was placed on an antidepressant.

The preceding case example illustrates a severe affective disorder in an early latency child[3] and also demonstrates the variety of self-destructive means a child may devise. This case illustrates full melancholic symptomatology in early preadolescence.

---

[3] Early latency: 6–8 years; middle latency: 8–10 years; late latency: 10–12 years.

Issues related to the child's psychiatric history and ongoing treatments are also explored during the elaboration phase of the interview.

Data related to the presenting problem become the core organizer of the interview process. All data gathering will have the presenting problem as its reference point and as its integrative core.

Extending the Exploration

The extending the exploration phase is equivalent to the review of systems conducted when completing the history and examination in the field of physical medicine. During this phase, the examiner extends the exploration to other areas and attempts to find threads connected to the presenting problem.

For example, the parents of a 12-year-old girl with anger dyscontrol may tell the examiner that their daughter is aggressive at home. The examiner explores whether the child also loses control at school or in the neighborhood. Has she ever had any other problems at school? If so, what kind? The examiner explores how this child does academically. How are her peer relationships? The examiner pursues any leads pertinent to the evolving hypothesis. For example, the exploration may branch into questions related to oppositional behavior, conduct problems, gang affiliation, or drug use.

It is always helpful to approach sensitive areas (e.g., suicidal or homicidal behaviors, drug abuse) from many different angles. Examiners should never be satisfied with a single denial to a question related to a sensitive issue. The same issue must be pursued from different perspectives. Sometimes rephrasing the question or using different language makes a big difference. The use of vernacular language may be quite appropriate in this regard.

Sometimes, despite careful exploration the examiner will not find corroboration for some clinical impressions (intuitions). In cases of suicidality, homicidality, psychosis, and other areas, the examiner must remain cautious because his or her clinical impressions may be correct despite a lack of clinical proof. When the examiner has an uneasy feeling despite the patient's denials regarding a major issue (e.g., suicide, homicide, drug abuse), he or she should heed this clinical sense. The examiner should attempt further clarification of the clinical incongruencies because they may indicate that the patient is withholding (voluntarily or involuntarily) relevant information or that other lines of inquiry may need to be explored. For example, some children tenaciously withhold sensitive information. Children are adept at keeping certain secrets (e.g., suicidal intentions, homicidal plans, psychotic experiences, drug abuse, physical or sexual abuse, and sexual activity) (see Ron's case in the "Closing the Interview" section later in this chapter). The examiner also needs to be aware of countertransference responses because tactful utilization of these responses may be helpful in the diagnostic process (see Chapter 11).

A number of areas need to be explored in every child or adolescent interview. These areas include the child's relationships with family members, the kind of discipline the child receives, the child's history of physical or sexual abuse, his or her school life (e.g., academic performance, school difficulties), and his or her friendships. The child's drug use, conduct difficulties, and sexual behavior also are commonly explored.

Substance abuse must be evaluated privately because adolescents will not want their parents to know about this aspect of their lives. It is not enough to ask an adolescent, "Have you used drugs?" This question is too general. This type of question gives the adolescent an easy way out; he or she may respond with a fast denial. The examiner needs to conduct a detailed inquiry, using questions such as the following: What drugs have you tried? Do you drink wine coolers, beer, or liquor? How many times a week do you drink? How often do you get drunk? What kinds of problems have you gotten into because of alcohol? Do you drive after drinking? Have you received any citations for driving while intoxicated? Is there a history of pathologic intoxication? What other drugs do you use when you drink? Have you been sexually involved when you've been drinking?

The examiner should inquire individually about the following substances of abuse: marijuana, amphetamines, cocaine, crack, LSD, sedatives, steroids, inhalants, and other hallucinogenic and mind-altering substances. The examiner should ask the patient systematically, "When did your use of [drug] start?" "How much do you use, and how often do you use it?" and "When was the last time you used [drug]?" This methodical inquiry needs to be repeated with each drug the patient admits to using (11).

The examiner also must attempt to ascertain whether the child has ever experienced any signs of withdrawal and whether the child has ever been delirious or psychotic under the influence of drugs. Furthermore, the examiner should explore impairment and lapses of judgment during drug use. For example, the examiner can use questions such as "When you use [drug], do you get sexually involved?" The examiner must explore whether the adolescent has used intravenous drugs and whether the adolescent has been sexually involved with HIV-infected individuals. If the examiner has not inquired about sexually transmitted diseases, this is the opportunity to do so.

The patient's sexual behavior should be explored. It is not enough to ask the patient, "Have you ever had sex?" It is better to assume that adolescents are sexually active. Issues related to protected sex and history of pregnancy need to be explored. Sexually active adolescent females must be asked, "Have you ever been pregnant?" A valid question for sexually active adolescent males is, "Have you ever impregnated a girl?"

Because children are protective of their caregivers, denials to direct questions such as "Have you been physically abused?" need to be considered carefully.

During the exploratory phase, the patient's medical history is investigated. A history of head trauma, seizures, congenital problems, or neurological problems may be relevant in the diagnostic process. A selected family and developmental history also may be illuminating.

Completing the Mental Status Examination

During the completing the mental status examination phase, the examiner finishes exploring areas of the patient's mental status that were not covered earlier. In the process of exploring the presenting problem, the examiner has the opportunity to assess a number of areas of the mental status examination. These findings may not need to be explored again formally if the examiner has a solid understanding about them already. For example, if during the interview the examiner has noticed that the child or adolescent gives accurate details of his or her own history, including dates and precise locations, the examiner can safely assume that the patient's recent memory is probably intact. If the child is in advanced math classes (e.g., calculus) at school, the child's calculation ability may not need to be tested, unless there are good reasons to doing so. In the same vein, if in a prior exploration the examiner determined that the child had hallucinatory experiences and the examiner ascertained the nature of those perceptions, it may not be necessary to inquire about them again.

When the examiner turns to the exploration of the patient's sensorium and intellectual capacities, it is helpful and sensitive to mark the transition to a different kind of questioning by telling the child that the next series of questions will test his or her memory, orientation, and so on, and by saying, for instance, "These are questions that are asked of all children." Children who have neuropsychological deficits may be sensitive to this examination. If, despite reassurances, the patient remains apprehensive or exhibits narcissistic mortification, this line of exploration will need to be interrupted or postponed.

Closing the Interview

When the examiner has a sense of closure regarding his or her understanding of the presenting problem and has elucidated the extent and context of the child's symptoms, the evaluation may come to an end. When the objectives of the evaluation have been achieved, the examiner can ask the patient how he or she can help. This provides a window into the patient's insight into the illness, and into the patient's motivation to change. It is always helpful to ask the family or the child if there is anything that the examiner has not asked or that needs to be discussed further; for example, "Is there anything we have overlooked?" "Is there any thing else that may help us to understand your child and your family better?" Many times the family or the child will add another significant piece of information that will help the examiner in the diagnostic assessment, as in the following case example:

> Ron, a 15-year-old Caucasian male, was brought in for a psychiatric evaluation because of suicidal behavior. The previous night, after an altercation with his stepfather, who had a legitimate complaint about Ron's behavior, Ron ingested six aspirin tablets with the intention of killing himself. The following morning, seeing that the aspirin hadn't affected him, he ingested 30 more aspirin tablets. Ron did not tell the family about either of the overdose attempts. He began to feel dizzy in school later that morning and told a friend what he had done. The friend reported the incident to the school nurse, who called the family immediately; this prompted the psychiatric evaluation.
>
> During the assessment, Ron minimized the two overdose attempts, denying their significance. Throughout the interview, Ron denied suicidal ideation and previous suicide attempts. When the family interview was about to end, and the examiner asked Ron's mother if she wanted to add anything, she called the examiner aside and showed him a cassette recorder: Ron had made a recording the night before, after he had taken the first six aspirin tablets. He wanted to leave a recording of what it was like to die by overdose. The value of this recording was immense; it corroborated the examiner's impressions that Ron had been very serious about killing himself.

In the previous case example, the examiner was cautious about the patient's denials and listened to his clinical sense (see "Extending the Exploration" earlier in this chapter and Chapter 11).

The examiner should follow the family or the child's lead regarding further discussion that needs to be pursued privately. Some parents feel they cannot talk about certain concerns in front of the child; likewise, many children feel they cannot discuss certain topics in front of their parents. Furthermore, some children are intimidating and even abusive to their parents. These observations are of obvious clinical relevance. The examiner should exercise caution when an adolescent wants to discuss issues without the parents present. The examiner should also be aware of the danger of misalliances, for example, when an adolescent asks the examiner to keep confidential information related to suicidality, homicidality, and unlawful or drug-abusing behaviors.

The interval between the closing of the interview and the interpretive phase may bring some surprises. Either the family or the child may make further disclosures, and the examiner should be ready to capitalize on them.

Because many psychiatric evaluations are conducted under stressful conditions and both the child and the parents are subjected to heightened anxiety, the examiner needs to be cautious about making premature diagnostic closures. The examiner must remember that the collected data may not be complete or may be distorted; this happens more often than not.

Interpreting the Results

In the interpretive phase, the examiner communicates to the family and the child his or her clinical impressions of the evaluation and the recommendations or treatment plan to be followed. The interpretive phase poses special challenges and unique opportunities for the examiner. A major challenge relates to the care required in presenting the findings and in drawing preliminary conclusions from the child and family interviews. The examiner initiates an active discussion of the observations and impressions, making a balanced account of the child's and family's strengths and difficulties and taking special care when discussing family factors that may contribute to the problem(s). The examiner needs to be careful not to be critical or negative. He or she also needs to convey to the child and the family a sense of hope. The examiner must remember the adaptive value of symptoms and that the child and the family are trying to cope with problems the best they can. If the examiner keeps this in mind, he or she will be able to come across as a balanced and sensitive professional.

As the examiner is presenting the conclusions to the family, he or she must pay attention to the responses the assessment and recommendations generate. After giving diagnostic and therapeutic suggestions to the parents, the examiner will notice whether they agree with the diagnosis and treatment plan and whether they regard the ideas presented as helpful. For example, "Do they show any eagerness to carry it out, or do they doubt it will work? Are they silent, uncomprehending, sullen, unenthusiastic or, perhaps, even hostile?" (12, p. 19). If parental conflicts have not appeared earlier, they may surface at this time. During this phase, resistance that may have been latent may reveal itself in full strength.

The examiner will continue making diagnostic observations until the child and the family depart from the diagnostic setting; all along there will be additional opportunities to observe patterns of behavior that may relate to the presenting problem. These observations will also alert the physician to difficulties or complications that may be encountered as he or she implements the treatment plan.

In the following case example, a parent displayed overt infantilizing behavior toward her 17-year-old daughter. The examiner became aware of the dependent relationship between mother and daughter and handled these observations tactfully.

> Julie, a 17-year-old Hispanic female, was evaluated after an overdose of ibuprofen and acetaminophen. Julie had no psychiatric history and at the time of the examination denied she had

tried to kill herself. She acknowledged only that she had broken up with her boyfriend and that she had been under a great deal of pressure at school. She had a long history of poor academic performance. She had failed ninth grade for the second time; however, she claimed to be very popular and asserted that she had lots of friends.

During the examination, Julie's mother held her daughter in her lap and held her daughter's hand throughout the interview. Julie's mother reported that she had completed her "baby's" homework during grammar school and middle school.

When the parents returned after the examiner performed the mental status examination on Julie, the father voiced the mother's irritation toward the examiner because of the way he went about ascertaining the intentionality of Julie's suicide attempt. The mother's reservations made the examiner aware that the psychiatric examination was posing a threat to the mother's dependent relationship with her daughter. Aware of this situation, the examiner was careful not to be critical of the closeness and special relationship between them.

In the interpretive phase of the evaluation, the examiner mentioned that Julie had a great sense of frustration at school and asked whether learning problems or cognitive deficits might be an issue. The mother promptly reassured Julie that she loved her no matter how she did at school. She comforted her daughter, suggesting that there were other ways to be successful in life. The mother then began to ask the examiner questions about her overprotective behavior and asked if her parenting behavior was right. She cried, expressing fears and concerns regarding Julie's suicide attempt.

The examiner told the mother that Julie had very little chance to learn what kinds of things she could and couldn't do if her mother kept doing things for her. Julie's mother had felt all along that Julie needed more help and attention than did other children. She was confused and upset over her daughter's suicide attempt and began to question how much of what happened was her fault; she was willing to do whatever the examiner recommended.

Julie was not willing to participate in individual psychotherapy but was willing to try family therapy. Thus the examiner recommended this modality. By the time the mother left the office, her attitude and relatedness toward the examiner had turned around. The outcome would no doubt have been different if the examiner had been critical of Julie's mother and her infantilizing behaviors.

The examiner needs to balance individual and family issues with cultural and other broader concerns. The examiner need not be either too serious or too formal; sensitive humor enlivens and lightens the interview process. Above all, the examiner needs to instill understanding and hope in the patient and the family and must serve as a model for problem solving.

The interview is a professional activity of unique importance in the diagnostic process. Its productivity will depend on the examiner's skill in creating an accepting and trusting atmosphere that promotes warm and productive rapport.

■ MODALITIES OF THE PSYCHIATRIC EXAMINATION

The psychiatric examination is considered *comprehensive* when most of the possible areas of psychopathology are reviewed; it is considered *focal* if only selected areas of the patient's life, or of the mental status examination, are explored.

Unstructured Interviews

The interview is *unstructured* if the examiner does not follow a prefixed scheme to conduct the interview process. In this modality, the examiner does not follow a prearranged path in the exploration of the relevant issues or in the manner in which he or she completes the mental status examination. This modality gives the examiner a great deal of flexibility; he or she adapts the examination to the relevant issues or to the most salient aspects that emerge during the examination. The examiner attempts to follow a coherent thread in the flow of emerging data and takes advantage of the child's emotional abreactions to understand the nature of the child's internal conflict.

In unstructured interviewing the examiner emphasizes the process and the vicissitudes of affect and attempts to help the patient see connections between the content of the interview and troublesome emotional factors that the patient may be experiencing. In this modality the empathic and emotional processes are emphasized, and building rapport and establishing a solid therapeutic alliance are the examination's major objectives. The patient's relatedness to the examiner becomes more important than the data and the thoroughness of the examination. The unstructured modality does not cover all the relevant areas of a psychiatric examination in a consistent and systematic fashion and frequently leaves important areas unexplored. Furthermore, in unstructured interviewing, significant room exists for subjective inferences regarding observations and diagnosis.

Structured Interviews

The *structured* interview seeks consistent and systematic data gathering and high levels of reliability in the psychiatric examination and diagnostic process. In the most structured form of interview, the examiner uses a standardized set of questions. The examiner stays with the predetermined format of the examination, without deviating, until the interview is completed. Structured interviewing has a unique role in research (i.e., to ascertain change in any given diagnostic category resulting from, or secondary to, a given intervention), in epidemiological studies (i.e., to establish incidence and prevalence of psychiatric disorders), and in developmental studies (i.e., to compare contemporary examination data to baseline assessments in order to ascertain developmental change). In structured interviewing, the degree of the examiner's inferences is decreased significantly.

Structured interviews could be classified as either highly structured or semistructured. Examples of highly structured interviews include the Diagnostic Interview for Children and Adolescents (DICA) and the Diagnostic Interview Schedule for Children (DISC). Examples of semistructured interviews include the Schedule for Affective Disorders and Schizophrenia for School Age Children (K-SADS), the Child Assessment Schedule, and the Interview Schedule for Children (13, pp. 460–463). These comprehensive diagnostic instruments vary in the degree of training required to administer them and in their degree of reliability, sensitivity, and specificity for certain diagnoses. In clinical practice this classification of structured interviews is blurred. For example, relatively inexperienced clinicians have administered semistructured instruments "in a highly structured fashion, with little variation from the suggested wording . . . and experienced clinicians have varied the wording of highly structured interviews without apparently changing the performance of the interview" (13, p. 463). Lay examiners have also been able to make judgments about answers that it was thought could be made only be made by clinicians (13, p. 463).

Structured interviews have a number of limitations that make them unsuitable in clinical practice. For example, the protocols are rigid and time-consuming. When these protocols are given to children and their families, they are left with the impression that the examiner is more interested in completing the test instrument than in listening to their concerns.

Other structured instruments have a more restricted psychopathological scope. Such instruments include the Schedule for the Assessment of Conduct, Hyperactivity, Anxiety, Mood, and Psychoactive Substances; the Interview for Childhood Disorders and Schizophrenia; and the Social Adjustment Inventory for Children and Adolescents (13, p. 463). On the overall importance and relevance of structured interviews, Angold comments, "Though structured interview techniques have many advantages, they will aid the clinical processes only when used skillfully and sensitively" (14, p. 54).

In clinical practice, behavioral rating scales, checklists, and symptom inventories are commonly used. Parents, teachers, children, clinicians, childcare workers, and others can administer them. Table 1–2 lists the advantages and limitations of behavioral rating scales (15).

A variety of parent rating scales exist: some rating forms focus on a particular type of disorder, such as hyperactivity (e.g., Conners's Parents Questionnaire), or a few broad-band disorders, such as personality disorder and conduct disorder (e.g., Quay and Peterson's Behavior Problem Checklist). Others (e.g., Achenbach's Child Behavior Checklist, Lessing et al.'s IJR Behavior Checklist, and Miller's Louisville Behavior Checklist) include a broader variety of problems (15, pp. 4–5). Teacher rating scales are similarly varied in scope. There are also self-rating scales such as the Children's Manifest Anxiety Scale, the State-Trait Anxiety Inventory for Children, and the Beck Depression Inventory.

■ STRATEGIES FOR EVALUATING PREADOLESCENTS

The interviewing space needs to be inviting to children and spacious enough to allow small children to play comfortably on the floor. It should contain a medium-sized table and appropriate chairs for playing and other diagnostic and therapeutic activities. For a small child or for a preadolescent, sitting at a table feels more natural than sitting in a chair, face to face with the examiner. A variety of materials and toys should be readily available to the child. Table 1–3 lists the basic toys necessary for the psychiatric assessment of preadolescents.

Engagement with the preadolescent is fostered when the child is addressed directly and is made an active participant of the diagnostic process from the very beginning. A common strategy is for the examiner to begin by asking simple questions to the preadolescent during the family meeting. For example, while taking notes, the examiner could ask the preadolescent how his or her name is spelled, what the current day or date is, and so on. The

TABLE 1–2.   **Advantages and limitations of rating scales**

Advantages

1. They are convenient and economical.

    The basic instrument is usually printed.

    The relevant observations can usually be made under a variety of conditions without rigid standardization of the observational interval, setting, or inputs to subjects and raters.

    They can be completed quickly.

2. They can be completed by diverse informants without specialized training. Parents, teachers, children, clinicians, and childcare workers can complete appropriate versions.

3. They can cover a wide range of data, from specific behaviors to inferential judgments based on diverse and subtle cues occurring over long time periods.

4. They provide scores that are easy to analyze.

5. High test-retest and interobserver reliability can be obtained when similar raters observe the subjects under similar conditions.

Limitations

1. Exclusive reliance on predetermined items may cause important characteristics to be overlooked. Provision should therefore be made for adding items as a scale is being developed and for inviting individualized descriptions of behavior that cannot be accurately captured by predetermined items.

2. Rating scales compare individuals in terms of item and scale scores but may not provide ideographic (individualized) descriptions of persons apart from their specific pattern of scores.

3. Rating scales are affected by the cooperation, knowledgeability, and candor of the rater, although gross distortions are clinically informative and can usually be detected by comparisons with other data.

4. Rating scales are subject to misuse by being overinterpreted or interpreted too literally in isolation from other data about the case. Ratings from different informants should therefore be compared with each other and with other types of data about the case.

Source.   Based on Achenbach 1995 (15, pp. 3–4).

child's demeanor and responses provide important information about the child's alertness and intelligence.

The examiner may also reach an agreement with the child regarding the family member to whom questions should be addressed. The preadolescent may be told that he or she is going to be asked the questions and that if a question becomes too difficult to answer or if he or she doesn't want to answer the question, the parents will be asked to answer it. This strategy gives the child a prominent role in the interview and helps to create a positive working and diagnostic alliance. Usually the family agrees with this arrangement, and the child and the family begin to provide diagnostic data. Another important aspect of this approach is the centrality it gives to the child's problems and concerns. When a mental status examination outline exists, the child may be "invited" to help the clinician fill in the requested information. Often the child takes an interest in this cooperative enterprise.

A face-to-face interaction in an "adult-like setting" is an awkward situation for the preadolescent. The examiner should be sensitive to the child's anxiety about the new situation and environment. Even with the best of preparation, the child will arrive with fears and negative expectations about the interview. A format in which the child and the examiner sit at a table gives the child a sense of comfort. It helps the child to feel at ease if the interview is conducted in a specially furnished playroom. The younger

---

TABLE 1–3. **Toys required for a diagnostic examination**

Playhouse with furniture and a toilet

Family of small dolls with a dad, a mom, and children

Set of wood blocks, set of plastic building blocks or Legos, plasticine or Play-Doh

Paper and pencils for drawing or writing

Puppets

Set of telephones

Action figures representing men with associated weaponry

Table games and other structured games (e.g., checkers, Parcheesi)

---

the child, the greater will be the need for nonverbal approaches such as play or the use of nonverbal media (e.g., drawing, puppetry, games; see Chapter 2). The nature of the media will depend on the child's developmental level and on the examiner's style, preference, and technical experience.

After the child is properly situated in the office, the examiner will attempt to engage the child. After some engagement is achieved, the examiner will tell the child what he or she already knows about the presenting problems and then will discuss with the child these concerns. Most children will start a verbal engagement when they are invited to discuss what is already known; more often than not, they will express their thoughts about the problems without major difficulties. The exploration will proceed from there.

It is not advisable to ask the child questions about issues the examiner already knows; this is disingenuous. It is better to disclose to the child what has already been learned about the problem and to encourage the child to present his or her point of view.

Communication Issues

Care must be taken not to ask leading questions (e.g., "You didn't want to kill yourself, did you?") or to ask questions that would result in yes or no answers (e.g., "Do you sleep well every night?"). The examiner should ask open-ended questions (e.g., "What did you intend when you overdosed?" or "How is your sleep?") and must pay close attention to the patient's response, including the associations it generates and the patient's flow and change of affect.

In general, open-ended questions are more productive than are close-ended ones. "Closed questions, in contrast, may inhibit emotional expression not only because they suggest a very brief factual reply but also because they suggest that the examiner has already decided what is important and relevant" (16, p. 413).

Interpretations that affirm and validate interventions are also productive. Interpretations and expressions of sympathy explicitly indicate the examiner's interest and attention with respect to emotions, feelings, and attitudes. Expressions of sympathy are also likely to be reinforcing in that a sympathetic tone and direct statements of concern show that the examiner cares. When such caring responses follow the expression of emotions or feelings, the informant is likely to be encouraged to go on showing feelings. Many interpretations carry the same message. Interpretations might draw the informant's attention to feelings that had been below the surface (16, p. 413; see also Rose's case earlier in this chapter).

Declaratory statements often elicit more information and create less resistance than do questions; this is particularly true if the questions explore issues the patient is not yet ready to communicate. For instance, when a patient is displaying a particular emotional state, it is better to say, "You look angry [or scared or nervous]," than to ask, "Are you angry [or scared or nervous]?" A statement such as "I understand you have problems at home" is a far better opener than the question "Do you have problems at home?" A question like "Do you have any problems?" will certainly start the interview on the wrong foot.

If the examiner knows that the child has a particular problem, he or she should state the problem up front. It is good practice to present the issues directly and get to the heart of the matter from the very start. For example, the examiner could start by saying, "I understand you have problems controlling yourself," or "It seems that you do not want to live any more."

In communicating with the preadolescent, the examiner needs to calibrate to the child's developmental and cognitive level the complexity of the vocabulary used. Although smart and verbally advanced children may have sophisticated language skills and a rich vocabulary, this is not the rule for most children, even those from well-educated families. The examiner should avoid using technical jargon. For example, simple terms such as "sad" and "feel bad" are better than "depressed" and "guilty." In contrast, most children are familiar with the term "suicide." In fact, inquiring about the meaning of this term is a smooth way to explore suicidal intentions or suicidal behavior in small children. Table 1–4 lists several terms often used in adult psychiatric evaluations and the less complex equivalents appropriate for use with preschoolers and early latency children.

When we look carefully, the words "upset," "scary," "nasty," "sad," "bad," and "good" carry more affect than do their more sophisticated synonyms; the latter are most frequently used at the service of intellectualization or isolation of affect. The examiner needs to pay equal attention to the use of idioms; even the most common idiom may be beyond a child's cognitive developmental comprehension. Preadolescents and even early adolescents tend to be concrete and often interpret idioms literally.

There is no taboo subject in any diagnostic interview; there is no area that cannot be discussed with children or adolescents if it is done with appropriate language and judicious timing.

Interviewing in Displacement

When interviewing preschoolers and early latency children, the examiner frequently encounters difficulties in exploring issues directly. When the examiner senses that the child is too self-conscious or too guarded, he or she may interview the child in displacement by addressing a fantasy character's issues rather than the patient's issues. The following case illustrates this point:

> Roland, a 9-year-old Caucasian male born with paralysis of the left side, was evaluated for aggressive behavior at home and at school. He initially refused to answer any questions regarding why he had been brought for a psychiatric examination. Roland's residual neurological sequelae were obvious: besides the paralysis, he displayed conjugated gazing to the left and nys-

TABLE 1–4.　**Appropriate terms for young children**

Common term	Appropriate for young children
Frightened	Scared
Frightful	Scary
Cruel or malicious	Mean
Anxious	Nervous
Angry or frustrated	Upset
Sexual nature	Nasty
Irritable	Grouchy or cranky
Feel guilty about . . .	Feel bad about . . .
Compulsive feelings or activities	Urges
Depressed	Feel down or feel sad
Self-concept	Feel good or feel bad about yourself
Feel hopeless	Feel like not caring anymore
Learning problems	Trouble learning or hard to learn

tagmus with rapid eye movements to the right. His voice was infantile and had an immature and unmelodious quality.

Roland was disgruntled and unhappy. He asked for his mother. The examiner empathized with Roland's distress over being away from his mother. Because Roland refused to indicate why his mother had brought him for the evaluation, and having announced that he wanted to talk about dinosaurs, the examiner went along with that idea.

Roland started by saying, "The baby dinosaur was angry." The examiner replied, "The baby dinosaur was angry at his mother." Roland agreed and continued, "The baby dinosaur was really mad and felt like hitting people." The examiner said, "If the baby dinosaur loses control and hits people, he is going to get in trouble." The examiner added, "The baby dinosaur was angry, in part because he was not with his mother," and he asked if there were other reasons why the baby dinosaur was angry. While this conversation continued, Roland kept attempting to stretch the fingers of his paralyzed left hand with his right hand. Roland was angry as he attempted to move his limp hand. The examiner said, "It seemed that the baby dinosaur was angry at his mother because he had problems with his left arm and left leg." Roland responded, "I'm very angry at my mother." The child then began to bite himself, saying "It's better to bite myself than to bite my mother."

The examiner addressed issues of Roland's defective self-concept and his feeling of rejection; he also suggested that Roland blamed his mother for the problems he had with his left side. Roland acknowledged that he had problems controlling his anger and that this was one of the reasons that he had been brought for the psychiatric examination.

In the preceding case example, the child was resistant to discussing the nature of his problems. Once the examiner followed the child's lead and approached his emotional problems in an indirect manner, using the mechanism of displacement, he was able to move into a direct exploration of the patient's painful subjective difficulties.

In the next case example, the child was very uncommunicative and resistant at first but became more open after the displacement mechanisms were respected and utilized.

Saul, a 7-year-old African American boy, had been referred for psychiatric evaluation because of aggressive and unruly behaviors. There was also a question regarding the presence of psychotic behaviors because he displayed a series of atypical behaviors at home and at school. He lived with his mother, a sister who was a couple of years his senior, and his maternal grandmother. Saul had threatened to kill his sister, mother, and grandmother with a knife. Saul's parents had been divorced for over a year, and his father had broken off all contact with the children. Saul and his sister missed their father a lot and were very angry that their father did not seem to care about them.

Saul reported seeing his grandfather, who had died 18 months earlier. Also, the family had overheard Saul talking to himself (as though to other people) when he was alone. Apparently he believed that people talked about him and that God was telling him to be good.

During the psychiatric examination, Saul was very unhappy. He appeared downcast and was overtly angry and defiant. He displayed poor eye contact and was uncooperative with the examiner. When the examiner asked him questions, he refused to answer them. He demonstrated unhappiness after each question, no matter how empathic the examiner tried to be. For instance, the examiner commented on how sad it must be for Saul that his father didn't show any interest in calling him. Instead of being more forthcoming with his communications, Saul became more defensive and less verbal.

Saul brought to the second diagnostic interview his school project on caterpillars. He began to talk about his project. The examiner picked up Saul's lead and followed the content and process of his narrative. Saul continued discussing his project and demonstrated an interest in the caterpillar's life. The examiner asked Saul what the caterpillar's family life was like. Saul explained that the caterpillar lived with his mother and sister alone. The examiner asked what happened to the caterpillar's father. Saul became sad and said that the father had gone away and had not come back. The examiner commented that the caterpillar must be very sad because it could not see its father anymore. Saul began to cry. At this point, the examiner said, "It is very hard for you not to see your father. You miss him a lot and are very angry that you can't see him." This interpretation brought the child's concerns from the displacement to the reality of his life.

In these and similar cases, the examiner's comments and interpretations through displacement build a bridge to the child's emotional difficulties in real life and to the feelings the child has in diverse areas of his or her life. Issues that the child has refused to acknowledge directly are accepted via the comments and interpretations made through displacement.

Interviewing through displacement is developmentally appropriate for preadolescents because this mechanism is prevalent among children in this age group.

■ STRATEGIES FOR EVALUATING ADOLESCENTS

It is helpful to start the adolescent evaluation with the parents and the adolescent together. The benefits of such a meeting are multiple. For example, the examiner hears the parents' concerns directly, and the examiner has the opportunity to observe how the adolescent relates to the parents and how the parents or family members relate to one another. During the family meeting, most of the preliminary exploration and overall assessment of the presenting problem and the adolescent's level of functioning are completed. The examiner explores the adolescent's school and family functioning, the parents' knowledge of their child's behaviors such as drug use, and other serious concerns. As these issues are addressed, the adolescent's participation is invited and encouraged. How conflicts between the parents and the adolescent are handled gives the examiner a sense of the intensity of the conflicts between them and of the problem-solving capacities within the adolescent and within the family.

After the parents express their concerns, the examiner asks them to leave. The adolescent is then given the opportunity to expand on, or to present his or her side regarding, the parents' concerns. The adolescent will be asked to talk about issues the parents may not have any knowledge about, for example, suicidal thoughts, school truancy, alcohol or drug use, illicit activities, sexual life, gang participation, cults, and other issues related to the presenting problem. During the individual interview with the adolescent, a comprehensive mental status examination also is completed.

If the adolescent is not cooperative and displays hostility or resistance from the very beginning of the interview, the examiner may need to consider a different approach. Katz (5) proposes four basic strategies to deal with the adolescent's immediate resistances, included as Strategies 1–4 in Table 1–5. These strategies parallel the recommendations given in Chapter 10.

The following case example illustrates the effectiveness of reversing roles with the patient:

TABLE 1–5.   **Strategies in the psychiatric examination of adolescents**

1. **Clarify your role as a stranger.** When the examiner detects an immediate distrust, he should respond with ready acceptance of the distrust, pointing out to the patient that he knows he is a stranger, that the patient has no reason to trust him.

2. **Analyze the situation to the patient.** When the examiner finds himself in trouble with a patient, it is helpful to analyze the situation to the patient and enlist his or her assistance. Often the patient has information that can be helpful.

3. **Seek opportunities to empathize with the patient.** The examiner should demonstrate as quickly as possible his powers as a therapist, the power to see things from the patient's point of view, the power of understanding what's going on in the patient.

4. **Offer immediate help to the patient.** Each adolescent who comes unwillingly to the office is being faced with the evidence of his or her helplessness. The examiner offers power in the form of knowledge, and help, if appropriate, by intervening in the patient's situation.

5. **Reverse roles with the patient.** The examiner asks the adolescent to take the examiner's role while the examiner takes his or her role. The examiner (as the adolescent) presents his or her concerns and seeks help from the adolescent.

6. **Support adaptive behavior.** The examiner validates, praises, and promotes normative behavior.

Source.   Strategies 1–4 are adapted from Katz 1990 (5, pp. 74–79).

Damian, a 16-year-old African American boy, was brought by his mother for a psychiatric evaluation because she felt she could no longer control him and was concerned that he was getting into progressively more trouble. Damian's parents had divorced 6 years earlier. The father kept custody of Damian and his younger brother after the divorce, but the children spent summers with the mother on a regular basis. Both parents had remarried.

Damian's father sent him to live with his mother 4 months earlier. Damian had very serious difficulties with his father, including physical fights on four occasions. The father had called the police and placed both children in shelter homes for a couple of weeks. Damian also had difficulties at school: he had been found with illegal substances on school grounds and was on probation. The father was so angry and frustrated with Damian that he didn't want anything to do with him.

Since being with his mother, Damian had displayed problems at home and at school. He flunked the previous school year because of poor attendance, and he had been truant from school on a regular basis. At home he was unruly, defiant, and confrontational, and he sought isolation. Damian left home without permission whenever he felt like doing so. He frequently sneaked out at night and had stayed out all night a number of times. His mother had found spray cans in his room and suspected that he was using other drugs. Damian adamantly denied he was abusing illegal substances. He had obtained a very well-paid summer job, but he was fired for unexplained absences.

The mental status examination revealed a very defensive and uncooperative adolescent who looked older than his stated age. He remained distant and uninvolved for most of the examination. He said at the outset, "I do not belong in an asylum. I am not crazy. I am not hearing voices or seeing things." He added, "I don't need any help. I want to go home." He said, "I want to go to Arizona," where his father lived. When the examiner asked Damian how he felt when his father sent him to live with his mother, he became tearful. He said he was surprised, adding, "I couldn't believe it." Damian mentioned several times that he missed his friends and indicated how unhappy he was living with his mother. The examiner asked Damian about his parents' divorce. He responded, "My life has been wrecked ever since the divorce." He felt that he could be mean to his parents because of the pain and misery they had put him through. Damian became even more tearful as he talked about how his parents' divorce had affected him.

When the examiner began to talk about the options for handling Damian's problems, Damian became defensive again and asserted that he had no problems and that he wanted to go home. Because he did not seem amenable to any recommendations, the examiner opted to ask Damian for help.

The examiner asked Damian to switch chairs. After the

chairs were switched, the examiner said to Damian, "Now you are the doctor. What would you do to help a child who is getting in trouble all the time? How would you help a youngster who cannot get along with either parent and who flunked the previous year? How can you help a child who doesn't like school?" Damian became reflective and then suggested that the child has to learn to get along with his mother, has to stay at home, has to ask permission to leave, and so on. Although Damian had been negative about receiving any psychiatric services, he now agreed to come back for an extended evaluation.

■ PROCESS INTERVIEWS

The *content* of a communication refers to the explicit aspects of the communication. The *process* refers to the implicit aspects, to the way the communication is presented. To assess the communication process, the examiner pays special attention to the way the patient communicates. The way things are conveyed may be more important than what is said. For example, the patient may be saying one thing with his or her words and a very different thing with his or her voice or body language. The examiner should inform the patient about any discrepancy between verbal and nonverbal behaviors and should make the patient aware of any atypical nonverbal communication. Any incongruity between verbal and nonverbal behaviors requires elucidation. Every time an abreaction of affect occurs, the examiner should ask the patient about the thoughts or memories that brought on those emotions. When the patient interrupts his or her own narrative or when unexpected transitions occur in the patient's train of thought, the examiner should ask about these interruptions or transitions. It matters a great deal whether the patient has noticed these events.

In the process interview, the examiner notices how things are said and presented. The following case example illustrates process interviewing (see also Kurt's case example in Chapter 4):

Donna, a 16-year-old Caucasian girl, was evaluated for protracted depression and suicidal behavior. According to Donna, her depression went back to when she was 7 or 8 years old, and she had felt suicidal for a long time. Donna's mother and maternal grandmother had received diagnoses of schizophrenia. A maternal aunt had raised Donna since early childhood. Donna had received both inpatient and prolonged outpatient treatments, with limited success.

At the time of the evaluation, Donna's aunt was in the process of giving up her guardianship rights to the state because she could not handle Donna and could no longer afford to pay for Donna's psychiatric services. Donna had been involved in a lesbian relationship with an adolescent female 3 years her senior and had displayed significant behavioral problems at school and at home. Donna also had problems with substance abuse and had abused marijuana, cocaine, LSD, and other mind-altering drugs.

Donna had been a bright and articulate child who had excelled at school. Her academic performance had suffered during the previous year. She was described as a gifted and creative adolescent.

Donna was a fairly kempt and groomed but rather unattractive adolescent; she was withdrawn and maintained poor eye contact. Her psychomotor activity was low. She appeared distant and was not spontaneous; there was an air of apprehension and fear about her. Her mood was very depressed, and she exhibited marked constriction of affect, both in range and in intensity. She rarely smiled.

Donna used sophisticated language, and her responses were filled with intellectualization and isolation of affect. When the examiner asked Donna questions, she often took a long time to answer, and she hesitated noticeably while responding. When the examiner asked Donna how she felt about her aunt, whom she called "mother," giving up her guardianship rights to the state, Donna gave a bland and unemotional response.

The examiner gave Donna feedback about the way she communicated and presented her thoughts. She expressed surprise and claimed that in all the time that she had been in treatment nobody had commented on the way she thought or how she came across. She said, "My thoughts are in a different channel from other people's. I always feel empty." When the examiner asked Donna why her thoughts were in a different channel from other people's, she said, "I need to build a barrier around people." Donna was able to discuss her apprehensions and paranoid feelings and her difficulties trusting and feeling close to people. The content of Donna's delusional depression is presented in a case example in Chapter 3. The process interview is illustrated further in Chapter 4 (see Kurt's case example).

■ PHYSICAL CONTACT

There are no rigid rules regarding physical contact. Each clinical situation requires consideration of the child's developmental level, but the clinician may wish to keep some key points in mind when making decisions regarding appropriate physical contact.

In general, the examiner should exercise restraint in the initiation of physical contact with a child except when the child is a toddler or a preschooler in need of guidance toward the office. Such guidance is achieved by holding the child's hand or making ongoing contact with the child's shoulder in a comforting and reassuring manner.

The examiner may respond to any physical contact related to social courtesies (e.g., handshaking). With older adolescents, the examiner may initiate handshaking upon greeting the patient. Younger children sometimes initiate affectionate contact. For example, they may seek comfort by body proximity or by holding the examiner's hand. Children may want to show appreciation and make affectionate body contact. If the contact is genuine and appropriate, it is accepted and appreciated. The examiner should remind the child that he or she can express emotions with words; words of appreciation are as good as hugs or other physical expressions of affection. Spontaneous embracing to express gratitude or to say "good-bye" is uncommon in loved and well-cared-for small children. For small children in need of reassurance and support, a tap on the shoulder or a delicate tapping on the head may be sufficient.

With children older than mid-latency age, the examiner should exercise clinical judgment as to when it is appropriate to receive or accept physical contact, when it should be avoided, or when limits need to be imposed. Caution should be exercised when the examiner and the patient are not of the same sex and when allegations of sexual abuse have been made; in such a case, no matter how young the child, physical contact should be avoided and discouraged.

When the child is female and the examiner is male and he detects promiscuous relating or inappropriate sexualization, he needs to exercise caution and set limits on boundary violations. The examiner should be particularly alert to any kind of physical contact with an overtly seductive female child or adolescent. The same caution applies to situations in which the examiner is female and the patient is male. Examiners of both sexes may also be the focus of homosexual behavior by children or adolescents who have been abused or by patients who are struggling with consolidation of their sexual identities.

In children who have not been sexually abused, there will be moments when the examiner may want to convey affirmation, approval, or reassurance by a gentle touch or when the doctor and patient converge in emotional rapport; in this case, sensitive contact could be appropriate and developmentally fitting.

Physical contact is obligatory in some situations. For example, the examiner must hold a small child who is beginning to harm himself or to display aggressive behavior toward the examiner. A firm hold may be necessary in these circumstances; the examiner should let the child know that he will not be allowed to either harm himself or hurt the doctor. If the patient is an adolescent who gets out of control, the examiner should warn the patient that if the aggressive or intimidating behavior persists, the evaluation will be terminated immediately. If the patient persists, the examination should end at once. If the adolescent gives signs of being on the verge of losing control and asks to leave, he or she should be given this opportunity without objections. The examiner should inform the parents that the adolescent has left the evaluation in a state of dyscontrol. Again, caution should be used if the patient has a history of sexual abuse or assaultive or violent behavior. The examiner should establish procedures to follow in the event that he or she is at risk or in danger. The examiner must take precautionary actions if a patient is out of control and is at risk for self-harm or for harming others.

Physician contact with preadolescent and adolescent patients during the physical and neurological examination merits special comment. There is obligatory contact during this process. Some child and adolescent psychiatrists delegate to pediatrician colleagues or other physicians all aspects of physical examination and medical care, but there are multiple arguments in favor of the evaluating and treating psychiatrist conducting the physical examination.

After conducting hundreds of physical examinations on preadolescents and adolescents, we have seen only two occasions when patients have misperceived the physical examination experience. In one case, a 12-year-old early adolescent schizophrenic girl said to the examiner: "I know you have the 'hots' for me. I know that because of the way you touched my breasts." Reality testing was used to address her misperceptions. In the other case, a 9-year-old overanxious girl felt very anxious during the physical examination and complained about it afterward. For most female patients, and for children in general, the physical examination is an uneventful experience with no detrimental psychological consequences. These indispensable procedures pose no significant risk for building a therapeutic alliance with the doctor.

The observations gathered during the physical and neurological examination are invaluable for achieving a comprehensive and integrative view of the patient. Findings frequently shed light on the diagnosis (e.g., evidence of a neurocutaneous disorder), aid in the examiner's understanding of the problem's etiology (e.g., evidence of self-inflicted injuries), or demonstrate the extent of a given identified problem (i.e., marked gynecomastia in an adolescent who has doubts about his sexual identity). In other cases, the physical examination puts the process of assessment and treatment in a very different direction (e.g., when the physician observes ample evidence of physical abuse or signs of drug addiction even though the patient has denied physical abuse or drug addiction throughout the interview). The examiner should explore methodically the history of every traumatic or surgical scar. These are but a few examples of the usefulness of conducting the physical examination during a comprehensive psychiatric examination. Neurological examination findings are equally valuable in patients with neuropsychiatric disorders.

The benefits of having the physical examination performed by the same physician who conducts the psychiatric examination far outweigh the risks (see Table 1–6 for a summary of benefits and risks). Some basic precautions minimize the potential negative risks even further: the physician should always conduct the examination in the presence of the nurse or, better yet, in the presence of one of the patient's parents. When evaluating female adolescents, the examiner should always invite the mother to be present during the examination. It is helpful to tell the patient what is about to happen during the examination (e.g., "Now I'm going to examine your ears and your eyes. Now I'm going to examine your belly."). The physician should remember that boys with a background of sexual abuse are as anxious about the physical examination as are girls with the same history. Some patients may object adamantly to a physical examination. If there is no medical emergency, the patient's refusal should be respected.

Special sensitivity needs to be demonstrated when examining the female thorax (i.e., when listening to heart sounds and when exploring the hypogastric and inguinal areas). Pelvic examination,

TABLE 1–6. **Benefits and risks of the evaluating psychiatrist performing the physical examination**

Benefits	Risks
Invaluable observations:	Privacy concerns
Findings shed light on diagnosis	Risk of sensual contact
Findings highlight magnitude of the problem	Concerns with therapeutic alliance
Findings reorient the focus of the examination	

when indicated, should be referred to a gynecologist. If the examiner is male and a female patient asks that a female physician conduct the physical examination, this request must be granted.

■ ACTIVITY, STRUCTURING, AND SUPPORT DURING THE PSYCHIATRIC EXAMINATION

The examiner strives to create the optimal level of activity (i.e., prompting and questioning) needed to elicit from the patient and the family any information relevant to the diagnostic assessment. Excessive prompting will stifle the patient's spontaneity and may render the interview mechanical and emotionally sterile. This may leave the child and his or her family dissatisfied, feeling intruded upon, or even misunderstood. When the interview has been too structured, the patient or the family may leave feeling that they could have said more, if they'd been given the opportunity. In contrast, in unstructured interviews, the data may be partial, incomplete, or irrelevant to the diagnostic goals, if the patient is not given enough guidance and structure. Not too much activity, not too much passivity; the ideal is definitely in the middle (see the "Modalities of the Psychiatric Examination" section earlier in this chapter).

Structuring entails controlling a number of variables during the interview. The examiner may need to control factors such as the interview space (e.g., limiting the child's actions or movements to a restricted area), the type of play and the toys used, the nature of the probing (e.g., using open-ended questioning or structured interviewing), and the degree and quality of nonverbal behavior (e.g., physical contact with the examiner). With verbal children, the examiner may direct the content and the process of the communication. Active structuring and limit setting (see next section) is needed with hyperactive, impulsive, aggressive, self-abusive, seductive, or disorganized children (e.g., with psychotic and neuropsychiatric patients).

The quality and degree of structure needed varies in each interview, depending on the child's developmental level, the quality and intensity of psychopathology, the child's dystonicity of symptoms, the child's willingness to participate in the interview, and the interest the child shows in working on his or her problems. Without appropriate structuring, a safe, effective, and productive interview cannot be achieved.

The examiner must convey to the child and the family that the interview will be conducted in a safe atmosphere where all verbalization will be permitted and encouraged. Any personal or physical aggression will be discouraged. The child needs to know that if he or she were to lose control, the examiner will help the child to regain control. If the child expresses aggression or self-abusive behaviors, the examiner will notice the context in which these behavior originated. The examiner's priority will be to help the child regain control and to return the interview to its exploratory mode. As mentioned earlier in this chapter, during an episode of dyscontrol a child could use as a weapon any item found in the examiner's office. As a result, the examiner must consider carefully the office decor and the items available to the child in the examination space. The examiner must actively monitor safety conditions throughout the psychiatric examination.

The child needs to be supported, or confronted, as needed. There is no contradiction if the examiner is supportive and empathic during some parts of the interview and challenging and confrontational during other parts. The examiner should demonstrate empathy toward the child's emotional pain and circumstances, but at the same time the examiner must confront the child's maladaptive behaviors. The examiner should help the patient assert self-control when an impulsive action is about to be carried out and should appeal to the child's adaptive functioning when he or she entertains any impulsive or destructive action. Balancing empathy and confrontation is an important skill for dealing with children and adolescents. With certain clinical presentations (e.g., acting-out behaviors, externalizing disorders), sensitive confrontations are always required; with internalizing disorders (e.g., anxiety, depression), in contrast, empathic interventions are the most helpful and productive.

■ LIMIT SETTING DURING THE PSYCHIATRIC EXAMINATION

Novice examiners have significant difficulty maintaining a safe and unencumbered diagnostic process. Impulsive children frequently violate space or personal boundaries. Children may become destructive or aggressive during the diagnostic examination, posing a risk to the safety of the diagnostic process. In these circumstances, the examiner needs to convey unambiguously that these behaviors must stop.

The examiner needs to convey that he or she is in charge of the psychiatric examination process at all times. Inexperienced examiners fear that setting limits during the diagnostic interview will make the child less cooperative or that setting limits will decrease the chances for building a diagnostic and therapeutic alliance. This is a groundless concern. Rather than decreasing trust in the examiner, appropriate and opportune limit setting gives patients a sense of security. Children and adolescents with impulse-control difficulties hope to find someone who will help them with this problem.

Appropriate structuring and timely limit setting are fundamental requirements in any diagnostic interview. Failure to assert limits and to delineate boundaries poses risks for the patient and the examiner and may imperil the entire diagnostic enterprise. The therapeutic alliance may be jeopardized if the patient perceives the examiner as not capable of establishing or maintaining a sense of safety during the examination. The following case example illustrates inadequate management of risk and boundary problems during a diagnostic interview:

> During the live patient interview portion of a mock oral board examination, a first-year fellow in child psychiatry encountered a 13-year-old Caucasian girl who displayed marked hyperactivity, impulsivity, and immaturity from the beginning of the interview. The child started off by making fun of the fellow's name. She also began to smile inappropriately, fidgeted a great deal, and stared at one of the ceiling corners. The fellow kept busy writing down the child's answers to his questions but often

missed important nonverbal behaviors.

The child kept squirming and tilting her chair backward. At one point, she got up, picked up a stick that was leaning against the wall in a corner of the room, and began to swing it from side to side. The stick made contact progressively with a piece of furniture, the child's chin, and the fellow's boots, legs, and knees. Finally, the child pointed the stick at the fellow's tie, directly at his neck, in a teasing, provocative, and dangerous gesture. In a bland and unconvincing fashion, the fellow said to the child that what she was doing was dangerous; however, he hesitated in asking her to put down the stick.

In the preceding case example, the hazardous development was predictable once this impulsive child picked up the stick. An experienced clinician would have anticipated the child's impulsivity, immaturity, inappropriate social behaviors, and her potential for aggressive behaviors. The most appropriate and timely intervention would have been to ask the child to put down the stick as soon as she picked it up from the corner.

Many examiners have had experience with children who bring to the interview knives, lighters, and other potentially dangerous items. In one way or another, these children have made the examiners aware of the presence of these items. They may have displayed and used these objects in a clearly provocative and dangerous manner. More often, the child psychiatrist will be asked to evaluate potentially dangerous adolescents. In these cases, the examiner needs to be alert in identifying (and anticipating) moments of potential danger during the examination. Limit setting needs to be enforced when the patient displays inappropriate familiarity with the examiner or when the patient behaves in a physically or sexually inappropriate manner toward the examiner.

■ CARRYING THE PSYCHIATRIC EXAMINATION

The concept of *carrying* relates to the process of assisting the patient during the psychiatric examination; it facilitates a good and productive flow of verbal communication. It implies a number of skills—including engagement, appropriate management of silences, and use of humor—and a good balance of exploratory and supportive approaches. This active assistance is of particular importance when interviewing primitive, resistant, or neuropsychologically impaired patients.

When the interviewee has cognitive or neuropsychological limitations, major challenges include aiding the patient in the initiation of verbalization, helping him or her with a sensitive management of silences, and prompting him or her to be introspective. The more impaired the child, the greater will be the need for communication assistance and the greater the examiner's responsibility to assist actively with the function of carrying the interview.

■ ENACTMENTS DURING THE PSYCHIATRIC EXAMINATION

Enactments are nonverbal dramatizations of internal emotional conflicts that may occur if the patient is either unaware of the problems or has difficulties communicating them in verbal language. Enactments represent active conflictive areas in which the patient needs assistance in verbalization and understanding. The examiner needs to transform nonverbal communication (e.g., gestures, actions, motor displays) into an explicitly verbalized problem. Here are some examples:

> Members of a gang had raped a 12-year-old Hispanic girl. When interviewed 2 years later, the girl was sitting by a metallic table that had in it multiple holes. As she discussed the rape, she stuck her fingers in and out of the holes, in an obvious copulatory gesture. This adolescent felt terrible about herself and had attempted to kill herself a number of times because she felt like "damaged goods" after the rape. The girl exhibited active symptoms of posttraumatic stress disorder. The enactment indicated how active and disorganizing the gang rape incident still was for her.

> A 14-year-old Caucasian boy with a history of neuropsychological deficits, low intellectual functioning, and significant language difficulties was seen in consultation for persistent regressive behavior and enuresis. The examiner had been in-

formed that the child seemed to enjoy urinating on himself. During the interview the boy repeatedly twisted and compulsively tightened the edge of his shirt around his fingers. This behavior appeared to be an enactment of the child's effort and conflict surrounding his enuresis.

A 13-year-old boy with a history of bipolar disorder was evaluated for depressive features after the manic state began to recede. When the patient was actively manic, he was busy all day long, lifting weights without feeling tired or experiencing muscle pain. He had an inordinate amount of energy. At the time of the interview, while talking about how much better he was feeling, he began to display his muscles and began contracting his biceps in both arms; he would touch the bulk of each bicep in a clearly exhibitionistic manner. The examiner reminded the patient about the feelings he had while in the manic state and pointed out to him that he might be missing the abundant energy he had before. This helped the patient understand some of his depressive feelings.

A 13-year-old Caucasian boy with a history of marked impulsivity and overt manic features was evaluated for issues regarding sexual identity: he had conspicuous gynecomastia and clearly effeminate traits. During the assessment, the boy placed his hands under his sweatshirt and formed with his fists two prominences on his upper chest, simulating female breasts. When the examiner asked, "What are you doing?" the boy responded, "Mountains." The examiner understood the patient was enacting, in a seductive and histrionic fashion, his concerns about his sexual identity in general and his gynecomastia (i.e., the "mountains" he had in his body) in particular.

■ PROSPECTIVE INTERVIEWS

Patients sometimes refuse to talk about the past. Children who have been heavily traumatized are very apprehensive about, if not resistant to, "opening up old wounds." In these situations, the examiner may attempt to carry out a *prospective interview,* in which the questions are addressed to the patient's future. Even though the patient refuses to reveal anything about the past, as the patient begins to talk about the future, he or she will provide informative clues about his or her problems and personality organization. Consider the following case example:

> Harold, an African American boy, was 2 months shy of age 18 years at the time of a psychiatric evaluation. He had a horrible childhood history, including gross neglect and frequent physical abuse by his alcoholic and drug-abusing mother. His father had been in and out of jail for theft and other crimes. Harold received serious and extensive burns on one occasion when his mother threw scalding water on him. Harold had moved frequently between his mother's house and his maternal grandmother's house. He yearned for his mother's love and couldn't understand why she didn't show any affection for him. His poverty and problems with enuresis led to frequent teasing by his peers; the enuresis also led to frequent whippings by his mother.
>
> From a very young age, Harold felt different, "sort of unique," among his peers. Peers remarked that he didn't "speak like blacks." He remembered feeling depressed all his life. He was 14 years old when he started thinking about suicide. He had a number of psychiatric hospitalizations after suicide attempts. His middle adolescence had been quite stormy: he had frequently been depressed and suicidal and had begun drinking, taking drugs, and stealing. He continued to crave his mother's love.
>
> At the time of the evaluation, Harold was living with a maternal aunt but still hoped to live with his mother. He described himself as a deep thinker and was actively involved with music, writing, and poetry. He had begun to understand that the lack of his mother's responsiveness probably was not his fault.
>
> Harold was able to develop rapport with the examiner and was able to display some degree of relatedness during the interview. His eye contact was intermittent, but he didn't use body language when he spoke. Harold had a British-like accent that was somewhat unusual given his background. His mood was euthymic (Harold was taking venlafaxine and had a very positive response to the medication.) His affect was markedly constricted in both range and intensity. He was not suicidal nor did he exhibit signs of psychosis. He was articulate and seemed thoughtful in his responses. Sensorium was intact, and intelli-

gence was judged as average if not better.

Although Harold would talk about any topic proposed for discussion, the examiner felt that a prospective interview would provide significant information about his ego strengths, resilience, and ideals. The examiner asked Harold to discuss his future plans. He said that he wanted to finish regular high school instead of opting for a GED. He wondered if he could become a social worker or a counselor to help other kids. He also discussed his interests in music and in writing. He didn't have any close friends but had begun to appreciate that different people have different things to offer. Efforts to gain his mother's love were still a high priority, even though he realized that his mother was a very troubled person and that he was not the reason why his mother had failed to love him. When asked to express his feeling about having a family, he said he would like to have a family of his own. Then he became more thoughtful and added that he worried about having a son because he didn't know what kind of father he would be. He said he was scared of becoming angry and losing control. In the past, when he felt very angry, he had felt like killing someone.

Harold verbalized his inner preoccupations in a matter-of-fact way, exhibiting prominent isolation of affect and a lack of affective modulation in his speech. He credited the antidepressant for improving his mood. The adaptive pragmatics of communication (he had to learn to appear normal, although deep inside, he was depressed) he exhibited at the beginning of the interview began to fade, and as the interview proceeded he became progressively apathetic and downcast. Harold appeared to be making good strides; however, he was at high risk for psychiatric relapse and future maladaptation. He required close psychiatric follow-up.

It is impossible to talk about the future without disclosing problems in the present and difficulties from the past. With the prospective interview strategy, the patient's defensiveness or resistance may be bypassed (see Chapter 10).

■ REFERENCES

1. Mrazek DA, Mrazek P, Klinnert M: Clinical assessment of parenting. J Am Acad Child Adolesc Psychiatry 34:272–282, 1995

2. Young JG, Leven L, Ludman W, et al: Interviewing children and adolescents, in Psychiatric Disorders in Children and Adolescents. Edited by Garfinkel BD, Carlson GA, Weller E. Philadelphia, PA, WB Saunders, 1990, pp 443–468

3. Winnicott DW: Therapeutic Consultations in Child Psychiatry. New York, Basic Books, 1971

4. Leon RL: Psychiatric Interviewing: A Primer. New York, Elsevier North-Holland, 1982

5. Katz P: The first few minutes: the engagement of the difficult adolescent. Adolescent Psychiatry 17:69–81, 1990

6. Brown GW, Rutter M: The measurements of family activities and relationships: a methodological study. Human Relations 19:241–263, 1966

7. Rutter M, Brown GW: The reliability and validity of measures of family life and relationships in families containing a psychiatric patient. Soc Psychiatry 1:38–53, 1966

8. Cox A, Hopkinson K, Rutter M: Psychiatric interviewing techniques II; naturalistic study: eliciting factual information. Br J Psychiatry 138:283–291, 1981

9. Cox A, Rutter M, Holbrook D: Psychiatric interviewing techniques V; experimental study: eliciting factual information. Br J Psychiatry 139:29–37, 1981

10. Nurcombe B: Malpractice, in Child and Adolescent Psychiatry: A Comprehensive Textbook. Edited by Lewis M. Baltimore, MD, Williams & Wilkins, 1996, pp 1134–1145

11. Senay EC: Diagnostic interview and mental status examination, in Substance Abuse: A Comprehensive Textbook, 3rd Edition. Edited by Lowinson JH, Ruiz P, Millman RB, et al. Baltimore, MD, Williams & Wilkins, 1997, pp 365–367

12. Reisman JM, Ribordy S: Principles of Psychotherapy With Children, 2nd Edition. New York, Lexington Books, 1993

13. Costello AJ: Structured interviewing, in Child and Adolescent Psychiatry: A Comprehensive Textbook. Edited by Lewis M. Baltimore, MD, Williams & Wilkins, 1996, pp 457–464

14. Angold A: Clinical interviewing with children and adolescents, in Child and Adolescent Psychiatry: Modern Approaches. Edited by

Rutter M, Taylor E, Hersov L. Oxford, England, Blackwell Scientific, 1994, pp 51–63

15. Achenbach TM: Clinical data systems: rating scales and interviews, in Psychiatry, Revised Edition, Vol 2. Edited by Michels R, Cooper AM, Guze SB, et al. Philadelphia, PA, Lippincott-Raven, 1995, pp 1–14

16. Hopkinson K, Cox A, Rutter M: Psychiatric interviewing techniques, III: naturalistic study: eliciting feelings. Br J Psychiatry 138:406–415, 1981

2

NONVERBAL TECHNIQUES FOR INTERVIEWING CHILDREN AND ADOLESCENTS

The child must be encouraged to express problems in his or her own words, to verbalize psychological, family, and social problems in a personal way. According to Warren and colleagues, "Understanding the child's experience is important for a comprehensive diagnosis and for designing treatment programs" (1, p. 1331).

As an alternative to verbal exploration, the examiner occasionally needs to use nonverbal techniques to access the child's psychological world. The value of nonverbal diagnostic techniques varies in relation to the effectiveness of each technique in drawing out relevant information from the child's internal world. Nonverbal techniques may enhance trust and communication between the child and the examiner. The specific techniques used depend on the interviewer's style and the child's developmental level. For example, some interviewers prefer diagnostic activities in the *microsphere* (the circumscribed therapeutic playing space of the office), whereas others prefer the larger field of the *macrosphere* (including space outside the office, e.g., in the playground). Some examiners select artistic media, whereas others prefer sports-oriented activities.

The best choice seems to be one that best stimulates the child's skills or talents, the one that most appeals to the child, the one that is closest to the child's favorite activities, or the one most appropriate to the child's developmental state. A developmental fit will be the most motivating to the child.

Nonverbal techniques are productive when 1) new material is presented, 2) the nonverbal productions complement prior verbalizations, or 3) the nonverbal productions add depth or new dimensions to the evaluation. Nonverbal techniques are particularly helpful when the child's capacity to speak is inhibited markedly (e.g., in elective mutism) or when the child is very anxious or very resistant to disclosing private feelings, or a secret such as abuse, that to press for verbal communication may be counterproductive.

■ DRAWING TECHNIQUES

If verbalization is gold, drawings are silver. Drawings, complemented with a sensitive exploration of their content, can illuminate the child's major issues or concerns. Drawings also give a good indication of the child's level of intelligence and creative and artistic talents and may indicate whether neuropsychological deficits are present. Drawings also aid in identifying body image difficulties and a variety of psychological conflicts or psychosocial stressors.

An added advantage of drawings is that they may serve as visible and concrete evidence that may be presented to parents who do not want to believe that anything is wrong with their child. A drawing may be used as a springboard for a discussion about sexual abuse or violence within the family when the drawing clearly represents or suggests these themes. When the examiner analyzes drawings, he or she needs to keep in mind that "drawings by young children are representations and not reproductions, that they express an inner and not a visual realism. The drawings make a statement about the child himself and less about the object drawn. The image is imbued with affective as well as cognitive elements" (2, p. 9). Table 2–1 lists the types of drawings used in a diagnostic interview, in the order in which they are solicited.

Male children regularly draw male figures when they are asked to draw a person; if a boy draws a female figure, sexual identity conflicts may be present. This is not the case for girls. The family

TABLE 2–1.	**Sequence of diagnostic drawing**

1. Free drawing
2. Draw a person
3. Draw a person from the opposite sex of the previous one
4. Draw the family doing something together (kinetic family drawing)
5. Optional drawings: a tree, a house, a car

drawing, called the *kinetic family drawing,* offers the examiner insight into family dynamics and particularly into the child's perceived role within the family. Whereas the person drawings may indicate the child's cognitive development, the family drawing elicits "mobilization of feelings that, while rendering the family drawing less valuable as an indicator of intelligence, confers upon it significance as an expression of the child's emotional life. The family drawing, then, can be viewed as an unstructured projective technique that may reveal the child's feelings in relation to those whom he regards as most important and whose formative influence is most powerful" (2, p. 100).

In the following case example, the use of drawing was instrumental in breaking through a mother's denial about her child's problems:

> Tom, a 9-year-old African American boy, was referred for evaluation because he was becoming progressively more aggressive in school, with both teachers and peers. Tom had been suspended many times because of this behavior and was frequently sent home, creating significant disruption for his mother, who was on active duty with the military. Tom's mother could not understand the school's concerns; she declared categorically that her son did not have any problems at home. Tom had earlier been given the diagnosis of attention-deficit/hyperactivity disorder and had taken medication for a short time without any benefit.
>
> Tom's parents had divorced one year before the evaluation, and Tom missed his father a great deal. Tom's mother described the child's father as very dependent and unreliable.

During the family interview, many aspects of the child's overall functioning were explored systematically. When asked how Tom was doing at home, his mother responded in a protective and defensive manner. To his mother's surprise, Tom reported, without prompting, that on one occasion he had pulled a knife on his brother when the latter found him attempting to harm himself with the knife. Tom added that he had thought about killing himself many times. He then revealed that he frequently abused himself by punching himself in the face or by throwing himself to the ground. This information alarmed his mother. Throughout this portion of the assessment, Tom remained very quiet and calm. He looked affectively frozen, if not emotionally blunted. Tom did not show any evidence of hyperactivity nor of overt distractibility during the examination.

When the examiner asked Tom about the things that he enjoyed doing, he said that he liked drawing a lot. The examiner pursued this interest by giving Tom some white paper and pencils and asking him first to draw whatever he wanted. He was then prompted for additional drawings.

Tom's first drawing was of a big, female figure with an open mouth and pointed teeth who was holding a child's head in her right hand. The female figure had beheaded the child, whose head was dripping blood. One of the child's eyes had popped out, and the female figure was eating the other eye. Tom narrated all of this without emotion.

Tom's second drawing, in response to the examiner's request that he draw a person, was of a male person in profile who was using a machine gun to shoot at a smaller figure. The smaller figure appeared to be scared. The examiner asked Tom, "Why is that big guy shooting the smaller one?" Tom replied, "The small one 'crossed' the other guy."

Tom's third drawing, in response to the examiner's request that he draw a female or a girl, was, again, of a big, female figure, this time strangling a child. The female figure was smiling, and the child was faceless.

Tom's fourth drawing, a family kinetic drawing, showed Tom's five family members, all holding weapons in both hands. Each family member had a different pair of weapons: knives, axes, pitchforks, small saws, and big saws. The family had killed someone, whose body lay in front of the group, and was posing in front of an automatic camera that was set to take a picture of the whole scene.

Tom displayed no emotion as he explained his drawings. The morbid content and preoccupation with violence reflected in Tom's drawings were alarming. After Tom's mother saw her son's drawings, it was not difficult to persuade her that Tom was a very disturbed child. She was shocked after seeing the drawings and hearing Tom's descriptions of them. Tom's drawings broke through his mother's denial, and she became receptive to therapeutic recommendations.

The following case example demonstrates the effectiveness of using drawings to evaluate an electively mute preadolescent girl.

Tina, an 8-year-old Caucasian girl, had been referred by a counselor from the nearby mental health mental retardation (MHMR) center because of concerns about her regressive behavior. The counselor noted that Tina rarely, if ever, spoke.

Three months before the evaluation, it was brought to Tina's mother's attention that Tina's 12-year-old sister had been sexually molested by the mother's fiancé. After this disclosure, the mother broke off her engagement. Tina's mother also learned that her former boyfriend had fondled Tina. At the time of the evaluation, charges had been filed against the former fiancé in connection with the sexual abuse he perpetrated against Tina's sister.

Since the time of the disclosure, Tina had exhibited significant regressive behavior: she had become very clingy, shadowed her mother everywhere, and refused to sleep in her own bed. There was no evidence of other regressive behavior such as enuresis or encopresis. At school, Tina was known as a quiet child who seldom spoke, which had been a concern to her teachers. Tina was a very good student and had kept up her grades, even during the time of the observed regressive behaviors.

Tina's father had been physically abusive toward her mother in front of the children; he also had problems with alcohol. Although contact between Tina and her father was irregular, she seemed to enjoy his sporadic visits.

Tina was a very pretty girl with freckles and big, inquisitive eyes. Her eye contact was intermittent. She clung to her mother, clutching her mother's hands throughout the interview. The examiner attempted to engage Tina in a verbal exchange, but whenever she was addressed, she would signal her mother to answer for her. She never spoke spontaneously. Although Tina didn't respond verbally, she gestured to the examiner when she was asked a number of questions during the mental status examination. She denied that she had ever thought of suicide or that she ever had any hallucinatory experiences.

Tina's mother reported that Tina also had problems talking to her counselor. When her mother said that Tina spent a great deal of time drawing, the examiner asked Tina if she would like to draw. She showed interest immediately. Tina's drawings helped the examiner to understand the reasons for her regressive behaviors and the effect of the recent fondling.

For the first drawing, Tina was asked to draw whatever she wanted. She drew a big house with two curtained windows (Figure 1). Tina drew a girl at the right side of the house, holding a flower in one hand and a lollipop in the other. The girl in the drawing seemed to be smiling. The sky was sunny (actually, the sun was smiling), three birds were flying around, and there were a few clouds. At the other side of the house was a tree with fruit on it, and hanging from the tree was a bird feeder with three birds feeding. This was an altogether happy and positive drawing.

For the second drawing, Tina was asked to draw a person. She drew a good-sized girl who was smiling. On the girl's abdomen she drew a large black dot that she identified as the girl's bellybutton (Figure 2).

For the third drawing, Tina was asked to draw a boy. She had problems drawing the figure; she erased the head a couple of times. The boy was clearly smaller than the girl in the previous drawing. She didn't draw a bellybutton on the boy, and he had a rather pleasant smile (Figure 3).

For the fourth drawing, Tina was asked to draw her family doing something together. The examiner also asked the mother to draw, in parallel, the same drawing. Tina's drawing was full of movement: the family was holding hands while watching TV

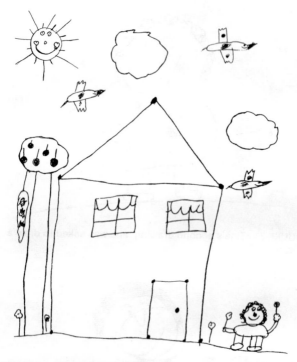

FIGURE 1.   **Tina's first drawing; she was asked to draw whatever she wanted.**

(Figure 4). In an interesting parallel, the mother drew herself and her children watching a movie at the theater (drawing not included here).

The examiner went back to the second drawing and asked Tina why the bellybutton was visible. Because Tina remained mute, the examiner ventured to say that the little girl felt pretty bad about what happened to her when her mother's boyfriend touched her on her private parts and that she feared that everybody knew or was going to know about it. The mother answered

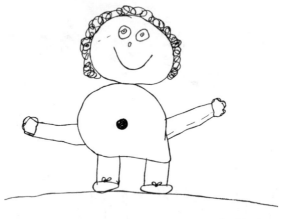

FIGURE 2. **Tina's second drawing; she was asked to draw a person.**

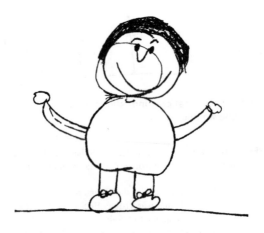

FIGURE 3. **Tina's third drawing; she was asked to draw a boy.**

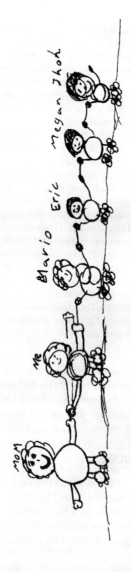

FIGURE 4. Tina's fourth drawing; she was asked to draw her family doing something together.

for Tina, saying that her daughter had told her how ashamed she felt about what happened. Because Tina didn't verbalize how she felt about the abusive incident, the examiner asked her to draw the way she was feeling about what happened. Tina's mother was asked again to draw in parallel to Tina. Tina drew a girl crying, tears running down both of the girl's cheeks (Figure 5). The mother again drew a picture similar to Tina's: a woman crying and looking quite sad (Figure 6).

The drawings were useful in getting information about the child's sense of herself, and in exploring the feelings she could not put into words. The drawings also showed that the girl was intelligent and creative. The first drawing demonstrated a positive self-image and the fourth demonstrated a good family relationship. The examiner felt that the regression was limited and that with ongoing counseling and maternal support, the impact of the fondling could be minimized. The examiner took into account that the elective mutism had preceded the abuse. Furthermore, Tina was demonstrating good evidence of resilience: she liked school and was doing well in her classes. Features of separation anxiety disorder were present, but features of a mood disorder were not. Tina was mandated back to her individual counselor who was told that Tina could be reevaluated if her regressive behaviors worsened or if other signs of emotional or behavioral deterioration appeared.

In the preceding case example, the parallel content of the mother's and daughter's drawings was remarkable. It was also interesting that the examiner involved the mother and the daughter in the process of drawing; the convergence of themes and feelings helped the examiner determine that the child was receiving good maternal care and that the mother was attuned to the child's needs.

■ PLAY TECHNIQUES

Play offers the examiner unique insight into the psychological conflicts experienced by preschoolers and young preadolescents. Although a diagnosis can be derived by interviewing the child, the data obtained lack information regarding the ongoing psychological conflicts that contribute to the child's overall destabilization.

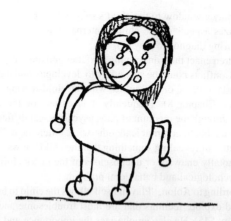

FIGURE 5. Tina's fifth drawing; she was asked to draw the way she was feeling about the abusive incident.

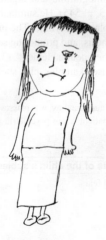

FIGURE 6. Tina's mother's drawing in response to being asked to draw in parallel to Tina's fifth drawing.

Why is play a window to the child's subjective world? Table 2–2 summarizes aspects of the child's internal world that can be inferred during diagnostic play (2).

Children enact their underlying anxieties and ongoing conflicts in play. Conflicts could be secondary to developmental delays, internalized conflicts, or difficulties with the child-rearing environment (see Chapter 8). Frequently it is easier for the child to express, through the medium of play, psychological difficulties he or she is unable to communicate otherwise. Often the difficulty is not a matter of revealing something that the child knows; children may be totally unaware or unconscious of the factors influencing their psychological and behavioral problems.

According to Ablon, "Play in itself allows the child to bring forward and explore feelings that are most troublesome and important" (3, p. 545). He also emphasizes the importance and salience of play in children's lives: "Play is a vehicle for symbolism and metaphor which the mind in turn utilizes to provide a scaffolding for structuralization, integration, and organization of affectively charged experience" (3, p. 545). He summarizes the overall functional importance of play by saying, "The innate capacity of play for organization, synthesis, and promoting self-regulatory process provides a powerful therapeutic element" (3, p. 546).

In the next three case examples, play sheds light on the child's underlying problems:

> Joel, a 5-year-old Caucasian boy, was reassessed after he was released from an inpatient acute psychiatric preadolescent pro-

---

TABLE 2–2. **Elements of the child's subjective world**

Conflicts, problems, and fears

Wishes and fantasies

Prior experiences

Traumatic experiences

Ongoing experiences

Problem-solving strategies

gram. He had been admitted to the program after he became unmanageable at the day-care center and at home. At the day-care center he was hyperactive and impulsive and frequently was aggressive and abusive to his peers. At home he was restless and defiant, talked back to mother, and displayed ongoing jealousy and aggressive behavior toward his 8-month-old sister. Joel's mother also reported that her son often displayed unusual behaviors such as precocious sexual behavior and strange verbalizations, including statements that there was a bad Joel inside of him. At times Joel appeared to be self-absorbed; at other times he seemed to be in a frenzy and unable to sleep. His mother reported that Joel experienced fluctuating moods; at times he looked miserable, cried easily, and said that he was a bad child.

These problems had been reactivated by the time the reassessment was conducted. When Joel's mother was asked about a possible history of physical or sexual abuse, she became indignant. What was striking to the examiner was the emotional distance between the child and the mother. She was eager to attribute the child's dysfunction to a biological problem and proposed that the child probably had a chemical imbalance; she disregarded other possibilities. The examiner's efforts to gather information about the child-rearing environment were met with noncontributory, vague, and evasive responses.

Joel's mother had recently separated from the child's father. She gave no importance to this event, even after reporting that Joel and his father seemed to have a good time together. She reported that when Joel spent time with his father, he didn't seem to display any of the troublesome behaviors she complained about. She had begun dating a man whom she believed was getting along well with Joel, and she hoped Joel would look up to him as a father, stating explicitly, "I wish Joel would forget about his real dad."

During the family interview, Joel made no contact with his mother. He displayed familiarity with the examiner, and at times he sought affection from him. When Joel's mother talked about Joel she displayed no concern or sense of empathy for what he might be experiencing.

When Joel was evaluated alone, he asked to play with toys.

He was offered a set of small animals, including a polar bear and a panda bear. Joel picked the polar bear and assigned the panda bear to the examiner; the polar bear was the mother, and the panda was the child. Joel told the examiner to make the panda bear call for its mommy. The examiner said, "Mommy! Mommy!" repeatedly, but the polar bear appeared to be completely indifferent to the panda's distress. When the examiner, in the role of the panda bear child, asked Joel, as the polar bear mother, why the mother didn't come to see him, Joel shouted, "Shut up," and added, "the mother is dead." He ordered the panda bear to continue crying and calling for its mommy.

This was a puzzling enactment (see Chapter 1 for more on the interpretation of enactments). When the examiner met again with the mother, he asked her to help him understand Joel's enactment. When she was told the content of the child's play, she confessed with great hesitation that she had been separated from Joel from the time he was 4 months old until he was 13 months old. She had been in prison for drug-related problems, and her mother had taken care of Joel. When she returned, Joel didn't recognize her, so she had attempted to gain the child's love, but for a long time she had felt that Joel didn't love her.

In the preceding case study, the revelation resulting from the child's play helped to explain the child's distance, the mother's emotional blandness, and the mother's parental inconsistency. The child's bonding with his mother was called into question. This developmental disturbance needed as much attention as the other disorders with which the child had been diagnosed (i.e., attention-deficit/hyperactivity disorder, oppositional defiant disorder, and probable bipolar disorder).

In the next case study, the child represents in play his concerns about body function and conflicts about elimination besides obvious problems with anger:

Chad, a 5-year-old Caucasian boy, was brought by his mother for evaluation. They had been staying at a shelter for battered women, where his mother had sought refuge with her two children from her husband's abusive treatment. Chad had attracted the attention of the shelter's administrators because of his hyperactive, disruptive, and aggressive behaviors toward his brother and even toward his mother. When it became clear that Chad was unresponsive to limits and discipline, his mother was advised to seek psychiatric consultation.

Chad's mother reported that his mood was very changeable. He had threatened to kill her, voiced a desire to die, and had also made veiled statements that he would kill himself. Chad had become progressively withdrawn, had lost weight, and repeatedly expressed wishes to see his father. Chad seemed to be preoccupied with defecation. His mother had overheard him singing gleefully, using words such as "ca-ca" and "butt hole." Chad had problems sleeping and at times appeared sad and withdrawn; at other times he seemed happy and hyperactive. His mother denied that Chad had been physically or sexually abused; however, Chad had witnessed his father abusing his mother many times.

During the session with the mother, Chad showed a significant degree of behavioral organization (see Chapter 3). He asked permission to use a number of toys and explored playing materials appropriately. Chad's mother was amazed to see him behaving so adaptively. She was equally amazed that after Chad was finished playing with the toys, he put them back where he had found them. At some point during the interview, Chad began to sing, using words such as "ca-ca," "butt," and "butt hole," as his mother had disclosed earlier. He seemed to be singing those words with a sense of joy.

Chad was a handsome boy. His speech was fairly well articulated; however, on occasion he exhibited speech difficulties. Although he appeared euthymic, he displayed some constriction in the affective sphere. Except when he was singing the scatological words, his affect was mostly appropriate. At times, the examiner sensed that Chad exhibited short-lived clang associations.[1] No psychotic symptoms were demonstrated, and no further evidence of thought disorder was observed. Chad moved around the office with a sense of familiarity and explored many

---

[1] *Clang associations* refer to the expression of words that rhyme (e.g., dog, fog, log). It is usually a serious symptom of thought disorder.

toy boxes and other items without any hesitation. Chad's mother attempted to guide and control him by telling him to ask permission before touching things. She was far more anxious than was Chad. Although Chad made contact with many play objects, he didn't concentrate on any item or use the toys to enact any elaborated themes.

During the individual assessment, Chad first played with animal toys. Sometimes his playing behavior was calm and sometimes it was playfully aggressive. He often paired off the toys for play. When he turned to the dinosaurs, he picked up the *Tyrannosaurus rex* first. This dinosaur attacked the other dinosaurs. From time to time, Chad would find delight in sticking another dinosaur's tail or one of its limbs into the *T. rex*'s mouth. After he enacted some aggressive scenes, Chad (still holding the *T. rex*) turned to the examiner and asked, "Where does the food the dinosaur eats go?" He asked if it went to the legs or to the bones. He seemed puzzled and intrigued. He repeated these questions a number of times, each time making direct eye contact with the examiner.

During the interpretive phase of the interview, Chad's mother added information of particular interest. She revealed that he had a history of chronic constipation. Chad would "hold on, " not moving his bowels for long periods of time. He would indicate a need to defecate by holding his legs together tightly and showing facial discomfort, but even then he would not go to the toilet. Finally, when Chad did go, his mother would help him in the act of releasing the hardened feces. She would hold and separate his legs (while he was sitting on the toilet) until he would painfully relieve himself. Chad had been encopretic from time to time.

In the preceding case example, the short play session shed light on the child's struggles in understanding the transformation of food, his corresponding difficulties with elimination, and his preoccupation with body functioning. What was the importance of this symptom in the overall psychopathologic picture? What was the connection between the constipation-encopresis and the other symptoms? The potty-training battle and other conflicts over con-

trol still seemed very active. How were the diagnoses of oppositional defiant disorder, attention-deficit/hyperactivity disorder,
and a probable affective disorder related to Chad's encopretic
behavior? Certainly the forceful child-mother transactions at the
toilet and the child's own preoccupations with food intake and
elimination provided a good starting point in understanding the
strong power struggle between the child and his mother.

The next case example shows how descriptive psychiatric observations, regular exploratory questions, and psychodynamic inferences from play observations are accomplished concomitantly
and complementarily.

> Susy, an adopted 8-year-old Hispanic girl, was referred for psy-
> chiatric evaluation for severe aggressive behavior. She had bit-
> ten a teacher's breast and had scratched some of her peers' faces
> to the point of bleeding. She had also been very obstinate and
> disruptive in the classroom.
>
> Her adoptive parents were divorced. Susy lived with her
> adoptive mother and other foster children (Susy's mother had
> served as a foster mother to many children). Susy was reported
> to be hyperactive, impulsive, and defiant. She had been adopted
> at age 5 years by the family that had cared for her since early in-
> fancy. She had not been expected to live because of severe respi-
> ratory difficulties shortly after birth. Her adoptive parents had
> been described as very inconsistent in limit setting and disci-
> pline. Susy had been given a number of psychotropic medica-
> tions, including stimulants, but none of them controlled her
> behavior effectively.
>
> During the play session, Susy selected a playhouse, a num-
> ber of small dolls (a mother, a father, a son, and a daughter), and
> miniature furniture. As she opened the house and began to ex-
> plore its contents, she would start to say something but never
> finish. This happened several times. When the examiner asked
> Susy about this behavior, she appeared preoccupied, as if expe-
> riencing internal perceptions. Susy did not respond to the exam-
> iner's comments. The examiner said, "I wonder if you are
> hearing something." When Susy continued to be unresponsive,
> the examiner said, "It seems that you are hearing voices. Can

you tell me what the voices are telling you?" She acknowledged that she was hearing voices but didn't reveal anything about their content. Susy also became distracted several times by noises coming from outside the office. She would ask the examiner where each noise came from and what was happening outside the office. Susy asked if her mother was coming.

After Susy explored some other elements of the playhouse (she particularly enjoyed turning on and off the working house light), she began to play with the dolls. She picked up the daughter doll and said it was her. She gave the father doll to the examiner and the mother doll to the female resident who was observing.

Susy brought her doll to the examiner's father doll and made her doll "kiss" the father doll and whisper something in its ear. The examiner asked Susy what her doll was saying to the father doll, but she refused to tell. Susy then took her doll to the mother doll, which the resident had placed on the house patio, and made her doll "kiss" the mother doll. Susy's doll whispered something in the mother doll's ear and again refused to tell the examiner what the whispering was about. Susy used her voice in an endearing manner and showed significant excitement during these dramatizations.

Susy's doll then wanted to get into the pool on the patio, but she said the water was too cold. She stated a number of times that she wanted to get into the pool and each time she would touch the water and say that it was cold. Susy took the father doll from the examiner and put it in a reclining chair on the patio. She sat the mother in another chair. Susy then placed her doll upstairs in the playhouse and turned the light off, saying that it was night. She said, "It was scary," more than once, but she would not tell the examiner what was scary in that room. She put her doll into bed and soon after brought the son doll (representing her brother) to sleep in the same bed. The examiner commented on the boy and the girl sleeping in the same bed, but Susy didn't respond.

Susy then said it was morning time and she brought her doll back downstairs, where she began playing with the mother doll. Susy had the mother doll ask the daughter doll to go upstairs to fix the bedroom because she had "made a mess." The daughter doll refused to go, and with a commanding voice, Susy made the daughter doll order the mother doll to go upstairs and fix the mess herself. The examiner asked Susy what was going on. Susy made the daughter doll begin to whine and fret and laid the doll down on the floor. The examiner asked Susy if the daughter doll was having a temper tantrum, and she agreed readily. The doll continued to lay on the floor, fussing and whining. The examiner restated that the doll was having a temper tantrum, and again Susy agreed. After this, Susy made the daughter doll go to the mother doll and kiss her. The daughter doll said she wanted to go to McDonald's. She displayed another temper tantrum when the mother doll said no. At this point, the examiner noticed a number of scabs and scars on Susy's arms and asked her what had happened. She said that she had scratched herself. The examiner said, "It seems that you scratch yourself when you have temper tantrums." She agreed.

Susy's next play scenario related to going to school. Her doll exited the house by the front door, was picked up by the school bus, and then came back home. Her doll kissed the mother and father dolls again. After 30 minutes of playing, the examiner said, "We are going to stop playing." Susy continued to play as though the examiner hadn't said a word. The examiner said, "We have to stop. We need to pick up now." Again, Susy didn't seem to listen. In a firmer manner, the examiner said, "We are not playing anymore. We need to pick up." Susy protested and asked, "Why?" The examiner began to help her to put away the house and other toys. Only then did she acknowledge that the playing was over.

In the preceding case example, the enactment of this child's strong oppositional traits was apparent throughout the session. In particular, observations during this session suggested the presence of psychotic features. The child's play also hinted at the child's fears (e.g., possible sexual abuse), her affectionate manipulations, and her difficulties with mood dysregulation and anger dyscontrol.

Gardner has described a number of playful and engaging techniques that can be used when working with resistant children who have difficulties with direct verbal communication or who require nonverbal engagement (4). Examples include the Mutual Storytelling Technique and the Talking, Feeling, and Doing Game.

■ REFERENCES

1. Warren SL, Oppenheim D, Emde RN: Can emotions and themes in children's play predict behavior problems? J Am Acad Child Adolesc Psychiatry 34:1331–1337, 1996
2. Di Leo JH: Children's Drawings as Diagnostic Aids. New York, Brunner/Mazel, 1973
3. Ablon SL: The therapeutic action of play: clinical perspectives. J Am Acad Child Adolesc Psychiatry 35:545–547, 1996
4. Gardner RA: Psychotherapeutic Approaches to the Resistant Child. New York, Jason Aronson, 1975

USE OF THE AMSIT IN DOCUMENTING THE CHILD AND ADOLESCENT PSYCHIATRIC EXAMINATION

In every diagnostic interview, the examiner must document the patient's mental status examination. The AMSIT is an acronym representing the components of the mental status examination: **A** (appearance, behavior, and speech); **M** (mood and affect); **S** (sensorium); **I** (intelligence); and **T** (thought). The AMSIT allows systematic documentation and organization of data collected during the psychiatric examination of adults. It was originated in the early 1970s by David Fuller at the University of Texas at San Antonio (1). The AMSIT has undergone a number of improvements. The latest version was written in 1997 (Table 3–1). Medical students, interns, general psychiatric residents, and fellows in child and adolescent psychiatry are expected to be proficient in the AMSIT.

The psychiatric examination provides data needed to establish a psychiatric diagnosis and to develop a comprehensive treatment plan. A comprehensive psychiatric evaluation of the child includes an inquiry into the child's presenting problems, his or her developmental course, and the nature of the family context or rearing environment. The developmental progression (which refers to the acquisition of abilities or skills at a given age) and the developmental context (which refers to psychosocial factors and the nature of the rearing environment) are fundamental concepts in the field of child and adolescent psychiatry.

TABLE 3–1. **David Fuller's outline of the AMSIT for adults**

Appearance, behavior, and speech

Physical appearance: apparent age, place, sex, and other identifying features; careful description of the patient's dress and behavior

Manner of relating to examiner: placating, negativistic, seductive, trusting, understanding of examiner's expectations, motivation to work with examiner, and so on

Psychomotor activity: increased, decreased, or neither increased nor decreased

Behavioral evidence of emotion: tremulousness, perspiration, tears, clenched fists, turned-down mouth, wrinkled brow, crying, evidence of anxiety, and so on

Repetitious activities: mannerisms, gestures, stereotyped behaviors, waxy flexibility, echopraxia, compulsive performance of repetitious acts

Disturbance of attention: distractibility, self-absorption

Speech: volume, rate (pressured or slowed), clarity, spontaneity; presence of mutism, word salad, perseveration, echolalia, neologisms, clang speech, repetition of stereotyped phrases

Mood and affect

Mood: position on seven-point depression-elation continuum; presence of angry, fearful, or anxious mood

Affect: range, intensity, lability, appropriateness to immediate thought

Sensorium

Orientation: for person, time, and place

Memory: recent and remote

Concentration

Calculating ability: valid only if patient is adequately educated

Intellectual function: estimate current level of function as above average, average, or below average based on general fund of information, vocabulary, and complexity of concepts

(continued)

TABLE 3–1.   **David Fuller's outline of the AMSIT for adults**
                (continued)

Thought

  Coherence

  Logic

  Goal directedness: presence of tangential or circumstantial thoughts

  Associations: presence of loose associations, blocking, flight of ideas

  Perceptions: presence of hallucinations, illusions, depersonalization, distortion of body image

  Delusions: currently held delusions

  Other thought content: noteworthy memories, other thoughts and feelings, poverty of thought, suicidal or homicidal intent

  Judgment

  Insight: how much and how little understanding the patient has about his or her condition

  Abstracting ability: similarities are more reliable than proverbs

---

Although the psychiatric examination of the child is a valuable component of the diagnostic process, it is only part of the process. The examiner must remember that the examination removes the child from his or her natural environment; thus, the child's family and other aspects of the child's psychosocial environment also need to be evaluated.

A child's mental status is an active, dynamic process, and it changes from one moment to the next. For example, a child who is withdrawn one moment may be active and engaging a moment later, and vice versa. In general, children and adolescents are environmentally reactive: whatever is going on around them influences their mood and other psychological processes. This reactivity may mislead the examiner who is determining the existence or severity of a given disorder. The AMSIT is a valuable tool for preparing consistent documentation of the psychiatric examination. The following sections describe the components of the AMSIT, as it pertains to child and adolescent psychiatry.

■ APPEARANCE, BEHAVIOR, AND SPEECH

Table 3–2 summarizes the specific areas of the AMSIT that are related to appearance, behavior, and speech. Keen, disciplined, and systematic observations must be made during this section of the AMSIT. Methodical inspection and careful observation account for approximately Two-thirds of the work involved in arriving at a diagnosis. A "clinical eye" and expertise give examiners an advantage in this area.

First impressions are significant. The examiner should consider the following questions: What is my first impression of the child (or the family)? Is the child likable? Is there anything odd about the child? Is there any sense of detachment, apprehension, or even danger? The answers to these questions are important in the overall assessment of the child and his or her family. While the examiner is assessing the child and the family, they are assessing the examiner: Is the doctor likable? Does the doctor come across as reassuring, or as critical and severe? Does the doctor appear to be comforting? Does the doctor seem willing to help?

Physical Appearance

The examiner should note whether the child appears to be his or her chronological age or looks younger or older than the stated age.

TABLE 3–2. **Elements of the appearance, behavior, and speech section of the AMSIT**

Physical appearance	Psychomotor activity
Gait and posture*	Involuntary movements*
Exploratory behavior*	Behavioral evidence of emotion
Playfulness*	Repetitious activities
Relatedness	Disturbance of attention
Eye contact	Speech
Behavioral organization	Disturbances of speech melody
Cooperative behavior*	(dysprosody)*

*Denotes topics that are considered in the AMSIT for children and adolescents.

The examiner should observe the child's nutritional state, his or her sense of vitality, and the presence or absence of secondary sexual characteristics. Marked slimness, cachexia, heaviness, or obesity will be readily apparent. In children showing such characteristics, issues related to eating disorders need to be explored, no matter what the presenting problem may be.

The examiner should note the presence of dysmorphic features in any of the following areas: facial complexion, shape and configuration of the eyes (e.g., slanted or mongoloid; different-colored irises), breadth or shape of the forehead, setting or configuration of the ears, and texture and docility of the hair (e.g., "electric" hair). The shape and configuration of the head should be noted. The examiner should also note any other unusual facial or cranial features.

The examiner should pay attention to the child's attire and physical presentation. Children with deviant social behavior often wear striking and unconventional attire. The examiner should note the child's footwear, hairstyle, and hair color. With female patients, the examiner also should note the use of nail polish and the quality of any makeup used. Revealing or see-through garments may indicate a defiance of norms and the transgression of social conventions. Children who wear such garments may also demonstrate precociousness, sexualization, or evidence of antisocial behavior. Rings and perforations are in style among some youth. If the examiner observes perforation of the nose, eyebrows, or tongue, he or she might also inquire about perforations elsewhere on the body, including the navel, nipples, or genitals. Children with sexual identity conflicts often present with ambiguous attire or with makeup that is more appropriate to the opposite sex. Masculine females frequently present without makeup; their attire and demeanor betrays their intentions of wanting to be male.

The examiner should observe any visible skin for the presence of tattoos; for signs of recent injuries or self-abusive or suicidal behaviors; or for evidence of old injuries such as multiple scarring of the knuckles, wrists, or forearms. These marks may be indicative of chronic self-abusive behavior or impulsive aggressive tendencies. If the patient's upper limbs show evidence of self-abusive behavior, the examiner should explore whether the patient abuses other parts of the body (e.g., legs, chest, breasts, genitals). The examiner should ask the child about all visible scars: each scar has a history to tell. The possibility of nonvisible scars needs to be kept in mind even if no scars associated with self-abusive behavior are visible.

Alert examiners may detect vein tracks or other signs of drug abuse. An attentive interviewer will detect evidence of hair pulling (trichotillomania) of the scalp or of the eyebrows and will observe signs of nail biting, nose picking, skin picking, and other compulsive traits. If the patient has an obvious disability, the examiner should note it and observe the limitations that it imposes on the patient and how he or she copes with it.

Gait and Posture

As the examiner enters the waiting room and then guides the child to the interviewing room, he or she should note the child's gait, including the child's grace, smoothness, and coordination. Does the child waddle, shuffle, or tiptoe? Does he or she move with agility? Does the examiner detect any unusual movements associated with the child's gait? For these and related observations, see Chapter 7.

Does the child sit or stand erect, or does he or she slouch? Some children are unable to keep an erect posture while sitting or standing. Does the child lean on the chair, the table, or on any other available support? Some children look hypotonic, or sluggish. Children with a background of early deprivation display unusual and ungraceful postures and may seem hypoactive or even apathetic. Children with chronic regressive states are likely to lean on the chair or to lie down on the sofa or on the floor, even though they exhibit no neuromotor impairment. The same is true for children with severe melancholic features. In severe psychomotor retardation, the child's inactivity may reach a catatonic state.

If the child is catatonic, the examiner should evaluate the degree of akinesia, including lack of blinking, persistence of unusual postures, vacant staring, or flatness of the emotional display. The examiner may also observe echopraxia, echolalia, and other automatic imitative behaviors. The examiner may test the patient for *cerea flexibilitas* (in which the patient maintains whatever body position he or she is placed in).

Some children come across as weak, anergic, or as temperamentally being hypoactive or hyporeactive. These children lack enthusiasm, and it is difficult to keep them motivated about anything.

Exploratory Behavior

Some children demonstrate no reticence when entering the examiner's office. Some children appear fearless in new circumstances and do not show any restraint in unfamiliar settings..These children often show a sense of familiarity with the examiner, even though this is the first time they have met him or her. Some children look around first but seem comfortable even though they are in a new environment. Others are apprehensive about coming into the office and need the active encouragement or assistance of a parent or other caregiver to help them in. These children show evidence of *behavioral inhibition*:[1] they hide behind their mothers and stay near them or they hide their faces with their hands to avoid eye contact. Other children fret or show wariness and need reassurance before any diagnostic engagement.

Playfulness

Playfulness is a quintessential characteristic of childhood. It should be present in well-adapted, so-called normal children. If the examiner encounters an overtly serious child, he or she needs to

---

[1] *Behavioral inhibition* is an enduring temperamental trait present in 20% of children, characterized by inhibition in situations of novelty, shyness, fear, and by a high level of psychophysiological arousal (e.g., high stable heart rates, muscle tension, pupillary dilation, high levels of cortisol and catecholamines) (2).

seek explanations for this demeanor. If the child lacks the quality of playfulness, the examiner will probably observe other evidence of developmental deviations, for example, lack of behavioral organization and exploratory behavior (both are discussed later in this chapter). The examiner may also observe inhibition, passivity, and separation problems.

Once the child engages in play, the examiner should attend to the content and process of the child's play. The examiner should note the nature of the child's enactments (see Chapter 1), the degree of the child's affective involvement (i.e., the child's emotional involvement with the examiner and the child's overt affective display), and the manner in which the child involves the examiner in the play. Frequently, children enact themes related to the major psychological issues that preoccupy or surround them (e.g., major anxieties or conflicts going on in their families).

Relatedness

Relatedness refers to the child's manner of relating to the examiner. Normal preschool and preadolescent children are reserved when they meet strangers. After they have gotten a "feeling" for the situation and have been reassured, they relate more warmly. Adolescents may be expectant and hesitant. Once the child feels comfortable, he or she will become more spontaneous and engaging. Anxious children need more time and more reassurance to feel at ease and to develop rapport. Schizoid children will appear distant and uninvolved. These children will not warm up to the interviewer, no matter how much effort is made to engage and comfort them. Psychotic children will show oddness and inappropriateness in relating, or they may display signs of self-absorption, evidence of response to internal stimuli, or inappropriate affect.

Some children show immediate familiarity with the examiner and, for that matter, with any stranger. Such children demonstrate boundary problems and will require ongoing structure to behave adaptively. Children who demonstrate promiscuous relating may also show evidence of seductive or even overt sexual behavior.

Management of these behaviors requires active limit-setting throughout the diagnostic interview (see Chapter 1). Other children behave in a hostile and aggressive manner or even in a paranoid fashion. These children are hyperalert and suspicious.

Eye Contact

Eye contact is a fundamental interactive behavior. It is a universal nonverbal behavior that increases attachment and rapport. Warm eye contact is a basic element of interpersonal engagement, and its absence indicates a significant relational problem. Children who display poor eye contact also display problems in interpersonal social behavior. These children avoid eye contact when they are anxious or when attachment or neuropsychiatric difficulties are present.

The more deviant the nature of the eye contact, the more serious the likelihood of profound developmental psychopathology in the social-relational area. Examples of deviant eye contact include the "see-through" eye contact observed in autistic children and the "staring" eye contact observed in paranoid and psychotic children. Seizure disorders and dissociative states must be considered in the differential diagnosis when staring is observed.

Behavioral Organization[2]

The examiner should note the patient's degree of adaptability and organizational behavior. Some children, no matter what is happening around them, are able to initiate or create adaptive activities or to immerse themselves in generative activities (e.g., play). Other children, even in the most propitious circumstances, are unable to generate constructive or productive activities and depend on the alter-ego functions of responsible adults for their organized and adaptive behavior. Children who lack behavioral organization will

---

[2]*Behavioral organization* refers to the degree to which the patient's behavior is self-structured. It indicates a capacity for generative activities (e.g., play) independent of the current circumstances. Children who lack this capacity need active structuring throughout the evaluation.

also show other deficits, such as an inability to focus, the absence of an organized approach to problem solving, or a lack of self-soothing functions.

Some children exhibit behavioral disturbance as soon as they enter the psychiatrist's office. They are fidgety, restless, and hyperactive. These children need active structuring throughout the evaluation. The structuring may include verbal redirection, limit setting, or even physical redirection or restraint.

Cooperative Behavior

The examiner should note the child's active and cooperative participation during the psychiatric examination. This quality is associated with the child's understanding of the presenting problems, the dystonicity of the symptoms, and his or her motivation to change.

Problems with compliance or with following directions are common and challenging complaints in the field of child and adolescent psychiatry. When faced with a child's oppositional behavior, the examiner should attempt to determine whether the behavior stems from a need to control, a power struggle motivation, or a sense of personal incompetence. In the latter case, when children are aware of their real or perceived incompetence (or mastery limitations), they will be reluctant to try a given task because they know, or believe, they cannot do it. Many so-called oppositional children have significant unidentified language disorders. These children often have major language receptive problems and cannot understand expectations or given commands. They may also have neuropsychological deficits that interfere with their ability to understand a task or its solution. The examiner should also determine whether these patients have any hearing problems.

Psychomotor Activity

Disturbances of psychomotor activity are probably the most commonly encountered disruptive behaviors in clinical settings. Psychomotor disturbances are caused by a multiplicity of medical, neurological, and psychiatric conditions. Attention-deficit/hyperactivity disorder (ADHD) is one of the most prevalent psychiatric diagnoses, and some of its features are among the most common behavior problems cited by school teachers. The triad of hyperactivity, distractibility (inattentiveness), and impulsivity commonly occurs as a primary disorder, a complicating comorbidity, or a secondary manifestation. When the examiner observes signs of ADHD, he or she should search for evidence of common comorbid disorders associated with this condition (e.g., oppositional defiant disorder, conduct disorder, depressive disorders, anxiety disorders, developmental language and learning disorders).

The examiner should distinguish between a child who exhibits hyperactive behavior (e.g., fidgetiness, aimless behavior) and a child who is driven by goal-directed behavior. The examiner should test the child's response to redirection or structure to determine whether the hyperkinesis is responsive or impervious to structuring or limit setting. The examiner also should attempt to determine whether the child's impairments are secondary to ADHD, one of the commonly associated conditions, or both.

Agitation and sensorium disturbances should alert the examiner to the possibility of delirium. Because delirium is a potentially life-threatening process, it should be considered in the differential diagnosis of hyperactivity, agitation, and restlessness in children.

Mania and akathisia should be considered in the differential diagnosis of agitation and restlessness. Manic patients are quite hyperactive. The examiner should pay attention to other manic manifestations, such as pressured speech, loose associations, and grandiosity. If akathisia is suspected, the examiner should determine whether the patient uses neuroleptics or selective serotonin reuptake inhibitor (SSRI) antidepressants and should look for other extrapyramidal symptoms (EPS) or other signs of neurological dysfunction.

Involuntary Movements

The examiner should observe whether the child displays tics of the face or the limbs, or muscle twitching or jerking. These signs should immediately raise the examiner's suspicion that the child may have Tourette's syndrome. Other involuntary movements (e.g., choreic or dyskinetic movements) may indicate a movement disorder, cerebral palsy, or other neurological conditions (e.g., Sydenham's chorea, Huntington's disease, Wilson's disease). The examiner should also be attentive to the child's production of vocal tics or guttural noises such as grunting, throat clearing, involuntary noises (including shrilly noises), or barking.

With children who are taking neuroleptic medications, the examiner should be alert to the presence of involuntary movements associated with acute dyskinesia and the orolingual and choreiform movements associated with tardive dyskinesia. Any of these findings require full neurological clarification. SSRI antidepressants can also induce EPS reactions (3).

Behavioral Evidence of Emotion

The examiner should observe any affective or emotional manifestations and pay special attention to the flow and vicissitudes of the child's emotional display. The examiner should note whether the child's emotional display is enduring or whether it is variable and unstable.

Anxiety disorders and depressive disorders are common afflictions treated in clinical psychiatric practice. Common signs or features of anxiety include the presence of specific and unspecific fears, thumb sucking, nail biting, hair pulling, frequent scratching, skin flushing, and bowel sounds. Cracking of the knuckles or the back is common in anxious adolescents. Preadolescents may exhibit manifestations of primitive anxiety and fear (e.g., urinating, passing gas, or defecating) during the interview.

Separation anxiety complaints are common. Children with these disorders refuse to separate from their mothers, stay close to their caregivers, and display limited curiosity and exploratory behavior. Equally common in anxious children are inhibitions in social settings, "freezing" in social situations, and elective mutism. Common features of melancholia include a sad face, a downcast demeanor, crying, and limited level of activity. Melancholic signs are commonly accompanied by negative cognitions such as helplessness, hopelessness, and worthlessness and by suicidal thoughts or behavior. Tiredness, sleep and appetite disturbances, and anhedonia are other components of melancholia. In contrast, euphoric mood coupled with restlessness, distractibility, a sense of grandiosity, and pressured speech should make the examiner suspect mania or hypomania. In general, mania and melancholia are *infectious moods,* meaning that the examiner is "contaminated" by the patient's prevailing mood. Often the examiner evolves a countertransference that is concordant with the child's prevailing mood (4, pp. 135–137). In addition, the examiner needs to recognize signs of fear, confusion, perplexity, hostility, seductiveness, and many other emotional states.

Repetitious Activities

The examiner should pay attention to the presence of repetitive motoric activities. On the most benign end of the spectrum are continuous hand-rubbing, frequent preening, and other behaviors associated with anxiety and tension. In the middle of the spectrum are behaviors such as thumb sucking, nail biting, and knuckle or spine cracking. At the most pathological end of the spectrum are behaviors such as rocking, arm flipping, and other autistic behaviors. When careful inspection does not reveal the presence of overt repetitious activities, the examiner should proceed with sensitive probing to rule out the presence of less obvious compulsive activities (see Chapter 4).

Disturbance of Attention

Although hyperactivity is commonly associated with inattentiveness and impulsivity, disturbance of the attentional processes sometimes occur without hyperactivity or impulsivity. In general, disturbances of attention reflect distractibility (a lack of a capacity for selective and sustained attention). Distractible children move from one activity to the next without finishing any of them.

Attention comprises many functions, including selective attention, sustained attention, intensity of attention, inhibitory control, and attentional shifts. The selection and organization of responses to stimuli depend on high-level executive functions (5). Attention is a fundamental function in information processing and cognitive and language functioning. Attention disturbances are implicated in the etiology of schizophrenia.

Speech

The speech area of the mental status examination is rich in findings and rewarding in the overall diagnostic process. The findings in this area range from overt aphasias with associated neurological findings to the less specific developmental language disorders. If a child does not seem to understand what the examiner is attempting to convey or when the child's responses seem to miss the point (e.g., when non sequitur responses are given), the examiner should suspect a receptive language disorder. The examiner must ascertain whether a hearing loss is present in these cases.

As the child speaks and responds to the examiner's questions, special attention should be paid to the spontaneity and flow of the child's speech, the richness of the vocabulary used, the child's abstraction capacity, the quality of the grammar used, and the child's ability to communicate emotion and meaning.

Children with receptive language difficulties look lost and confused. The examiner should consider the following questions: Is the patient attempting to communicate at all? Is the patient gesturing or attempting to use other nonverbal behavior? Is the patient capable of developing rapport? Is the patient attempting to connect with the examiner? The answers to these questions will assist the examiner in differentiating autism from other communication disorders.

Limited lexicon, grammatical mistakes, inappropriate use of prepositions, and problems with syntax are common in children with expressive language delays. Their speech and language are usually immature. Expressive language disorders may be associated with psychosocial developmental immaturity.

The examiner should also note the naturalness of the patient's speech and the quality of the communication process used. Odd speech, affectation in the communication (i.e., pedantic talk), or unusual features of the communication process or of its contents, such as echolalia, neologisms, or bizarre productions, should raise the suspicion of a thought disorder (e.g., schizophrenia).

The examiner must attend to the volume and rate of the speech as well as to the quality of its articulation. The examiner should note whether the patient's speech is loud, pressured, or slurred and whether evidence of mispronunciations, stuttering, or other unusual speech qualities is present.

The examiner should note the amount of time that elapses before the patient initiates a verbal response. Some patients take a rather long time before beginning any response, whereas others blurt out responses impulsively before the examiner finishes the question or before he or she has completed a thought.

Disturbances of Speech Melody

Disturbances of speech melody (called *dysprosody*) are prevalent in severe aphasias and developmental language disorders. The examiner should pay attention to these speech qualities because they are revealing. Disturbances of the musicality and rhythm of the speech indicate that an injurious event affected the child's neuro-linguistic development in early periods of language and speech formation.

Instead of the soft, childlike, sweet, and melodious quality of the typical child's speech, the examiner may hear a grave, hoarse voice that resembles an adult's or elderly person's voice. The child's voice may have a high-pitched tone, or, in male children, the child's speech may have an effeminate quality (see Carlos's case example in Chapter 10). Dysprosody is a striking finding.

Children who have pervasive personality disorders or other severe neurodevelopmental disorders also exhibit problems with voice melody and voice inflection. For instance, when they attempt to make a statement, they may raise their voice as if asking a question.

■ MOOD AND AFFECT

Cummings's definitions of mood and affect are clear and succinct: "Mood is an internally experienced pervasive emotion. Affect is the outward emotional display" (6, p. 168). In this section of the mental status examination, the examiner notes the child's predominant affect and the subjective states that accompany it. He or she may also observe the quality and intensity of affective expression.

Among the most valuable and clinically relevant aspects of the AMSIT is the expectation that the examiner will consider the presence of depression or mania in every psychiatric evaluation. The AMSIT expects the examiner to rate the patient's depressive or elated affect on a seven-point numerical scale. The scale includes depression at one extreme, euthymia at the center, and mania at the other extreme. Every AMSIT should assess the patient's degree of affective expression or mood disturbance.

Loved and well-cared-for children are, by nature, bubbly and expansive. The examiner should describe any deviation from this state. Thus a serious child may already be demonstrating emotional disturbance. A serious countenance may be part of a restrained, euthymic state in an adult, but this is not necessarily the case in children.

Reactivity to environmental factors complicates both the identification of affective disturbance and the determination of its severity. Many depressed children react positively to reassurance and may even engage in playful interactions. These observations may mislead the diagnostician.

The examiner should note the child's spontaneous affective display and any changes of affect that occur during the interview. The examiner should describe the intensity and the range of the affective expression. It is equally important to observe if the affect is appropriate to the thought content or if it is inappropriate either to the thought content or to the interviewing context.

Silliness and inappropriateness of affect are common in immature and regressed children. These affective states may represent early forms of hypomania. Some children are openly silly, whereas others display overt euphoria. Affect disturbance is common in so-called borderline disorder, in Asperger's syndrome, and in schizophrenia.

Other mood and emotional states may be as prominent and as important as those associated with depression and mania. Anger, anxiety, fear, and other states of emotional arousal are common phenomena observed in clinical practice.

The examiner should differentiate depression related to a psychiatric disorder from depression related to neuropsychiatric dysfunction. Harris warns, "In the assessment of affect, apathy must be distinguished from depression. Moreover, the experience of emotion must be clarified because in some conditions, such as certain right-hemispheric dysfunction presentations or in pseudobulbar palsy, the physical expression of affect (e.g., facial expression, voice tone) may be impaired although inner experience may remain intact. Finally, with some frontal lobe lesions and in some metabolic encephalopathies, severe apathy may be noted in the absence of depression" (7, p. 31).

■ SENSORIUM

Orientation

Children of normal intelligence, even early preadolescents, frequently know the day of the week, the month, and the year of the evaluation. Less precision should be expected with the date, but even so, alert and bright children will be very close to the correct date. It is telling when the examiner asks the child questions regarding orientation, and the child turns to the mother for guidance or expects her to give the response. The examiner needs to look beyond the overt dependency and explore cognitive problems or generalized difficulties with orientation in time and space. Significant deviations from orientation to time are common in children who have cognitive impairments and in children who have neurodevelopmental disorders such as learning disorders and right-hemispheric dysfunctions. The same can be said of orientation to place.

Memory

Disorders of memory result from problems with encoding (i.e., registration secondary to attentional disturbances) or from difficulties with decoding or retrieval (see Chapter 7). "The impairment of new learning, or *anterograde amnesia,* is a defining attribute of organic amnesia" (8, p. 448). *Retrograde amnesia* refers to impairment for memories acquired before brain damage (8, p. 448). The examiner should notice the accuracy of the child's recall and the coherence and relevance of details included in the child's narrative. Memory problems should be suspected when, in response to the questions posed by the examiner, the child looks confused or uncertain or seeks support for his or her answers from significant others.

A child of normal intelligence will be able to talk about important recent events. For example, if the child is a sports enthusiast, the examiner may test the child's tracking of recent sporting events and the accuracy of the recall.

The task of remembering three different words is a classical and practical short-term memory test. The examiner should select unrelated words. This challenge becomes more demanding if one of the words is abstract (e.g., honesty, fairness).

Concentration

Concentration reflects the patient's ability to focus and sustain attention in cognitive tasks. An adolescent with normal intelligence and without specific learning disabilities in arithmetic should be able to demonstrate proficiency with the serial sevens test (e.g., "take 7 away from 100 and keep taking 7 away from the result"). The response to this challenge is considered satisfactory when the adolescent gives five or six accurate responses. For an early latency child, this may be a formidable challenge, in which case the examiner may choose a less difficult task such as serial threes (e.g., "take 3 away from 20 and keep doing so from each answer you get").

The repetition of digits forward and backward is a traditional test of concentration and immediate memory. Adolescents with good concentration and good immediate recall should be able to repeat five or six numbers forward and up to four or five digits backward. Younger children should be expected to be proficient with fewer digits (see Chapter 7).

Calculating Ability

If the examiner is testing the child's concentration and calculating ability with serial sevens, and the child finds the task too difficult, the examiner could try easier challenges such as serial threes (as described in the preceding section) or could present simple calculation problems such as $6 + 7 = ?$ or $9 + 4 - 3 = ?$ Even these simple tests may be very trying for children who have cognitive limitations or for those with specific developmental learning disorders.

Overall Conclusion

The AMSIT requires the clinician to make an overall assessment of the patient's sensorium based on the entire examination or specific findings. A significant impairment of the sensorium should raise the suspicion of delirium, which requires diligent exploration of the central nervous system. Because delirium can be fatal, its elucidation and treatment are medical and neurological emergencies.

■ INTELLECTUAL FUNCTION

Even experienced clinicians err in their estimation of a patient's intelligence level. Children may appear retarded although they are not, or they may come across as being brighter than they really are. Factors that may mislead clinicians in this assessment include the presence of comorbid conditions and the presence of language or learning disorders.

In ascertaining intellectual functioning, a detailed developmental history is required. A record of the child's achievement of milestones and the time at which the child began to produce speech are of particular importance. The child's history of academic progress or academic retention is also relevant. The fact that the child has a history of grade retention does not mean the child is intellectually impaired. Similarly, the fact that a child is promoted year after year does not mean he or she is devoid of cognitive or learning problems.

Sometimes teachers may perceive bright students as retarded. For example, a child was referred for an evaluation because his teacher believed he was too "slow." The child came across to the examiners as extremely bright, creative, and imaginative; and his IQ score was about 142. Comprehensive psychometric testing, complemented, when indicated, with neuropsychological testing, will assist in the clarification of language or learning disabilities.

■ THOUGHT

The basic caveat in the identification of thought disorders is that the presence of severe language disorders can confuse the clinical picture. Developmental and academic histories are very helpful in preventing this confusion, as are the child's affective expression and his or her efforts to communicate. Table 3–3 lists the topics covered in the thought section of the AMSIT.

There are no typical symptoms that make the diagnosis of schizophrenia unequivocal. It was formerly thought that first-rank symptoms (the Schneiderian criteria) were associated only with schizophrenia. Akiskal and Puzantian demonstrated the presence of first-rank symptoms in affective disorders with psychotic features (9).

Some clinicians still confuse the concepts of psychosis and thought disorder. *Psychosis* refers to problems with reality testing and the presence of hallucinations or delusions; *thought disorder* refers to disorders of the process of thought production, thought concatenation, and thought organization.

Coherence

The examiner should note the threading and convergence of the patient's thinking. The examiner should consider the following relevant questions: Are the child's thoughts threaded together to express the intended idea? Does the narrative make sense? Is the narrative clear? Are the topic or themes connected to one another? When the child speaks, can the child's train of thought be followed?

Logic

In assessing the child's logic, the examiner should consider the following questions: Does the child respect the laws of reasoning? Does the child respect the laws of time and space, of the contradiction of the opposites (i.e., if you state something, you rule out or exclude the opposite) (see Troy's case study, Note 2, in Chapter 4)? Do the child's conclusions derive from established premises? Are

---

TABLE 3–3.   Elements of the thought section of the AMSIT

Coherence	Perceptions
Logic	Delusions
Metaphoric thinking	Content of thought
Goal directedness	Judgment
Reality testing	Abstracting ability
Associations	Insight

cause-effect relationships respected in the child's arguments? According to Caplan, illogical thinking is based on a defective control of cognitive processing and represents a negative sign of childhood-onset schizophrenia (10, p. 610). This defect appears to reflect frontal lobe impairment (10, p. 611; see Chapter 4).

Metaphoric Thinking

Adolescents sometimes use metaphors to describe their conflicts or concerns; it is useful to stay within the metaphor and to make interventions that use the patient's metaphoric language. This approach parallels the process of interviewing in displacement (see Chapter 1). The following case examples illustrate the use of metaphors:

> Tim, a 15-year-old Caucasian adolescent, was evaluated for rebellious, aggressive behavior and anger dyscontrol. He said to the interviewer that he "felt like a bull." This metaphor was helpful in understanding the patient's sense of being "untamable" and out of control and it clarified the child's narcissism and his concerns about losing control. When the interviewer stressed that the patient was behaving like a bull, the adolescent responded with satisfaction. This approach improved the therapeutic alliance and made the patient more receptive to the examiner's recommendations.

> Sharon, a 15-year-old Caucasian adolescent, was referred for an evaluation because of her bulimic behavior, which had continued for more than a year. She was preoccupied with her looks and compared herself unfavorably to her more attractive mother, who had been a beauty pageant queen in her younger years. She was also very preoccupied with boys and sex. She said, "When I was younger I could handle the 'small hormones' but now that I'm becoming older, I feel I can't handle the 'big hormones.'" Sharon was terrified of the idea of turning 18 and being on her own. Her concerns with the "big hormones" clearly indicated her difficulties with her emerging sexuality and the separation process involved in turning 18.

Goal Directedness

When observing goal directedness, the examiner should observe whether the child's narrative includes details that are relevant to the idea he or she wants to communicate. Does the child branch off into unimportant details? Does the child deviate from the point that he or she initially wanted to make? The examiner should listen for irrelevant or unnecessary details. While listening to the child's narrative, the examiner should consider the following questions: Does the child go into the substantive matter of the idea he or she wants to communicate? Does the child get lost in minutia unrelated to the core idea?

The most common disturbances in goal directedness are *circumstantiality* and *tangentiality*. In circumstantiality, the child's train of thought branches off into irrelevant details, but the child eventually gets back the main idea. In tangentiality, the child's main idea is lost and he or she goes off into extraneous ideas. The following example illustrates a thought disorder involving goal directedness:

Jennifer, an 11-year-old Caucasian girl, underwent a psychiatric evaluation for explosive and assaultive behavior that resulted in her biting and punching a teacher. In less than 6 weeks, she had three episodes of dyscontrol at school, all involving fights with peers. School administrators felt that they no longer could provide a psychoeducational program for Jennifer on school grounds, because she posed a serious risk to other students. Jennifer attended a day hospital program the previous year for similar reasons. She was described as moody and grandiose. She was her mother's only source of emotional support, and the mother and child were entangled in a dependent, symbiotic relationship.

During the mental status examination, Jennifer showed a mildly expansive mood and a clear thought disorder, exemplified by ever-present circumstantiality, tangential thinking, and loose associations. During the interview, the examiner asked Jennifer, an obese child, "What do you think of your weight?" She responded, "Okay. My belly is good for many things. The belly floats in the water. . . . I can bob other kids with my belly, it doesn't bother me. . . . I've seen 500-pound guys. They are huge . . . in Sumo wrestling in Japan . . . Yokosama. . . . It doesn't matter. . . . This big guy. . . . "

According to Caplan, "certain aspects of thought disorder, such as illogical thinking, are found in childhood psychiatric disorders other than schizophrenia. Looseness of the associations, however, seems to occur specifically in childhood schizophrenia" (10, p. 608). Caplan clarified that "to date, there have been no studies on thought disorder in representative samples of children with psychotic depression and manic disorder. Additional studies are warranted, therefore, to determine whether formal thought disorder is a nonspecific clinical manifestation of childhood psychosis or whether it occurs specifically in childhood schizophrenia" (10, p. 608). Caplan also asserted that loose associations are secondary to distractibility and represent a positive sign of childhood-onset schizophrenia (10, p. 610). She postulated that this defect is secondary to a disconnection between the prefrontal cortex and the subcortical regions (i.e., basal ganglia and thalamus) (10, p. 612).

Reality Testing

By mid-latency age, a child's *reality testing* (ability to differentiate reality from fantasy) should be established solidly; however, reliable reality testing can be demonstrated even earlier. This issue relates to how old the child is before he or she can distinguish fantasy from reality and how old he or she is before hallucinations or delusions can be observed. What follows is an example of reality testing disturbance in a preschooler:

Fabio, a 4½-year-old Hispanic boy, was referred for evaluation of aggressive behavior. He demonstrated murderous behavior toward his baby brother. He spontaneously verbalized that the "jungle," a monster-like figure, was coming to kill him, and he added that the jungle was going to kill his family, too. To protect himself against the jungle, Fabio would take a knife to bed with him. He saw the jungle and heard it. He said that he heard the jungle telling him that it was coming to hurt him. This is the youngest child with overt psychotic features (i.e., visual and auditory hallucinations) that the examiners had ever encountered.

By early mid-latency age, children can clearly differentiate between thoughts coming from inside their heads and voices coming from outside their heads. Consider the following case example:

Dionne, a 9-year-old African American girl who was referred for suicidal behavior, complained of hearing voices. When the examiner asked Dionne if she was hearing her own thoughts, she said, "A thought and a voice are different. A thought comes from inside of my head; a voice comes from outside of my head."

The following case example illustrates confusion of reality with fantasy and gross impairment of reality testing in a late preadolescent child:

Dwayne, an 11-year-old African American boy, was evaluated for explosive and assaultive behaviors. He had hit his female teacher and bitten her nose. The school was no longer willing to put other students at risk because Dwayne had lost control around his peers several times before. Dwayne had been seeing a child psychiatrist for over a year, had been in acute inpatient programs, and had taken various psychotropic medications without any significant effect. He lived with his father at the time of the evaluation. Before that, he lived with his mother in another state. His father took custody of the child when he learned that Dwayne was physically abused at his mother's house. Dwayne's stepbrother allegedly would encourage the family dogs to attack Dwayne. Dwayne had extensive scars on his back.

The mental status examination revealed a handsome African American child who was extremely dysphoric; he also displayed an apathetic demeanor. He was not spontaneous and did not respond verbally to any questions. He exhibited a disgruntled countenance and an ongoing sense of irritation. The omega sign (a persistent frown) was prominent. He appeared to be very depressed. Because his internal world was inaccessible to exploration, his thought processes could not be assessed. The dosage of his antidepressant medication was increased, and he was asked to come the following week for another diagnostic appointment.

When Dwayne came to the second appointment, this time with his father, he brought several pieces of chewing gum. Upon entering the office, he put a piece of gum in his mouth. This time he was talkative. He began narrating a fantasy story, and his father pointed out that the theme of the story was related to a movie he and Dwayne had watched a couple of days earlier. Shortly after this, Dwayne opened his mouth and showed the examiner that the gum was stuck on his lower molars. He didn't seem to know what to do. The examiner suggested that Dwayne could dislodge the gum with his finger.

At this point, Dwayne said that he had fought with Mike Tyson the night before. His father promptly explained that Dwayne had played a Mike Tyson boxing video game the night before. Dwayne went on, saying that he had "blown out Tyson's teeth" and so on. Suddenly Dwayne opened his mouth and indicated that the place where the gum had stuck was the place where Tyson had hit him the previous night. This was followed almost immediately by the revelation that he had bad dreams that night. Dwayne reported dreams of monsters eating his hands. He then showed the examiner his fingers and said, "I had some funny feelings where the monsters were eating my fingers." The nature and extent of this child's psychotic thinking had not been appreciated earlier. Dwayne was placed on neuroleptics with positive results.

Associations

Associations refer to the manner in which the child's thoughts are connected among themselves. As the child speaks, the examiner should follow the sequence of the child's thinking and the links between each of the child's thoughts. The examiner should note whether the child's thoughts flow smoothly. The examiner should also observe the transitions between thoughts and should note whether the patient returns to the original thought after digressing into other topics. Does the patient jump from one idea to the next without a clear thread linking the two ideas? The examiner should note the *affective prosody* (i.e., the emotional coherence of the thought content). *Ideo-affective dissociation* involves a noticeable incongruency between the expressed thoughts and the associated emotions.

The main disturbances of association are blocking, loose associations, and flight of ideas. *Blocking* refers to the interruption of the train of thought. It is detected when the child stops presenting the main idea and either becomes silent (i.e., making a prolonged pause) or, after a short pause, goes onto another thought that is not connected to the preceding, unfinished thought. When the examiner calls attention to this disturbance, the child has significant difficulty coming back to the interrupted idea. In general, patients are unaware of disturbances in their thought processes.

When a child's ideas are weakly connected to one another, the disturbance is called *loose associations.* In *flight of ideas,* the chain of thoughts is presented as an apposition of ideas that are not connected to one another. In the most extreme case, the ideas are so disconnected that no sense can be made of them. This condition is often described as *word salad.* In flight of ideas, the child presents his or her thoughts at a fast pace. The speech frequently may be increased in rate if not pressured. Correspondingly, the patient may acknowledge that his or her thinking is rushing or going very fast. In other words, the patient can't control his or her thinking. This symptom helps explain the impulsivity or lack of judgment exhibited by hypomanic and manic patients.

Perceptions

Normal perceptions are those that have consensual validation within a given culture. *Consensual validation* means that what a person sees, hears, or touches is similar to what another person sees, hears, or touches. Disturbances of perception occur when the objects of the perception do not exist, do not have consensual validation, or both. This process is called *hallucinating* and the experience itself, a *hallucination*. When the object of experience is present but is distorted in its nature or relation to the person, or when it is misidentified, the process is called an *illusion*.

Hallucinations may occur in any of the sensory modalities—visual, auditory, gustatory, olfactory, or tactual—or they may be visceral (i.e., in other body sensations) or experiential. *Complex partial seizures* represent a neuropsychiatric condition that must be considered in the differential diagnosis of perceptual disturbances and other psychotic disorders. In the following case example, the examiner ascertained the unsuspected diagnosis of complex partial seizures, through the use of systematic questioning:

Ralph, a 14-year-old mixed-raced adolescent, was admitted to an acute psychiatric care program for unrelenting suicidal ideation and serious conflicts with his mother. He had a background of gang involvement and other conduct disorder problems. Ralph lost his most important source of emotional support when his maternal grandfather died a short time before the admission. Ralph had been quite attached to his grandfather. His parents were divorced but still continued a bitter relationship. He was caught in a painful loyalty conflict because both parents were pressuring him to live with them. Ralph had witnessed his father physically abusing his mother and hated him for that. Ralph's medical background was positive for an episode of meningitis at age 15 months. He also had complained of "panic dreams" 2 years earlier, but a magnetic resonance imaging scan taken at the time was normal.

Ralph, who weighed 280 pounds, looked older than his stated age and appeared depressed. During the mental status examination, he denied hearing voices and denied visual hallucinations. When he was asked if he smelled any unusual smells, he readily reported olfactory and gustatory hallucinations: "An ugly smell, like a cadaver . . . a pretty bad taste, like rotten meat." While experiencing those hallucinations, he heard screeching, yelling, and beeping noises, and all of this was accompanied by a disturbance of consciousness and a sense of confusion for about 2 minutes. When this happened, he didn't know what was going on. At times he felt like he was going to faint and his legs would get weak. During the previous summer, while playing basketball, Ralph's legs gave way after he experienced the olfactory hallucinations. He had a feeling of "strangeness" and experienced profuse sweating, even during the winter. Additional exploration revealed that he had experienced déjà vu phenomena, dreams that foretold the future, and an urgency to urinate during these episodes. The diagnosis of complex partial seizures was substantiated, although it had not been suspected initially.

Commanding auditory hallucinations are of particular clinical importance. The examiner should explore how strong the hallucinations are and what the patient does when he or she hears the voices. Is the patient able to fight them and resist their commands? Invariably, parents are skeptical about the reality of preadolescents' perceptual symptoms and need to be educated about them (see Note 1).

A disturbance of perception may be centered in the sense of self, in the body image, or in aspects of it. *Depersonalization* denotes a sense of strangeness in the sense of self; that is, the patient feels he or she is not the same as before and feels strange. This experience may be accompanied by a sense of confusion or bewilderment. This phenomenon occurs in affective disorders and dissociative states and is commonly observed in psychotic children.

When a girl with anorexia nervosa looks at the mirror and sees a fat person, she has, among other things, disturbances of perception of body image. Disturbance of body image may be localized, as in the cases of *body dysmorphic disorder* (when the patient thinks something is wrong with a specific body part). When there is a sense of internal body damage, uncorroborated by medical evidence and impervious to reassurance, the distortion is called *hypochondria*.

Out-of-body experiences are reported with some frequency. *Autoscopic hallucinations* are an uncommon complaint in the field of child and adolescent psychiatry. A sense of the presence of a dead person or even experiences such as talking to or hearing from dead people are common experiences for children in bereavement.

Delusions

Delusional thinking refers to a belief or system of beliefs without consensual validation in a given culture. Hallucinations are far more common in children than are delusions. *Ideas of reference* refer to the beliefs that everything the patient perceives is related directly to himself or herself. The most common problems in this area relate to the belief that when people are talking or laughing, they are talking about or laughing at the patient. Some patients feel that others are following them. Others harbor persecutory delusions. These patients think that others are plotting to kill them or harm them in some way. Patients may see signs in the environment that somehow convey a secret or special message to them. Delusions of guilt are described in Chapter 4 (see case examples on Salim and Fred).

Children's concerns can sometimes be quite bizarre, as the following case examples show:

> Ted, an 8-year-old Caucasian boy, reported that monsters were coming at night to exchange his blood for a green liquid. He was so terrified that he asked his father to cover the opening under his bed with a board. Ted believed that the monsters lived under the bed and that nailing the board there would keep the monsters from coming out.

> Mat, a schizoid 10-year-old Caucasian boy, frequently worried that scorpions would come out from the showerhead or climb into his bed while he slept. This child was ostracized, ridiculed, and rejected by his peers.

Extreme forms of disturbances of body image or its functions occur when the patient complains that his or her body or body parts are damaged or, worse, that the patient's insides may be "rotting."

The following case examples illustrate the presence of such *somatic delusions*:

> Donna, a sophisticated and talented 16-year-old Caucasian adolescent, was evaluated for intense and unremitting suicidal ideation. She had a long history of depression, dating back to when she was 7 years old. She had been a patient in a number of psychiatric hospitals. In explaining her sense of hopelessness, she reported that her "insides were rotten" and that parts of her were "dead inside." She acknowledged that 90% of her suicidal intent stemmed from that belief.

> Ming, a 16-year-old Asian American adolescent and the mother of a 13-month-old infant, exhibited a severe major depressive episode with psychotic features. Besides auditory commanding hallucinations ordering her to kill herself, she had a deep-seated belief that she had cancer. No amount of reassurance or medical evidence could persuade her to the contrary.

In clinical practice, after observing the patient's thought processes, the following *chain inquiry* is useful: 1) systematic questioning regarding the presence of auditory, visual, olfactory, gustatory, tactual, and other atypical perceptions such as depersonalization and out-of-body experiences; 2) systematic questioning of referential and persecutory ideation; and 3) systematic questioning regarding beliefs of thought intrusion or thought withdrawal. This line of inquiry may be completed with a full exploration of obsessive-compulsive symptomatology.

Other Thought Content

In addition to the concerns that the patient expresses, the examiner should note the presence of the following: 1) suicidal and homicidal ideation, 2) obsessional thinking, 3) compulsive activities, 4) alcohol and substance abuse, 5) gang involvement, and 6) other significant content not included elsewhere.

Judgment

The AMSIT demands that the assessment of the patient's judgment be based on observations and on the patient's response to specific situations presented during the psychiatric examination. A child is assumed to have good judgment if he or she gives a satisfactory answer to questions such as "What do you do if you are in a theater and you see smoke?" or "What do you do if you find a stamped envelope?" The determination regarding impairment of judgment needs to take into account the patient's history of chronic impulsivity and the patient's lack of forethought before carrying out impulsive actions. The patient's history tells far more about the patient's judgment than do his or her responses to standard questions. A clever and manipulative child may be able to give the right answers to hypothetical questions posed by the examiner, even though the child displays poor judgment in the real world.

Abstracting Ability

The assessment of the child's *abstracting ability* (i.e., his or her capacity for categorical thinking) needs to take into account the child's cognitive development. A common but incorrect assumption is that when a person reaches late adolescence or adulthood he or she has reached the cognitive developmental stage of formal operations. As such, this person should be capable of abstract thinking, as tested by similarities and interpretation of proverbs. However, not everyone reaches this state of cognitive development. Children who are in the process of acquiring this cognitive sophistication should not be expected to perform well in this area, although some bright children do. In general, preadolescents and some adolescents tend to be concrete.

This area is often assessed by paying close attention to the patient's language and the sophistication of his or her responses. The examiner should also note the richness of the child's vocabulary and the manner with which the child discusses problems. For example, does the child use rich, complex, and metaphorical language?

Insight

It is difficult to make judgments about a child's insight. Pre-adolescents begrudgingly acknowledge their problems, and adolescents more often than not only pay lip service to recognition of personal problems and express no willingness to change. Judgments about the presence of insight are based on the degree of the patient's dystonicity over the symptoms and the explicit desire to change.

■ NOTE

1. Hallucinations may be more prevalent in children than is currently thought. Schreier quotes Garralda (1984), who distinguishes nonpsychotic children who hallucinate from psychotic children: "They are not delusional; they do not exhibit disturbance in the production of language; they do not evidence decreased motor activity or signs of incongruous mood; and they do not present with bizarre behaviors or social withdrawal" (11, p. 623). Long-term follow-up of hallucinations has little prognostic significance. In Schreier's view, "hallucinations of critical voices or of those demanding that the patient do horrific acts to the self or to others do not predict severity or necessitate a poor prognosis" (11, p. 624). The presence of a single voice seems to indicate a good prognosis. The presence of internal versus external voices does not have any predictive value. Hallucinations may persist for several years without a major role in the child's functioning (11, p. 624). Schreier has found an association between nonpsychotic hallucinations and migraine (11, p. 624).

■ REFERENCES

1. Fuller D: The AMSIT (student handout). University of Texas Health Science Center at San Antonio, Department of Psychiatry, 1998
2. Kagan J: Galen's Prophesy Temperament in Human Nature. New York, Basic Books, 1994
3. Pies RW: Must we consider SSRIs neuroleptics (guest editorial)? J Clin Psychopharmacol 17:443–445, 1997
4. Racker H: Transference and Countertransference. London, Hogarth, 1968

5. Taylor E: Development and psychopathology of attention, in Development Through Life; A Handbook for Clinicians. Edited by Rutter M, Hay DF. Oxford, England, Blackwell Scientific, 1994, pp 185–211

6. Cummings J: Neuropsychiatry and behavioral neurology, in Comprehensive Textbook of Psychiatry/VI, 6th Edition. Edited by Kaplan HI, Sadock BJ. Baltimore, MD, Williams & Wilkins, 1995, pp 167–187

7. Harris JC: Developmental Neuropsychiatry; Assessment, Diagnosis, and Treatment of Developmental Disorders, Vol 2. Oxford, England, Oxford University Press, 1995

8. Zola S: Amnesia: neuroanatomic and clinical aspects, in Behavioral Neurology and Neuropsychology. Edited by Feinberg TE, Farah MJ. New York, McGraw Hill, 1997, pp 447–461

9. Akiskal HS, Puzantian VR: Psychotic forms of depression and mania. Psychiatr Clin North Am 2:419–439, 1979

10. Caplan R: Thought disorder in childhood. J Am Acad Child Adolesc Psychiatry 33:605–615, 1994

11. Schreier HA: Hallucinations in nonpsychotic children; more common than we think? J Am Acad Child Adolesc Psychiatry 38:623–625, 1999

EVALUATION OF INTERNALIZING SYMPTOMS

For didactic and organizational purposes, I distinguish in this book between internalizing and externalizing symptoms. The distinction often is not clear because of the intrinsic nature of a given disorder. For example, in bipolar disorder internalizing and externalizing symptoms are usually mixed. The distinction may also be blurred because of comorbid disorders (e.g., suicidal or depressive features in children who have conduct disorder). A mix of symptoms is the rule rather than the exception in child and adolescent psychiatry.

■ EVALUATION OF SUICIDAL BEHAVIORS

Pfeffer recommends that "all suicidal ideas and actions of children should be taken seriously and evaluated thoroughly and repeatedly" (1, p. 174). The evaluation of suicidal behavior entails the exploration of the what, how, when, where, and why of the suicidal behavior.

"What" refers to the nature of the suicidal behavior, including what the patient wishes to do and what he or she expects will happen if the action is accomplished. It is important not to stop the exploration after the patient discloses that he or she wants to commit suicide in a particular way. The examiner should continue exploring alternative plans the patient may have (consider Matthew's case example in Chapter 1). Having multiple suicidal alternatives correlates with the child's sense of hopelessness and despair and with the seriousness of the suicidal intent. It is equally important to know whether the child expects to be rescued.

"How" refers to plans the child has conceived or the steps the child may have already taken to kill himself or herself. Here the examiner assesses prior suicidal behaviors and the seriousness of current plans. The examiner should determine how close the child is to hurting himself or herself, so that necessary steps can be taken to ensure the child's safety.

"When" and "where" relate to the time and place planned for the suicide. Suicidal behavior may be connected temporally to significant events in the patient's life. Common precipitating events include a recent breakup with a girlfriend or boyfriend and conflicts with the family. The recent death of someone close to the patient is a frequent precipitating event, particularly if the person killed himself or herself or died suddenly. If one of the patient's close friends has committed suicide, the examiner should ask the patient whether he or she had prior knowledge of the event or whether the child ever made a suicide pact with the deceased. The examiner should explore the degree of guilt the patient feels over the friend's death. Patients who have a depressive background are particularly vulnerable to the contagion effects of a close friend's suicide (i.e., when a patient is particularly likely to commit suicide in response to a close friend's suicide). Anniversaries are times of emotional reactivation of painful memories and unresolved guilt, and these occasions may activate suicidal behavior or fantasies of reunion with the deceased. When the patient is deeply emotionally connected to a dead person (e.g., grandparents, other relatives, or friends), the presence of psychotic features should be considered.

The examiner should explore whether the patient is experiencing auditory, commanding hallucinations such as "voices" asking the patient to join the deceased. The voices may tell the patient to kill himself or herself or to commit other acts (e.g., to kill others). The examiner should determine whether the patient is able to suppress these commands or is helpless against their overpowering influence. When suicidal behavior is unrelenting, the examiner should explore the possibility of psychotic guilt or other obsessive or delusional features (see Donna's case example in Chapters 1 and

3). Schneiderman et al. (2) reviewed a number of studies to determine factors that increase the bereavement risk when a parent or child dies. These factors are listed in Table 4–1.

In relation to "why," the examiner should explore psychological factors that motivate the patient's suicidal ideation and behavior. Many emotional states activate suicidal behaviors: helplessness; emotional pain; anger; worthlessness or devaluation; shame or humiliation; emptiness; nihilism; rejection or abandonment; loneliness or feelings of being unloved; disappointment or feelings of failure; hopelessness, despair, or futility; fears of a mental breakdown; feelings that a handicap or a medical illness is unacceptable; self-hatred; guilt; and many other negative, self-blaming, disorganizing, and pain-inducing subjective states. Following Pfeffer, Table 4–2 addresses areas of inquiry that are pertinent in the evaluation of suicidal risk in children (1).

In the assessment of current suicidal risk, it is important to evaluate the child's current psychological status and to determine the

TABLE 4–1.　**Factors that increase bereavement risk after parental death**

Factor	Result
Type of death	Outcome is poorer in sudden deaths
Psychiatry history of the surviving parent	Poor outcome if surviving parent has a psychiatric history
Sex of the deceased parent	Poorer outcome when the mother is the deceased
Social supports	Better outcomes in higher quality social supports
Parent's involvement with the child prior to death	More symptoms when higher level of involvement prior to death
Age and sex of the child	No significant outcome factors
Socioeconomic factors	More depression in children in higher socioeconomic brackets

Source.　Based on Schneiderman et al. 1996 (2).

TABLE 4–2.	**Pertinent areas of inquiry in suicidal children**

Suicidal fantasies and actions

Consequences of the suicidal act

Circumstances at the time of the suicidal behavior

Motivations for suicidal behavior

Experiences and concepts about death

History of suicide within the family or in close friends

Exploration of depression and other affective states

Exploration of family and environmental circumstances

History of a recent loss (e.g., breakup with a loved one)

Use of alcohol or drugs

Source. Based on Pfeffer 1986 (1, pp. 187–188).

ongoing family and environmental conditions. Pfeffer warns that "the status of these variables may change rapidly, so that repeated, comprehensive discussion with a suicidal youngster is necessary" (3, p. 670). Pfeffer stresses the need to assess the family's level of functioning and the circumstances surrounding the child: "It is important to determine whether the family can provide a consistent, stable environment or whether there is a high intensity of stress, violence, and psychopathology and unavailability of relatives. Positive social supports are critical in diminishing suicidal risk among children and adolescents" (3, p. 670).

Because suicidal behavior and self-abusive behavior do not necessarily belong to the same psychopathological domains, they need to be examined separately. The management and prognosis of these behaviors are very different.

Explanations offered by the child or the family should not discourage the examiner from exploring the motivations or reasons for the child's suicidal behaviors. After serious suicidal behavior, children sometimes claim they were simply seeking attention. This explanation may be the parents', not the child's, interpretation of the event. Dissociative episodes are an uncommon explanation when the patient disconnects or denies the seriousness of suicidal experiences. The examiner should not ask the child, "Did you really intend to kill yourself?" This judgment is the examiner's to make, not the child's.

Revelations of abuse should not be disregarded after the patient recants them; the same holds true for statements that a suicidal behavior lacked intent.

The factors considered in the evaluation of suicide attempts are relevant to the overall assessment of suicidal behavior (4). Table 4–3 summarizes the areas the examiner should consider in evaluating a child's suicide attempts.

Berman and Carroll discuss family factors that contribute to suicidal behaviors: "The motives for suicide attempts of adolescents appear largely directed towards effecting change in or escape from an interpersonal system" (5, p. 60). On dealing with the close relatives of suicidal children, these authors say,

---

TABLE 4–3. **Factors to be explored in suicide attempts**

Precipitating events

Presence of depression, guilt, hopelessness, or anger

Presence of cognitive deficits (e.g., poor problem-solving strategies)

Presence of maladaptive coping (e.g., social isolation, drug abuse)

Interpersonal difficulties with girlfriend, boyfriend, or parents

Family conflicts, including family violence and physical or sexual abuse

Personal losses through death, divorce, or relocations

Peer rejection

Physical illness or other personal factors

Pact with a person who committed suicide or who is about to do so

Contagion or imitation with recent suicidal behavior

Source. Based on Spirito et al. 1989 (4, pp. 338–350).

As essential as it is to view parents as 'first finders,' to identify and provide assistance to the precipitously or potentially suicidal child, these parents may be least equipped to accomplish these tasks. Because of their own pathology; their intimate relationship with and, therefore, blind spots to their children; and/or the implicit and explicit blame levied by having a suicidal child, most parents deny, minimize, distort, etc. and only notice after (and, perhaps, only because of) a suicide attempt. (5, p. 60)

Gutstein addresses the influence of family factors in the precipitation of suicidal behavior in adolescents. He considers that suicidal behavior at this age represents for the child the hope for reconciliation with his or her family:

The child at risk in the isolated family learns that losses cannot be replaced and that separations, rather than being followed by reconciliation, lead to further isolation and alienation. This experience of *irreplaceability,* combined with the child's yearning for an exclusive, symbiotic relationship, and the family's rigid responses to developmental transitions, set the stage for the child's later suicide response to the adolescent crisis. (6, p. 247)

Gutstein concludes,

For these adolescents, perceiving the need for exclusivity and believing in the irreplaceability of key others, the anticipated loss of an exclusive relationship is experienced as a disaster. The suicidal threat or attempt may be made in a desperate effort to forestall the impending loss. The behavior may be precipitated by a loved one's actual or anticipated severance of a relationship. Its purpose is to influence the other not to make a choice exclusive of oneself, or to reverse an exclusive choice one is forced to make. When the adolescent believes that the loss has already occurred, then the act is no longer an attempt to change the other, but a more final and fatal decision. (6, p. 248)

The psychiatrist has a duty and professional responsibility to take all the steps necessary to prevent a patient from killing himself or herself. This goal needs to be tempered, however, by the psychiatrist's limited capacity to predict suicidal behavior. Shaffer offers a sobering reminder: "In even the most troubled patient, suicide is a rare event whose eventuality and precise timing defy accurate prediction. Although a well-supervised environment may significantly reduce opportunities to commit suicide, a determined patient may circumvent supervision by feigning recovery and denying suicidal preoccupations" (7, p. 172). To this he adds a humbling comment: "For both the clinician and the public health official the message could be that we do not currently have a scale that will predict either a further suicide attempt or ultimate death by suicide with any useful accuracy" (7, p. 173).

Goodyer also offers some caveats about the identification of suicidal behaviors:

> The presence of dysphoria may increase and maintain the risk for suicidal behavior in the population at large. Both clinical and community studies indicate, however, that in adolescents major depression is not a prerequisite for suicidal behavior. In addition, the association between thoughts and acts of suicide in this age group remains unclear.... By contrast, complete suicide appears to be commonly associated with features of major depression.... Such cases [completed suicide] appear likely to be comorbid for antisocial and interpersonal aggression. (8, p. 589)

Thus family factors related to suicidal behaviors need to be examined carefully and exhaustively. The examination of suicidal risk demands a thorough assessment of the family's functional level, family factors that contribute to precipitating events, the family's understanding of its role in the child's suicidal behavior, the family's commitment to ensuring the child's safety, and the family's determination to prioritize its emotional and financial resources for the treatment of the child's behavior and the improvement of the family's functioning.

When the child psychiatrist concludes that the child is actively suicidal and that the family cannot guarantee the child's safety (e.g., because of denial or minimization of the suicidal experience), measures should be taken to safeguard the child's life (e.g., hospitalization, involuntary commitment).

■ EVALUATION OF DEPRESSIVE SYMPTOMS

The identification of mood disorders (i.e., depression and mania) poses significant clinical challenges to the child psychiatrist. Mania poses more challenges than does depression.

Depression is polymorphic in its manifestation. Clinical depression varies in the nature and intensity of its presenting symptoms. The examiner should attempt to elicit as complete a picture of the depressive syndrome as possible by identifying a variety of symptoms associated with this disorder and by estimating their severity.

In exploring a patient's depressive mood, the examiner should inquire about the presence of sadness. Pertinent questions include the following: Do you feel sad? How often do you feel sad? When do you feel sad? How bad does it get? What is the worst it has ever been? How long does it last? When you feel sad, what do you feel like doing? When you feel sad, is there anything that helps you to feel better? Because crying is common in depressed children, the following questions should be asked: How often do you cry? When you feel like crying, what comes to your mind?

In general, small children feel depressed when they feel unloved, whatever the reasons may be. Serious family events—such as parental desertion, neglect, or discord; family violence; physical abuse; and other adversities—need to be identified.

Constitutional dysregulation of affect is an important factor in the origin of depressive affect. This problem starts very early in life and is manifested by irritability, temper tantrums, low tolerance for frustration, unhappiness, and limited response to soothing and loving care. The disturbance is enduring and creates a great deal of distress for caregivers because nothing seems to soothe these children. Children with a difficult temperament are usually a bad match for impatient parents, more so if the parents have mood dysregulations of their own. Akiskal describes the concept of *temperament dysregulation,* also known as *subaffective temperament* (9, p. 756). These concepts refer to specific constitutionally based affective dispositions (e.g., melancholic-dysthymic, choleric-irritable, sanguine-hyperthymic, and cyclothymic) that are manifested predominantly at the subclinical level. These dispositions "are distressing and disruptive and are in a continuum with major mood states" (9, p. 756). Thus moody behavior, angry outbursts, and explosive episodes must be explored. Marked irritability is a behavioral change that many parents report observing in their children. For example, children may start displaying verbally, if not physically, abusive behavior toward their parents and siblings. Other forms of aggressive acting-out, such as defiant and rebellious behaviors, are also common complaints.

Irritability is a prevalent mood in depressed children and often generates a stable dysphoric affect. Many children identify this mood as soon as they wake up in the morning. The following question may be helpful: When you first open your eyes in the morning, how do you feel? These children are hyperreactive: anything can set them off. Any demand is upsetting, and any expectation is too much for them. These children are prone to exhibit explosive behavior or to lose control. Parents frequently complain that these children are moody if not violent. Pertinent questions to ask include the following: How often do you feel grouchy (irritable)? What does it take for you to feel grouchy? When you feel grouchy, how long do you feel like that? Is there anything that makes the grouchy feelings go away? Do you have a temper? What happens when you lose your temper? These questions may be followed by exploration of potential aggression against the self (self-abusive behavior), against others (violent and assaultive behaviors), or against the physical environment (destructiveness, vandalism, and so on).

Guilt and its sources need to be identified. Children often feel responsible for things they have not caused. The following questions are helpful in identifying guilty feelings: Is there anything for you to feel bad about? Is there anything you feel you need to be punished for? In extreme cases, guilt takes a psychotic quality, as when the child feels responsible for the ills of the world and beyond. The following case example illustrates this *psychotic guilt*:

> Salim, the 8-year-old son of a Lebanese father and an American mother, was hospitalized for unrelenting suicidal ideation. He had overt psychotic features: he complained that aliens were after him. Salim's parents were divorced but maintained a bitter and hostile relationship. Salim's custody was still an issue, and he was caught in a loyalty conflict between his parents.
>
> When watching television programs about the country's most-wanted criminals, Salim would ask his mother to call the Federal Bureau of Investigations to tell them that he was the person they were looking for. He also blamed himself for the war in Yugoslavia, for worldwide pollution problems, and so on. These delusional beliefs were impervious to reassurance or to reality testing.

Other times, guilt is latent but can be brought readily to the surface, as illustrated in the following case example:

> Fred, a 12-year-old Caucasian boy, was admitted to an acute psychiatric setting because he set fire to the blankets and mattress where his younger brother was sleeping. His brother sustained second- and third-degree burns. During the interview, Fred appeared sad and downcast. The examiner told Fred that he didn't look happy and asked, "When was the last time you were happy?" Fred became tearful but tried not to cry. Upon seeing this emotional struggle, the examiner said, "Can you share with me what is going on in your mind right now? You are trying very hard not to cry." Fred attempted to control his tears but finally broke down and tears poured down his cheeks. Holding his head in his hands, he said, "I can't believe what I did to my brother." He continued sobbing and expressing sorrow, saying, "I burnt my brother. . . . "
>
> Fred began displaying signs of genuine emotion; the emotional abreaction was clearly associated with guilt. Fred revealed that he had heard voices commanding him to kill his

brother. This revelation helped the examiner conclude that Fred had a psychotic depression.

The concept of a bad parent is an alien concept for a child. It takes a great deal of psychological growth and cognitive development to appreciate that one's parents may have some flaws. Children who endure parental abuse usually blame themselves for the abuse. Similarly, if a parent abandons a child, the child usually feels that he or she did something that pushed away the parent.

Emotional withdrawal occurs in many depressed children. Depressed children seek solitude and withdraw from family and peer interactions. Parents report that such children do not participate in family activities or that they isolate themselves in their rooms, refuse to be with friends, and so on. Helpful questions include the following: Do you have any friends? How are you getting along with your friends? Do you have a best friend? How much time do you spend with your best friend? Do you enjoy your friends? What kind of groups or fun (social) activities do you participate in?

Anhedonia is evidenced when the child no longer feels happy, cannot have fun any more, or cannot join in pleasurable activities. Pertinent questions include the following: When was the last time you felt happy? In a given week, how many days do you feel happy? What kinds of things can you do to feel happy? The child's history will indicate whether previous interests in sports or in other activities are no longer important to the child. Formerly athletic children no longer display interest in their favorite sports. When invited to participate in games, they refuse, or when they do, their participation is perfunctory; they simply go through the motions.

Hopelessness needs to be identified. Signs of hopelessness include behaviors that indicate the child feels there is nothing to live for anymore or when the child begins to dispose of valuable belongings (e.g., giving away CDs or baseball card collections). Hopelessness is obvious in the presence of unremitting suicidal behavior or when the child considers multiple alternatives for committing suicide. Typically when the child is experiencing such feelings—no matter how good the options presented to the child are and no matter how positive some alternatives may be—the child's characteristic and disheartened response is, "I don't care" or "It doesn't matter."

Depressed children complain of being tired; this complaint is present from the moment they wake up and usually remains throughout the day. The sense of tiredness contributes to the depressed child's lack of motivation, loss of interest in school, and problems with concentration. Tiredness is also secondary to sleep problems that are common in depressed children.

Depressed children frequently have marked difficulty falling asleep (initial insomnia). When they do fall asleep, they frequently wake up during the night and have trouble going back to sleep (middle insomnia). Problems with terminal insomnia occur when depressed children wake up very early in the morning (e.g., at 4:00 A.M. or 5:00 A.M.) and are unable to fall asleep again. For depressed children, sleep is seldom refreshing. When the time to wake up arrives, depressed children prefer to stay in bed, in part, because getting up requires effort. Not surprisingly, many depressed children fall asleep during school or invert their biorhythm (i.e., by sleeping during the day and staying up at night). Many parents struggle every morning to get these children ready for school. Tardiness and absenteeism from school may be revealing. Frequently, parents are unaware of the presence or severity of their child's sleep difficulties. Tiredness in a child, without a known medical problem, should raise suspicion of a depressive disorder. In atypical depressions, children display hypersomnia and sleep a great deal.

Another contributor to tiredness is limited food intake due to a lack of appetite. Many depressed children lose weight even though they are not making any conscious effort to do so. Failure to gain weight in small children is an equivalent sign. Children with atypical depressions may show an appetite increase and may gain weight.

Deterioration in academic performance or behavior at school is a common complication of depressed mood. The child's grades suffer for a number of reasons: poor motivation (lack of interest), tiredness, or impaired concentration. This last impairment is common in depressed children. Bad conduct in school is a consequence of dysphoria (e.g., from irritability and low tolerance for frustration).

Hyperactivity, restlessness, and agitation sometimes occur in depressed children. These symptoms may be intrinsic to the disorder or may represent the expression of associated comorbid conditions such as attention-deficit/hyperactivity disorder (ADHD) or anxiety disorders. More frequently, depressed children display slowness in psychomotor activity. Children with prominent melancholic features exhibit a marked decrease in the psychomotor sphere; in extreme cases, the examiner may observe signs of catatonia (see Chapter 3).

Negative cognition (e.g., feelings of worthlessness, personal devaluation, and poor self-concept), concentration or memory difficulties, and suicidal ideation are common in depressive disorders. Suicidal ideation and suicidal behavior must be explored systematically in all depressed patients (see preceding section in this chapter).

In an attempt to deal with dysphoric affect, depressed children may start using alcohol or drugs. If they do not get the nurturing and understanding they need in their home environment, they seek a sense of belonging in alternative family groups, such as gangs or cults.

Because the length of the depression and the number of depressive episodes have diagnostic, therapeutic, and prognostic implications, the examiner should strive to determine these factors. Depressive disorders are commonly associated with anxiety disorders, oppositional defiant disorder (ODD), conduct disorder, substance abuse disorders, obsessive-compulsive disorder (OCD), and ADHD.

With depressed children, particular attention needs to be paid to psychotic features (i.e., auditory and visual hallucinations and paranoid features), which are common in severe depressions. Of particular importance is the identification of auditory hallucinations that command the patient to kill himself or herself. As mentioned earlier, if these perceptual disturbances are identified, the examiner should ask whether the voices also command the patient to hurt or to kill anyone else. Suicidal and homicidal auditory commands frequently coexist.

The *Diagnostic and Statistical Manual of Mental Disorders, Fourth Edition* (DSM-IV; 10), classifies depressive disorders as major depressive disorder (either single episode or recurrent), dysthymic disorder, and depressive disorder not otherwise specified (NOS; includes disorders that do not meet either the specific depressive disorder diagnostic category or the categories of adjustment disorders). DSM-IV also includes other depressive syndromes such as premenstrual dysphoric disorder, minor depressive disorder, recurrent brief depressive episode, postpsychotic depressive disorder of schizophrenia, and other less well-defined depressions (10).

In the differential diagnosis of depression, bipolar depression poses the biggest challenge. Accurate identification of bipolar disorder is necessary because of the risks associated with antidepressant treatments. The severe clinical course and complications associated with bipolar disorder increase the patient's risks of suicidality and psychosocial dysfunction (e.g., conduct disorder, substance abuse, school and family dysfunction). About one-third or more of the children given the diagnosis of depression eventually develop bipolar disorder. Bowden and Rhodes highlight the following features commonly associated with bipolar depression: positive family history of bipolar disorder, psychomotor retardation rather than agitation, psychotic or delusional features, hypersomnia, and a rapid onset rather than an insidious presentation (11, p. 431).

There is an important clinical caveat in the evaluation of depression in children. Some children do not display depression during the interview, but this does not mean that they do not have a depressive syndrome. Consider the following case example:

> Lillian, a 14-year-old Caucasian adolescent, was evaluated for episodes of running away, aggression toward her mother, and rebelliousness and defiance directed at her parents. Lillian had

threatened her mother a number of times and had become progressively more violent toward her. Lillian was markedly ambivalent toward her mother: when feeling close to her mother, she began to act out against her or ran away. Sometimes she ran away to avoid striking her mother.

Lillian's mother reported that her daughter had become increasingly dysphoric over the preceding 5 months, especially during the preceding 2 months. Lillian had become irritable, explosive, and even physically abusive toward her younger half-siblings. Her academic performance had deteriorated: she was getting D's and F's, although previously she had gotten A's and B's. She had lost about 20 pounds in 4 months. Lillian had begun to defy her parents' rules and had confronted her parents regarding curfew and other restrictions.

Lillian had befriended gang members and experimented with marijuana and drinking. She had no legal problems other than the charge of running away. Lillian was still a virgin; however, she confessed that her current boyfriend had put pressure on her to have sex. She was about 7 years old when her stepgrandfather had fondled her. He had been prosecuted and sent to prison for fondling Lillian and his other granddaughters.

Lillian reported that a number of her friends had died. Most recently, two teenage friends had been killed in a drive-by shooting. A rival gang member had killed her closest friend, a 16-year-old gang member whom she considered a brother. This had been a significant loss for her; she dreamed about her dead friend and mentioned him frequently in her writings, letters, and poetry.

Lillian had no psychiatric history despite two previous suicide attempts. In the latest attempt, she overdosed on many over-the-counter pills while under the influence of alcohol and marijuana. The first attempt occurred a year earlier, when she overdosed on over-the-counter medications. Lillian's 18-year-old sister had a stormy adolescence that included multiple hospitalizations and extensive psychiatric treatments. She had been given the diagnosis of bipolar disorder, which was being treated with lithium.

The mental status examination disclosed the presence of a 14-year-old female who appeared somewhat older than her stated age. She was not very attractive: she had a prominent forehead and a conspicuous overbite. She was anxious and fidgeted throughout the examination. Her mood was considered euthymic, and her affect was constricted in range and intensity. She denied suicidal and homicidal ideation. She appeared to be intelligent. Her language was unremarkable for receptive and expressive functions. Her sensorium was clear. Her thought content related to her conflicts with and anger toward her mother, the loss of her close friends, and issues related to her discontent with her body (she had a well-endowed bosom and was self-conscious about it). She exhibited no evidence of hallucinations or delusional thinking. She had some degree of insight, but her judgment was impaired.

Even though Lillian appeared euthymic during the mental status examination, her history and overall clinical picture, plus the family history of affective disorders, were compatible with a depressive disorder. Lillian displayed a number of atypical depressive features and was given the diagnosis of depressive disorder NOS.

Depressive disorders carry a serious prognosis in a variety of ways:

1. Affective disorders are frequently recurrent conditions.
2. Depressive disorders increase the risk of suicidal behavior.
3. Depressive disorders are frequently associated with comorbid conditions such as ODD, conduct disorder, substance abuse disorders, and anxiety disorders.
4. Depressive disorders have a detrimental effect on psychological and interpersonal development.
5. Depressive disorders interfere with school academic progress and with other adaptive functions.
6. Children with depressive disorders have a significant risk of developing bipolar disorders with added comorbid risks.

■ EVALUATION OF ANXIOUS SYMPTOMS

The following case example illustrates many issues common in anxious children. It also depicts the relationship between anxiety disorders and depressive disorders.

Glenn, a 9-year-old Caucasian boy, was referred for evaluation because of concerns about a progressive depression with ongoing suicidal verbalizations. Glenn, his mother, and her male friend sat down for the family evaluation, and Glenn began to present his concerns in a very coherent and articulate way. He became the main spokesperson for the group. As he was talking and responding to minor cues, Glenn's mother and her friend assented to most of what he said. Their nonverbal behavior indicated that they supported his disclosures and history presentation. At no point did Glenn's mother contradict him. He spoke with significant anxiety and with marked intensity. It is uncommon for a child to be so active during a psychiatric examination.

Glenn reported that he began to feel depressed about 2 months prior to the psychiatric assessment. He had become very "grouchy," and when upset, he would hit walls and stomp his feet. He was assaultive toward his younger brothers (ages 5 and 6). Glenn was moody and had problems falling asleep: he woke up in the middle of the night and complained of nightmares. Glenn also had difficulties with his appetite. He had been thinking about suicide with increasing intensity but had developed no plans. He cried on a regular basis.

There had been a tense custody dispute between Glenn's parents after their divorce 5 years earlier. Glenn's mother remarried but had been divorced from her second husband for more than a year. Glenn stated that he would rather kill himself than go to live with his father. Glenn's father had been very abusive to his mother; Glenn saw her being beaten many times. Glenn also witnessed his father attempting to kill his mother on more than one occasion (his father had shot, stabbed, and battered Glenn's mother in front of him). It was reported that Glenn's younger brothers were equally afraid of their father. Glenn's father allegedly shot Glenn's dog in the head right in front of him. There were also reports that Glenn had gotten drunk once after his father gave him alcohol. There were no indications that Glenn had tried or used any other substances.

Glenn worried a lot about his mother. He was afraid something bad could happen to her and was protective of her. His mother said that she had posttraumatic stress disorder (PTSD) secondary to physical, sexual, and emotional abuse perpetrated by Glenn's father. She worked at a nightclub. Glenn didn't like her job and worried about it. The mother came to the evaluation inappropriately dressed in revealing shorts and blouse.

Glenn's mother broke down when her son revealed that his father had sexually abused him. She needed a great deal of reassurance and support, both from her male companion and from the examiner. The mother had initially misrepresented the companion as a brother; he was her boyfriend. Glenn's mother appeared helpless and on the verge of tears throughout the interview. She changed the focus from Glenn's concerns to her own.

Glenn felt very close to his grandparents, but his mother had concerns about them because of their drinking. The most recent stressors for the family had been the family's recent relocation from Okinawa, Japan, and the mother's separation from her second husband.

Two years prior to the evaluation, Glenn had seen a psychiatrist after one of his younger brothers had been sexually molested by his stepfather's brother. Glenn had been diagnosed with "gastric ulcer" a year and a half before this psychiatric assessment; he was taking antacids on a regular basis. Glenn had been educated abroad because of his father's military career. Glenn had completed third grade in Okinawa and was currently attending advanced classes in fourth grade at the local school. Because of ongoing somatic complaints, Glenn was absent from school at least once a week. He enjoyed sports, including hockey and swimming.

The mental status examination revealed a handsome, well-dressed, and articulate 9-year-old boy, who appeared to be his chronological age. He was cooperative and was an excellent historian. He gave a coherent account of his problems and fears with minimal participation from his mother. He appeared depressed, tense, and anxious. His affect was increased in intensity but appropriate. He reported passive suicidal ideation with no plans. His thought processes were unremarkable; there was no evidence of delusional or hallucinatory experiences. His thought content centered on fears about his natural father, fears about his mother, worries that something bad would happen to him, and bad feelings in his stomach. Glenn's level of intelligence appeared above average. He appeared to have excellent verbal skills and good receptive language. His sensorium was intact, and his judgment and insight were good. Glenn had indicated to his mother that he needed psychological help.

In Glenn's case, a depressive disorder could be considered the predominant condition, and an anxiety disorder could be considered its major comorbid condition; however, the clinical picture could have been interpreted the other way around. Anxiety features had been the most prominent psychopathology throughout Glenn's life. Somatization had been a major problem, and a physician had diagnosed Glenn's anxious epigastric distress as gastric ulcer.

Not all anxious children are as forthcoming as Glenn. The examiner more frequently encounters patients who become electively mute during the psychiatric examination. Engaging them verbally may be trying. The examiner needs time and patience and may also need to engage the nonverbal child with nonverbal techniques (see Chapter 2).

The most commonly endorsed anxiety symptoms among preadolescents are excessive concerns about competence, excessive need for reassurance, fear of harm to an attachment figure, fear of the dark, and somatic complaints (12, p. 1112). In adolescents, the most frequently endorsed anxiety symptoms are fear of heights, fear of public speaking, blushing, excessive worrying about past behavior, and self-consciousness (12, p. 1113).

Children who develop anxiety disorders have antecedents of behavioral inhibition (see Chapter 3). This condition should be considered an enduring temperamental trait. Behavioral inhibition is indicated by a tendency to withdraw, to be unusually shy, and to show fear in the presence of novelty. Demonstrative physiological markers include higher stable heart rates in tasks that require cognitive effort; tension of the larynx and vocal cords; elevated salivary cortisol levels; elevated catecholamines; and pupillary dilation in cognitive tasks (12, p. 1111). Attachment difficulties in infancy probably predispose children to the development of anxiety disorders later in childhood (12, p. 1111). The following areas of symptomatology need to be explored on a regular basis in anxious children:

Separation anxiety.   Anxious children display separation difficulties. Frequently, school refusal problems bring these children to the child psychiatrist for the first time. These children are afraid of being alone and are clingy and dependent on their caregivers. For example, anxious children are unable to enjoy the thrills of a slumber party because they do not venture beyond their own homes. They have great difficulty sleeping in their own beds and often go to the parents' room to sleep with them. Separation anxiety is a nonspecific precursor for a number of adult psychiatric conditions including depression and a variety of anxiety disorders (12, p. 1114).

Worrying.   Worrying is a common symptom. Anxious children worry that something bad may happen to their parents or complain of vague or ill-defined apprehensions. For example, they fear that "something bad" may happen to them.

Fears.   Fears of the dark or of storms and other specific phobias are common.

Social phobia.   Social phobia is a common impediment for anxious children. They are very self-conscious and prone to experience embarrassment and shame. These children suffer a lot when asked to go in front of the class or when they have to speak in front of a group. Anxious children are doubtful, insecure, and have poor self-esteem; they need frequent reassurance and support; and commonly they have problems initiating and maintaining friendships. Social phobias, with onset in early and mid-adolescence, are characterized by excessive anxiety about social or performance situations in which the individual fears scrutiny and exposure to unfamiliar persons. In order for this diagnosis to apply, the anxiety should occur in peer situations, and the ability for age-appropriate relationships with familiar people must be evident (12, p. 1114).

Somatization.   Somatization is a common phenomenon in anxious children. Nausea, vomiting, and epigastric pain or distress frequently accompany anxiety disorders. As Glenn's case illustrated, these children are often diagnosed incorrectly with medical illnesses, such as peptic ulcers or irritable bowel syndrome. Anxious children also complain of chest pain, dizziness, headaches, and others somatic symptoms. Many anxious children with epigastric distress undergo unnecessary X rays and endoscopic procedures. Other anxious children make multiple visits to the pediatrician or family physician for somatic complaints. Panic symptoms are beginning to be recognized in pediatric populations.

Elective mutism.   There is an evolving consensus that elective mutism represents an anxiety disorder. Black and Uhde reported that "in 97% (of the cases), there was clear evidence of significant social, academic, or family impairment due to social anxiety, *other than that attributable to the failure to speak,* sufficient for a diagnosis of SP (social phobia) or avoidant disorder" (13, p. 854).

Physical and sexual abuse.   Many anxious children have a history of physical and sexual abuse and have been raised in environments in which marital discord and overt family dysfunction are commonplace.

Anxiety features within the family.   Children who have severe anxiety disorders often have other family members who exhibit incapacitating anxiety symptoms. The following case exemplifies this situation:

Aurora, a 9-year-old Hispanic girl, was evaluated for school refusal. She had prominent somatic complaints and, because of epigastric discomfort, had been diagnosed with a peptic ulcer. She had undergone endoscopy and an upper gastrointestinal series. Aurora's mother had a crippling anxiety disorder with prominent agoraphobic features. Her maternal grandfather had quit grammar school and never returned because of severe anxiety features; he had remained agoraphobic most of his life.

Mood disorders.   Anxiety disorders are commonly comorbid with mood disorders and vice versa. Judd and Burrows propose three models to explain the relationship between depression and anxiety: 1) the unitary model proposes that anxiety and depression are variants of the same disorder; 2) the dualist model advocates that depression and anxiety are different entities, and 3) the anxious-depressive position proposes a mixture of the two models, phenomenologically different from primary anxiety or primary depression (14, pp. 79–82).

■ EVALUATION OF OBSESSIVE-COMPULSIVE BEHAVIORS

OCD is two to three times more common than is schizophrenia. In adults it takes, on average, two decades from the onset of the disorder until it is appropriately diagnosed and treated. The lateness of diagnosing this entity is probably similar when the disorder starts in school age or adolescence. The delay in diagnosis occurs in part because patients are secretive about their symptoms, but examiners often fail to screen systematically for OCD symptoms. It is hoped that attention to early detection and prompt diagnosis and treatment may decrease the extended time between onset of symptoms and treatment relief.

When evaluating a patient for *obsessive symptoms,* the examiner should ask about unwelcome and recurring thoughts. Consider the following questions: Are there any thoughts that keep coming to your mind in spite of your efforts to get rid of them? What are they? Because of the irrational nature of the intrusive thoughts, many obsessional adolescents fear they are becoming insane. Some may respond affirmatively to the question "Do you fear you are going crazy?" The examiner should determine the context in which the symptoms worsen or reappear.

The most common obsessional symptoms are concerns about

dirt and germs, fears of an ill fate befalling loved ones, preoccupa-tions with exactness or symmetry, and religious scrupulousness (15, p. 337). Concerns over bodily functions, preoccupations with lucky numbers, sexual or aggressive preoccupations, and fear of harm to oneself are less common (16, p. 685). Obsessional think-ing related to forbidden, aggressive, and sexual content (e.g., per-verse sexual thoughts) is infrequent in adolescents but occurs more commonly in adults.

Prominent obsessive-compulsive symptomatology occurs in a variety of psychiatric and neurological disorders. Children with anxiety disorders experience prominent obsessional and rumina-tive ideation. This behavior is observed more readily in children who have prominent separation anxiety. Many adolescents with prominent separation anxiety will hide it from the examiner, fear-ing they will be ridiculed or considered immature. Depressed chil-dren frequently struggle with obsessional ideas about committing suicide and ruminate a great deal about their self-worth and lov-ability. Some aggressive children fear losing control of recurrent homicidal ideation. Obsessional features are also common in ado-lescents who have addictive tendencies or perverse proclivities. Transitory but pronounced obsessional and compulsive features are common in patients undergoing profound psychotic regres-sions (e.g., in schizophrenia and bipolar disorder). Frequently these transitory clinical pictures are misdiagnosed because of the prominent nature of the obsessive-compulsive features. Consider the following case example:

> Ramona, a 13-year-old Hispanic adolescent, presented for treat-ment in a florid manic state. She displayed conspicuous compul-sive traits, and her mother reported that Ramona was preoccupied with dirt and went around the house cleaning and vacuuming. She also spent an inordinate amount of time picking up things from the floor and tidying up.
>
> An alternative interpretation to Ramona's clinical picture is that she had bipolar disorder and OCD; however, such comorbidity is uncommon in bipolar disorder.

Obsessive-compulsive features are also prevalent in children who have eating disorders. Obsessional concerns with weight and body image, often of a quasi-delusional proportion, are prominent symptoms in severe cases of eating disorders. These symptoms need to be explored exhaustively. In children with OCD, the examiner needs to explore the possibility of Tourette's syndrome.

Because OCD features are common, Hollander and Benzaquen propose the concept of an OCD spectrum that is organized in three overlapping clusters (17). Table 4–4 illustrates this concept.

Normative obsessive-compulsive features that do not interfere with daily functioning are common developmental features during latency (more so at the beginning than at the end of this developmental stage).

Compulsive symptoms in children and adolescents center around cleaning, hand washing, and orderly and meticulous behaviors. When careful investigation does not reveal the presence of overt repetitious activities, the examiner should proceed with sensitive probing to rule out the presence of less obvious compulsive activities. The exploration of compulsive symptoms can be initiated by asking the following questions: Are there any silly habits that you cannot stop? Are there any habits you do in secret that you do not want people to know about? Commonly children respond by mentioning nail biting or hair pulling (trichotillomania). The examiner needs to continue exploring other compulsive features such as repetitive hand washing, doing and undoing behaviors (e.g., tying and untying shoes, dressing and undressing), checking behaviors, and an overzealous need for orderliness. Table 4–5 summarizes the compulsive features that Swebo et al. (15) identified as the most common in children with OCD. Skin picking has also been recognized as a compulsive symptom (see Britt's case example in Chapter 11). In children and adolescents, rituals are more common than are obsessions, and pure obsessional presentations are rare.

TABLE 4–4. **OCD spectrum**

Cluster	Characteristics	Examples
1	Marked preoccupation with bodily appearance and sensations and with associated behaviors performed in order to decrease anxiety brought on by these preoccupations	Body dysmorphic disorder Depersonalization disorder Hypochondriasis Anorexia nervosa Binge eating[a]
2	Impulse-style disorders	Intermittent explosive disorder[b] Pathological gambling[b] Compulsive buying[a] Sexual compulsions[b] Kleptomania[a] Pyromania[b] Trichotillomania[a] Self-injurious behaviors[a]
3	Neurological disorders with compulsive features	Autism Asperger's disorder Tourette's syndrome Sydenham's chorea Huntington's disease Torticollis Certain types of epilepsy

Note. An overlap is suggested between OCD and somatoform, dissociative, eating, tick, neurological, autistic, pervasive developmental, and impulse-control disorders.
[a]Symptoms more common in females; [b]Symptoms more common in males.
Source. Based on Hollander and Benzaquen 1996 (17, pp. 18–19).

Some children spend a great deal of time readying themselves for school in the mornings, and they may start to get poorer school grades if their compulsions to repeat behaviors interfere with their academic work. The following case illustrates many of the features commonly described in adolescents with OCD:

TABLE 4–5. **Common compulsive behaviors in children and adolescents**

Behavior	Percentage of cases involving this behavior
Excessive and ritualized hand washing, showering, bathing, tooth brushing, and grooming	85
Repeating rituals (e.g., going in or out of a door, up or down from a chair)	51
Checking rituals (e.g., checking doors, locks, appliances, emergency brake, paper route, homework)	45
Miscellaneous rituals (e.g., writing, moving, speaking)	26
Rituals to avoid contact with contaminants	23
Touching	20
Counting	18
Hoarding or collecting	11

Source. From Swebo et al. 1989 (15, p. 337).

Ann, a Caucasian adolescent, was 16 years old when her parents requested a psychiatric consultation. Ann's grades were deteriorating, her fears and inhibition were increasing, she was becoming socially withdrawn, and she demonstrated an increased need for her mother's assistance both in personal care and in homework assignments. Ann had been shy all her life, but her social isolation had been more noticeable lately. She began to refuse to leave home during the weekends and felt progressively uneasy in social situations. She was intelligent and had striking artistic talents. Her parents had noticed that her need for perfection had intensified during the preceding 3 months. This observation coincided with the observation that she got "stuck" more frequently in the mornings when she had to get ready for school. She often missed the school bus because it took her a long time to get ready in the morning.

Ann's problems in the morning started with difficulty finishing her shower. She would spend a great deal of time soaping herself over and over; she couldn't stop doing this. While dressing, she would get stuck buttoning her shirt and could not tie her shoes because she needed to tie them over and over again. Other times she got stuck putting her shoes on, because of her compulsion to align the creases in her socks with certain features of her shoes. To cope with Ann's worsening behavioral paralysis, her mother began to wake her up very early and had taken a progressively more active role in helping Ann to keep moving and not get stuck. Her mother's assistance included bathing her, dressing her, and so on. Ann's mother also participated actively in her homework, because Ann had similar difficulties finishing this task. The intensification of Ann's regressive and dependent behaviors was wearing thin her mother's patience. Ann was unable to explain her peculiar behaviors and denied any significant ongoing concerns. Ann's progressive incapacitation affected her whole family and her mother in particular.

The examiner should inquire about the presence of comorbid conditions because the majority of children with OCD have associated comorbidity. Frequently associated conditions are depressive and anxiety disorders (e.g., social phobias), disruptive behavior disorders, and developmental language or learning disorders. Compulsive personality disorder is uncommon. Soft neurological signs are observed in some children with OCD. The examiner should also determine whether OCD features are present in other family members because such features are common in close relatives of children with OCD.

Of great interest are observations that link streptococcal infections to the onset or exacerbation of OCD symptoms (18, p. 1268). Because of these observations, it will be progressively more important—in new cases of OCD or in reactivations of the disorder—to inquire about recent streptococcal infections.

■ EVALUATION OF PSYCHOTIC SYMPTOMS

Psychotic symptoms are rather uncommon in the overall psychopathology of childhood and adolescence. Affective psychoses (i.e., psychosis associated with mood disorders), dissociative psychoses (i.e., psychosis associated with PTSD or dissociative identity disorder), and psychoses associated with or secondary to addictive substances are commonly seen in clinical practice. Psychosis associated with complex partial seizures is probably more frequent than is schizophrenia. Very early onset schizophrenia (VEOS) disorder, formerly called childhood schizophrenia, is a rare psychiatric disorder. Not all psychotic symptoms have a progressive or negative prognosis (see Chapter 3, Note 1).

Clinicians seldom encounter schizophrenic preadolescents in inpatient settings. This means that even among the most seriously disturbed children, schizophrenia is an uncommon illness in preadolescence. VEOS is probably 25–50 times less common than is early-onset schizophrenia (EOS) with onset in adolescence.

VEOS and some forms of EOS are considered neurodevelopmental disorders. Harris summarizes the development of the concept of childhood schizophrenia: "The possibility of a genetically based neurointegrative defect in schizophrenia was initially proposed by Bender (1947) and later referred to as 'pandysmaturation' by Fish (1977). . . . Pandysmaturation seems to have neurodevelopmental origins rather than being the result of obstetrical complications" (19, p. 415). In Harris's opinion, "although childhood onset schizophrenia seems to be on a continuum with adult schizophrenia, it represents the more severe neurobiologic presentation" (19, p. 411). A common concept used to describe this disorder is one of multidimensional impairment (i.e., schizophrenic children demonstrate functional disturbance in many developmental domains). The schizophrenic process is insidious, and more often than not, the affected child comes to the child psychiatrist only after many years of developmental disturbance.

Examiners should ask the following questions of children in whom schizophrenia is suspected: Is there a history of schizophrenia in the family? Is there any history of difficulties in relating to others? The following questions are pertinent regarding the child's developmental history: How was the pregnancy? Were there any problems during labor and delivery? Any neonatal complications?

Was the baby responsive to the mother (or primary caregiver)? Did the child cuddle? Did he or she mold into the mother's arms? At what point did the major milestones occur? In particular, when did social smiling and stranger anxiety first occur? When did the child begin to talk? What was the child's socialization progress? What progress has the child made in the process of separation-individuation? What autonomous behavior is the child able to demonstrate? What self-care behaviors is the child capable of? Is the child able to sleep alone in his or her own bed? Does the child demonstrate consistent behavioral organization (see Chapter 3)? Is there any harmony in the progress of the developmental lines (see Chapter 8)? If the child demonstrates affect disturbance or mood dysregulation, the history and vicissitudes of these disturbances must be assessed.

Relevant questions regarding psychosocial development include the following: Does the child play with other children, or does the child prefer to be alone? Is the child able to share? How easy is it for the child to make friends? Is the child able to keep the friends that he or she makes? Is the child invited to birthday or slumber parties? Does the child behave or play in a gender-appropriate manner? Does the child demonstrate empathy or a concern for others? Does the child demonstrate any realistic self-esteem or self-worth? These questions are equally relevant in the evaluation of profound developmental disturbances such as autism and pervasive developmental disorders.

Fundamental observations during the psychiatric examination focus on the child's overall demeanor, the degree and appropriateness of the child's relations to the family and to the examiner, the propriety of the child's social behavior, the range and appropriateness of the child's affective display, and the nature of the child's thought processes. The following case example illustrates the clinical presentation of VEOS in middle latency age:

> Rick, a 9-year-old Caucasian boy, was given an emergency psychiatric examination after his mother saw him attempting to push his 6-year-old brother down the stairs. Rick had been seen

by a number of psychiatrists over the years in response to his teachers' expressed concerns about his unusual behaviors. Rick had trouble getting along with his peers and demonstrated profound emotional immaturity. He still carried around a teddy bear, sucked his thumb, and kept pretty much to himself, even on the playground. He frequently adopted unusual postures such as curling up into a fetal position or lying down under his desk. Most of the time he withdrew from group interactions. Although Rick had been tested in the past and was found to be of normal intelligence, his academic performance had deteriorated progressively over the previous few years. His parents had been told that Rick was hyperactive and he had been tried on stimulant medications. The medications had no beneficial effects; instead, Rick demonstrated more irritability and worsening of his persistent sleep disturbance. It would take him a long time to fall sleep, although he was able to sleep in his own bed. A few days before the evaluation, Rick's parents took him to a neurologist. There were no neurological findings, and an electroencephalogram (EEG) showed only nonspecific findings.

Rick would wake up at about 6:30 A.M. every morning, but he was very slow in getting ready for school. His mother provided a great deal of assistance with his hygiene and dressing, although Rick could do those tasks by himself. Rick was a fussy eater and was very thin. There were always questions about his health. In the past, Rick's food intake had been supplemented with Ensure. His mother also complained that her son got upset easily and would become enraged at minor provocations. Anger dyscontrol was a significant problem. He regularly focused his anger on his younger brother. Rick had become progressively more aggressive with his brother and had attempted to choke him. The day of the examination, Rick had also attacked his mother.

Six months before the evaluation, Rick had disclosed that he began hearing voices when he was 8 years old. He claimed he heard a mean voice telling him to do bad things like hitting and kicking his brother hard. This voice also told him to hurt his 17-year-old sister and asked him to be mean to the family dog. He said that sometimes he was able to make the voices go away, but sometime he wasn't.

Rick was born prematurely, and at birth, he experienced respiratory distress. He spent 11 days on a respirator and stayed in the neonatal unit until he was 4 weeks old. His language development was precocious: Rick began to talk by 8 months and talked in full sentences by the time he was a year and a half old. He did not start walking until after he was 12 months old. Rick's father had always felt very proud of his son's intelligence. When his mother expressed concerns about Rick to her husband, he disregarded her anxieties.

Rick's mother first became concerned about her son when he was 4 years old. At that time, she heard from other mothers and friends that there was something unusual about Rick. She heard similar concerns from the day-care center staff; in particular, she was told that Rick had problems socializing with other children. At times Rick complained that other kids made fun of him, in part, because he frequently told stories about aliens. His mother described Rick as introverted; he didn't initiate play with peers and tended to play by himself.

Rick had been on the honor roll in first and second grade, but his academic performance had deteriorated. At school Rick was described as oppositional and had problems doing schoolwork. There were no reports of physical aggression or explosive outbursts at school. Rick had required one-to-one teaching during kindergarten.

Rick's parents had been married for 12 years. This was Rick's mother's second marriage. She had two children from a previous marriage: a 21-year-old son and a 17-year-old daughter. The son had stayed with the father, and the daughter had lived with her mother until she was 15 years old, at which time she decided to live with her father. She moved back to her mother's home 4 months before Rick's psychiatric evaluation. Apparently, Rick took it very hard when his sister left: he became depressed, stopped eating, and cried a great deal. His mother reported that Rick had returned to normal after his sister came back. Rick's parents reported no history of physical or sexual abuse. Their marriage was described as stable. His mother reported being markedly stressed about Rick's problems to the point where she had feared hurting him.

The mental status examination revealed the presence of a

thin, almost emaciated, and peculiar looking boy who looked and acted younger than the stated age. Rick held his teddy bear, called Hypo, all the time. Rick smelled Hypo frequently and kept it close to his chest. Rick had big, unexpressive eyes and big ears. His eye contact was erratic. At times he stared blankly at the ceiling or the wall. From time to time he would display unusual eye movements, converging his eyes in a peculiar fashion. His posture was unusual. He slouched in the chair despite his parents' prompting him to sit upright. Rick would often bend over and seemed able to rest his chest on his lap. He also displayed unusual finger movements, mostly stereotypic, in both hands. He sucked his thumb sporadically. Rick would stay in abnormal positions for extended periods of time. He was also very fidgety.

Rick didn't display any spontaneous speech. When he was asked a question, there were prolonged latencies. Both the parents and the examiner would often need to repeat the question before he would start talking. His responses were simple and unelaborated, and he spoke in a halting and hesitating manner. Rick remained indifferent, if not detached, in his manner of relating to the examiner. He sometimes appeared vacant and distant. Rick's mood appeared euthymic, but his affect was constricted markedly and remained so throughout the psychiatric examination. The range and intensity of his affect were decreased markedly. No evidence of inappropriate affect was observed. It was questionable if an engagement was ever achieved.

When Rick was asked about the incident with his brother, he said that a commanding voice had told him to push his brother down the stairs. Rick said that he had been hearing four kinds of voices for a long time. A mean voice asked him to do mean things and got him in trouble all the time. Rick added that he wanted to block this voice but often could not. He described the second voice as the wacky one: that voice asked him to do funny and silly things (e.g., make noises). He said he could block this voice but did not want to. The third voice was a kind one. A fourth voice, a "weird one," sounded like a vampire that could predict the future. This voice told him to go to the bathroom, do either "number one" or "number two," and talked to him about eating. Rick reported visual hallucinations: he saw animals from time to time. Rick also believed that he had a person in his stomach that pushed his stomach to one side. Furthermore, he said that his teddy bear talked to him. Rick's responses to the examiner's questions were disjointed and rambling. Often it was hard to follow what he was saying. His sensorium was clear; there were no signs of any overt expressive or receptive language difficulties. For more information regarding further diagnostic assessment on this child, see Note 1.

Based on Rick's developmental history, his difficulties with interpersonal relatedness, the presence of stable regressive behavior, and his long history of psychosis, a diagnosis of VEOS was made. Rick fulfilled DSM-IV criteria for the diagnosis of schizophrenia: criterion A (psychotic symptom lasting more than 1 month), criterion B (social and occupational dysfunction), and criterion C (the disturbance has persisted for more than 6 months).

The preceding case example has features similar to those described in EOS: "With the early onset of schizophrenia, there is a higher frequency of premorbid developmental disorders; rates of 54% to 90% have been reported, depending on the study; the earlier the onset, the more likely the developmental disorder. Premorbid schizoid and schizotypal personality features are commonly reported; the child is seen by others as odd, anxious and socially isolated" (19, p. 411).

Rick is an interesting example of disharmony in the unfolding of the developmental lines (see Chapter 8). He exhibited precocious cognitive and linguistic development while other lines lagged farther behind or did not develop at all.

The diagnosis of VEOS should not be made without taking a comprehensive history, including a detailed developmental history, a detailed psychosocial assessment, a methodical psychiatric examination, a physical and neurological examination, and related tests and procedures. Complete psychological testing (psychoeducational and projective) is mandatory. Other testing and examinations may be deemed necessary in any given case (e.g., speech and language assessment, neuropsychological testing, further neurological examinations such as an EEG or neuroimaging studies).

Although the presence of thought disorder is necessary to make the diagnosis of schizophrenia, this criterion is not sufficient to make such a diagnosis. In the absence of any significant medical or neurological disorder, the child must show persistent developmental deviation or developmental arrest (or marked loss of the adaptive capacity), profound problems in interpersonal relationships, disturbance in affect and emotional development, and clear evidence of thought disorder.

Schizophrenia in childhood is associated with unspecific neurological findings, language disorders, cognitive impairments, ADHD, and other disorders. The child psychiatrist should exhaustively rule out medical and neurological conditions. Finally, the examiner needs to heed Volkmar's advice: "If psychosis is suspected, consideration of the patient's safety—and, as appropriate, that of others—should be the initial consideration" (20, p. 848).

The following case example illustrates schizophrenia developed in middle to late adolescence (i.e., EOS):

> Troy, a 17-year-old Hispanic adolescent, had been referred by the local school district because of concerns over bizarre behaviors that included inappropriate sexual verbalizations and open masturbation. He had been verbalizing homosexual intentions and spoke about having sex with a dog. It had been reported that Troy kept checking his "belly," even in front of people. Before the evaluation, Troy had inappropriately grabbed a teacher's hand. Teachers and classmates felt uneasy about him.
>
> Troy's mother complained that her son had problems with hygiene and personal care. She also reported that Troy frequently got angry and that he was self-abusive. According to his mother, Troy had demonstrated disturbed behavior for the past few years. Troy had undergone his first psychiatric evaluation the previous Christmas (one year before the current evaluation). Three months before the first psychiatric examination, he had spent 3 weeks in a program for adolescents at the local state hospital after he stopped eating.
>
> Troy was conceived out of wedlock, but the pregnancy had

been uneventful. Troy's father was described as alcoholic. His mother reported no significant problems with her son during childhood. Apparently, Troy was sexually abused (anal penetration) by one of his maternal uncles when he was 10 years old. There was also a history of physical abuse. Troy's mother reported that one of her brothers and an uncle were mentally ill. The precise nature of those illnesses could not be ascertained. Troy had tried a number of drugs in the past, including LSD, marijuana, alcohol, and tobacco products.

Troy's mother reported changes in his behavior after she had a stroke, 2 years before the evaluation. After the stroke, she was paralyzed on her right side for months. During that time, she had severe expressive language difficulties. She still had problems with word finding (the examiner also felt she had difficulties understanding the seriousness of her son's psychiatric problems).

Troy was born abroad but had been brought to the United States when he was about 5 years old. At the time of the psychiatric evaluation, Troy was living with his mother and his stepfather. The relationship between stepfather and stepson was not positive because the stepfather was in charge of limit setting, and he had to discipline Troy for his inappropriate behaviors, which included open disrespect and overt indiscretions toward his mother. Although he had opportunities to see his natural father, he had shown no interest in doing so.

During the previous year, the parents had noticed a progressive deterioration in Troy's behavior. Troy's mother had observed him masturbating openly and without any discretion or sense of propriety. Troy often made inappropriate sexual comments to his mother. When his attention was called to these improprieties, he blandly responded by saying, "There was nothing wrong with that." During the previous year, Troy had developed an infatuation with Salvador Dali's art; he spent a lot of time drawing surrealistic drawings of body parts with explicit sexual content. Troy took offense when his family called his attention to the impropriety of his art. His dream was to become an artist like Dali, and he daydreamed of exhibiting his artwork.

The mental status examination showed a tall, Hispanic male who looked younger than the stated age. He displayed an inappropriate smile throughout the examination. Troy's grooming and hygiene were poor. He wore baggy pants and a T-shirt with M. C. Escher drawings on the front and back. His medium-length black hair was tucked behind his ears, and his fingernails were painted black. Troy walked slowly, and his posture was stooped.

As soon as Troy and his mother entered the interviewing room, he sat down and began to touch and inspect his abdomen. His mother asked the examiner why Troy kept looking at and touching his belly. The examiner told the mother in a playful and humorous manner that maybe Troy thought he was pregnant. Upon hearing this, Troy smiled and, as though expressing a sigh of relief, said, "You see, mom, this doctor makes a lot of sense."

Troy remained aloof and distant throughout the interview, and the examiner could not develop a rapport with him. Troy was unfriendly and had very poor eye contact. He was also evasive and secretive. He looked mildly depressed, and his affect was grossly inappropriate: he displayed a silly, sardonic smile throughout the interview. The range and intensity of his affect were decreased. Troy was oriented to time and place. His memories were intact, and his intellectual functions appeared average.

In the area of thought processes, Troy was not logical and at times was incoherent. Troy exhibited very loose associations. He claimed that he heard and saw his own thoughts. He was markedly delusional; his delusions related to the end of the world and were blasphemous in nature. He made innumerable references to feces, body orifices, and primitive sexual misconceptions. For instance, he thought that Jesus was made of the "crap that comes from the butt." There was also repeated telescoping (e.g., merging, confusion) of psychosexual issues. He talked about a girl who was born from the butt of the cross. A repeated theme was that of a child who is being delivered vaginally to become the leg of his mother. He wondered if he was pregnant. He advanced that he would like to be a girl when he dies and wished he had his whole body full of penises and wished that girls had multiple vaginas. He wished he could die and have sex. He declared that Satan had sex with Jesus. In reference to the latter, he brought to the examination a picture he was proud of: a large poster, of good artistic quality, in which

Satan was sodomizing Jesus. He seemed pleased to be showing his artwork and was completely unaware of the offensive nature of its content. He seemed very surprised when the examiner asked him to think about the implications of such a picture in a very religious Christian community. He didn't see anything wrong with it. Troy stated that when he masturbated he became God; he also saw God. When he was questioned about suicidal ideation, he responded that he thought about it. When asked if he had any plans to kill himself, he was secretive and evasive. He denied any homicidal ideation. His judgment and insight were nil. For more information regarding further diagnostic assessment of this adolescent, see Note 2.

Troy fulfilled diagnostic criteria for schizophrenia. He had history of active symptoms (hallucinations and delusions) for more than 1 year (criterion A). Residual symptoms (i.e., affective flattening) and marginal educational and interpersonal functioning (i.e., significant compromise of the level of adaptive functioning, including a decline in self-care and marginal social adjustment) were also present (criterion B). Troy demonstrated serious impairment of reality testing, and he lacked insight and a sense of social propriety (judgment impairment). He also displayed a conspicuous thought disorder. Finally, the global disturbance had lasted for over 1 year (criterion C).

Cautions expressed earlier in this chapter regarding the diagnosis of VEOS apply equally to the diagnosis of EOS. A complete medical and neurological examination is mandatory before EOS can be diagnosed, because medical and neurological conditions can mimic schizophrenic disorders. Consider the following case example:

Myra, a 16-year-old Caucasian adolescent, was brought for a psychiatric examination by her natural mother, who had been followed by the examiner for paranoid and dysphoric features. Myra's mother complained that she did not show any initiative in taking care of herself and that she needed to be "on her" about basic personal care, including hygiene. At school, Myra refused to participate or to do any schoolwork; at home, she wanted to stay in bed or in her room most of the time. She had been evaluated by a psychiatrist a number of months before the current psychiatric evaluation and had received the diagnosis of chronic schizophrenia. Olanzapine had been prescribed for her, but her mother had interrupted the neuroleptic treatment because she was becoming overly sedated. Myra did not have a history of seizures or head trauma or a history of fainting or blacking out. She had no significant medical history.

According to Myra, she regularly saw Jesus and her dead baby brother. She had been experiencing those perceptions for 5 years. Both Jesus and her baby brother said to her, "You will be dying soon . . . you will be reuniting with your brother." Myra enjoyed hearing these voices, claiming that they were soothing. She wanted to join her brother in heaven and anticipated she would die in the year 2000.

The mental status examination revealed the presence of a quiet, withdrawn, nonspontaneous adolescent who appeared somewhat older than the stated age. Her psychomotor activity was decreased, and her speech was dysprosodic. She spoke in a monotone with no emotion. Her mood appeared depressed, and her affect was blunted markedly. Myra denied homicidal or suicidal ideation. She was illogical but goal directed. She endorsed auditory, visual, gustatory, and olfactory hallucinations. Besides hearing and seeing her dead brother and Jesus, she reported a periodic experience of "an awful smell, like a skunk" and "a taste, like throwing up." During those experiences Myra felt confused. She also endorsed strong and prominent paranoid delusions. She believed that many people wanted to kill her and that people had guns and knives for that purpose. Myra believed she had been in danger since she was 3 or 4 years old. Her sensorium was clear.

Because of the diagnostic impression of complex partial seizures, Myra was referred to a neurologist. His mother refused to comply with the consultation and also refused to consider neuroleptic medications, claiming that previous experiences with those medications had been negative. Because the examiner thought that the probability of a complex seizure was strong, he prescribed valproic acid. When the examiner saw Myra 2 weeks later, the sense of confusion and the olfactory and gustatory hallucinations had improved. Although Myra was still seeing her brother and Jesus, these experiences and the voices associated with them were less frequent than before. What was most striking were the changes in Myra's mood and in her emotional display. She was more expressive and displayed a broader range and richer intensity of affect. Her paranoid feelings had decreased, and she felt less suspicious and more at ease. The dosage of valproic acid was adjusted, and Myra's psychotic and paranoid symptomatology improved further. Although Myra fulfilled criteria for the diagnosis of paranoid schizophrenia, she most probably had a neurological disorder, a complex partial seizure disorder.

■ EVALUATION OF SCHIZOID SYMPTOMS

In the differential diagnosis of depression, questions regarding how to separate affective disorders from schizoid disorders are raised frequently. Close attention to the patient's history and affective display and close monitoring of the examiner's emotional reactions during the interview (see Chapter 11) are helpful aids in differentiating this diagnostic complexity.

The social developmental history is of great assistance in the differential diagnosis. The examiner should inquire into the child's early response to the caregiver. Did the child respond emotionally to the mother (or primary caregiver)? Did the child cuddle? Did he or she mold into the mother's arms? Did the infant anticipate, and express in nonverbal behavior, the mother's approach? Did the child demonstrate evidence of stranger anxiety or separation distress? Did the child exhibit exploratory behavior and a capacity to separate from the mother? Did the child approach or initiate contact with other children? Does the child demonstrate evidence of behavioral inhibition? Is the child able to play with other children? Do other children seek out the child? Does the child demonstrate social skills and communication pragmatics? Has the child been a loner? Does the child prefer to play by himself or herself? Attachment difficulties need to be considered in the differential diagnosis of schizoid disorders (21). The following case example is typical of children with schizoid disorders:

Kurt, a 14-year-old male Caucasian adolescent, had been admitted to a local state hospital after making a suicidal gesture. He had a history of extensive conduct disorder, including regular use of his mother's car without permission. He sneaked out at night regularly. During the interview, Kurt appeared meek and behaved oddly. He constantly attempted to hide his hands in the long sleeves of his sweater. His eye contact was erratic, and his speech was monotonous and dysprosodic. His mood was constricted markedly, and he did not seem to be in touch with his feelings. When he was asked to describe his mood, he said he was happy. He immediately corrected himself and said he was sad. There was no modulation of affect throughout the interview, except, for a short moment, when he declared that he missed home. At that moment, he became tearful, helpless, and childish. He did not endorse any psychotic features.

At no point during the interview did the examiner feel that he had made emotional contact with Kurt, and there was no countertransference response concordant with the diagnosis of depression.

Children with language disorders and other neuropsychological deficits—particularly children with nonverbal learning disabilities ue to problems in decoding and expressing affective communication—display difficulties in interpersonal communication and frequently create diagnostic confusion. Such difficulties complicate the identification and assessment of depressive affect. This observation is in agreement with Cummings's assertion that "right-hemispheric damage sustained in childhood may result in a schizoid type of behavioral pattern, perhaps because the inability to perceive or to execute emotional cues limits the child's ability to engage in interpersonal relationships" (22, p. 185).

When working with schizoid children, examiners may encounter difficulties in establishing rapport, peculiarities in the child's affective display, or some degree of inappropriateness of the child's affect. Some children with neuropsychological difficulties want to connect with others and are interested in people; however, they either do not know how to go about doing so or use means that put off other children.

When examining children with schizoid features, the evaluator senses their inability to link emotionally to others, their sense of isolation, and their difficulty warming up to social interactions. The examiner's subjective response is of immense diagnostic value. In general, when the patient is depressed, he or she stimulates depressive feelings in the examiner. As expressed by Akiskal and Akiskal, "The depressed person's dejection and pain tend to be communicated to the clinician and elicit emotional as well as intellectual empathy. Admittedly, this criterion is subjective, but is invaluable in the hands of experienced clinicians" (23, p. 43).

The examiner will find that schizoid children have long-standing difficulties with interpersonal relationships. These children typically are unable to initiate friendships. Commonly they are loners, and more often than not they are ostracized and ridiculed by peers. Schizoid children are frequently odd looking, and their affective communications are atypical. Often their affect is constricted, and at times their emotional display is inappropriate. Comorbid cognitive, language, and psychotic disorders are common. Soft neurological deficits (e.g., in gross and fine motor coordination) and other deficits may be present.

■ NOTES

1. Further diagnostic assessment on Rick:

   Physical examination. Positive findings: a very thin child with elongated fingers and inwardly curved fifth fingers on both hands.

   Neurological screening. Positive findings: dysgraphia, balance difficulties, apraxia (had difficulties putting on his shoes).

   Psychological testing. Positive findings: deficits in written expression. He obtained a superior score on letter-word identification and an average score on passage comprehension.

   Projective testing. Positive findings: deficits in perceptual accuracy consistent with impaired reality testing. Rick misinterpreted and/or distorted perceptual stimuli. Serious problems in thought processes were observed, mainly discontinuity; at times his thinking was incoherent and overtly concrete. There was evidence of significant social and emotional immaturity; this was reflected in his social ineptness and the problems in establishing and maintaining rapport with others. He showed very little interest in approaching and being close to others, and had a very unrealistic view of self and others. There was very little human content in the Rorschach responses while ambiguous and solitary "alien" beings were prominent. Also, Rick had a very inaccurate perception of how others perceive and relate to him and a poor awareness of the extent/significance of his problems. Aggression was poorly neutralized and there was also delay in the process of separation and individuation from the parents.

Occupational therapy assessment. Positive findings: poor to fair kinesthetic abilities; significant difficulties with visual-motor control and fine motor manipulation of objects. There were problems in sensory-motor processing. Sensory-motor testing revealed visual crossing midline problems (e.g., he ignored the right side of the page while copying geometric shapes until he shifted the paper to his left side).

2. Further diagnostic assessment on Troy:

Physical examination. Positive findings: there were multiple self-inflicted injuries in the anterior aspect of both forearms. Otherwise, the physical examination was unremarkable.

Neurological screening. Positive findings: Troy was left-handed. There was evidence of difficulties with praxis. Some degree of dysprosody was also present.

Psychological testing. Positive findings: Troy used a neologism during the examination. He used the word "insormal" to indicate incestuous relations between siblings that are approved by parents. He told the tester his idea for an art piece: to cut off one of his fingers and mount it on cardboard. Troy's thought processes were tangential and rambling. The thought content was consistently dominated by bizarre, morbid, and often perverse themes. He often condensed sexuality with religious symbolism and a personal sense of alienation. His ideas frequently involved the condensation or fusion of opposite qualities, activities, ideas and feelings (e.g., good/evil, procreation/killing, and pleasure/pain). He often seemed fascinated and perplexed by his bizarre musings, which took on a stereotyped and perseverative quality over the course of the evaluation. He said his main interests were in being "bizarre" and "weird."

Projective testing.   Troy's self-image was distorted and conflictive. He appeared to reject all conventional aspects of his identity and life, including identifications with the family, in favor of an intense identification with countercultural ideas and values (i.e., the "bizarre"). He entertained grandiose fantasies (e.g., "being famous someday and producing great works of art") while simultaneously being preoccupied with masochistic themes of humiliation and self-abuse. Troy was very conflicted about gender identification. He was comfortable with social isolation and alienation and appeared indifferent to others except as they provided stimulation for his fantasy life and nourishment of his fascination with the bizarre. Troy's inner life was characterized by pervasive boundary confusion in which conflicted ideas, tendencies, and feelings were resolved or negated in fantasy through the fusion or merger of conflicted opposites. His internal representations were poorly differentiated and lacked substance and diversity. Troy's intense fantasy preoccupation with sexual and religious conflicts may represent primitive denial and distortion defenses, which provided a means of dealing with early trauma. For example, he wondered aloud if death might consist of continuously repeated sexual activity with transvestites that creates "straight good feelings, no bad feelings or thoughts, just good." Troy's thinking disturbance impaired significantly his capacity for adaptive social and educational functioning and self-care, and adversely impacted his motivation for conventional pursuits. On the positive side, Troy's artistic abilities were well developed and represented a potential strength for him that should be further developed.

Cognitive testing.   Troy's level of intelligence was in the low average range. Troy was learning disabled in written expression.

■ REFERENCES

1. Pfeffer C: The suicidal child, in The Evaluation of Childhood Suicidal Risk by Clinical Interview. Edited by Pfeffer C. New York, Guilford, 1986, pp 173–192

2. Schneiderman G, Winders P, Tallett S, et al: Update on bereavement risk (letter). J Am Acad Child Adolesc Psychiatry 35:132–133, 1996

3. Pfeffer C: Attempted suicide in children and adolescents: causes and management, in Child and Adolescent Psychiatry: A Comprehensive Textbook, 1st Edition. Edited by Lewis M. Baltimore, MD, Williams & Wilkins, 1991, pp 664–672

4. Spirito A, Brown L, Overholser J, et al: Attempted suicide in adolescence: a review and critique of the literature. Clin Psychol Rev 9:335–363, 1989

5. Berman AL, Carroll TA: Adolescent suicide: a critical review. Death Education 8:53–63, 1984

6. Gutstein SE: Adolescent suicide: the loss of reconciliation, in Living Beyond Loss Death in the Family. Edited by Walsh F, McGoldrick M. New York, WW Norton, 1991

7. Shaffer D: Discussion of "Predictive validity of the suicide scale among adolescents in group home treatment." J Am Acad Child Adolesc Psychiatry 35:172–174, 1996

8. Goodyer IM: Depression in childhood and adolescence, in Handbook of Affective Disorders, 2nd Edition. Edited by Paykel ES. New York, Guilford, 1992, pp 585–600

9. Akiskal HS: Developmental pathways to bipolarity: are juvenile-onset depressions pre-bipolar? J Am Acad Child Adolesc Psychiatry 34:754–763, 1995

10. American Psychiatric Association: Diagnostic and Statistical Manual of Mental Disorders, 4th Edition. Washington, DC, American Psychiatric Association, 1994

11. Bowden CL, Rhodes LJ: Mania in children and adolescents: recognition and treatment. Psychiatr Ann 26 (suppl):430–434, 1996

12. Bernstein G, Borchardt C, Perwien AR: Anxiety disorders in children and adolescents: a review of the past 10 years. J Am Acad Child Adolesc Psychiatry 35:1110–1119, 1996

13. Black B, Uhde TW: Psychiatric characteristics of children with elective mutism: a pilot study. J Am Acad Child Adolesc Psychiatry 34:847–862, 1995

14. Judd FK, Burrows GD: Anxiety disorders and their relationship to depression, in Handbook of Affective Disorders, 2nd Edition. Edited by Paykel ES. New York, Guilford, 1992, pp 77–87

15. Swebo SE, Rapoport JL, Leonard H, et al: Obsessive-compulsive disorder in children and adolescents. Arch Gen Psychiatry 46:335–341, 1989

16. Towbin KE, Riddle MA: Obsessive-compulsive disorder, in Child and Adolescent Psychiatry: A Comprehensive Textbook, 2nd Edition. Edited by Lewis M. Baltimore, MD, Williams & Wilkins, 1996, pp 684–693

17. Hollander E, Benzaquen SD: Is there a distinct OCD spectrum? International Journal of Neuropsychiatric Medicine 1:17–26, 1996

18. March JS, Leonard HL: Obsessive-compulsive disorder in children and adolescents: a review of the past 10 years. J Am Acad Child Adolesc Psychiatry 34:1265–1273, 1996

19. Harris JC: Developmental Neuropsychiatry; Assessment, Diagnosis, and Treatment of Developmental Disorders, Vol 2. Oxford, England, Oxford University Press, 1995

20. Volkmar FR: Childhood and adolescent psychosis: a review of the past 10 years. J Am Acad Child Adolesc Psychiatry 35:843–851, 1996

21. Volkmar F: Reactive attachment disorders of infancy or early childhood, in Comprehensive Textbook of Psychiatry/VI, 6th Edition, Vol 2. Edited by Kaplan HI, Sadock BJ. Baltimore, MD, Williams & Wilkins, 1995, pp 2354–2359

22. Cummings J: Neuropsychiatry: clinical assessment and approach to diagnosis, in Comprehensive Textbook of Psychiatry/VI, 6th Edition, Vol 1. Edited by Kaplan HI, Sadock BJ. Baltimore, MD, Williams & Wilkins, 1995, pp 167–187

23. Akiskal HS, Akiskal K: Mental status examination; the art and science of the clinical interview, in Diagnostic Interviewing, 2nd Edition. Edited by Hersen M, Turner SM. New York, Plenum, 1994, pp 25–51

5

EVALUATION OF EXTERNALIZING SYMPTOMS

■ EVALUATION OF HYPERACTIVE AND IMPULSIVE BEHAVIORS

Although distractibility was traditionally considered the core feature of attention-deficit/hyperactivity disorder (ADHD), more recently researchers have proposed that the central deficit in ADHD is a problem of behavioral inhibition that involves a delay in internalization of self-control and self-regulation. The behavior of children who have ADHD is regulated more by immediate circumstances (i.e., external sources) and less by executive functions and considerations of time and the future (1, pp. 313–314). "ADHD *is far more a deficit of behavioral inhibition than of attention* (1, p. 313).

DSM-IV distinguishes three types of ADHD: inattentive, hyperactive-impulsive, and combined. The inattentive type predominates in pediatric populations, whereas the hyperactive-impulsive and combined types are more prevalent in child psychiatric populations. The ADHD types are associated with different clinical, comorbid, and prognostic courses. Children with the combined type have the highest rates of comorbid disruptive, anxiety, and depressive disorders. In comparison with the combined type, children with the inattentive type have similar rates of comorbid anxiety and depressive disorders but lower rates of disruptive disorders. Children with the hyperactive-impulsive type have the highest rates of externalizing disorders but lower rates of associated anxiety and depression, in comparison with the other subtypes. Children with the combined or inattentive types have higher rates of academic problems than do children with the hyperactive-impulsive type (2, p. 186). In comparison to the other types, children with the combined type have higher lifetime rates of conduct, oppositional, bipolar, language, and tic disorders; they also have the highest rate of counseling and multimodal treatments. There were few differences between the hyperactive-impulsive and the inattentive types, although children with the inattentive type had a higher lifetime prevalence of major depressive disorder (2, p. 190).

In evaluating children who have the hyperactive-impulsive type of ADHD, the examiner should inquire about the onset of the hyperactivity and impulsivity. Commonly the examiner will trace the origin of these symptoms to early preschool age. Some mothers report hyperactivity during the child's gestational or early neonatal life. There are often complaints that these children were hyperactive, willful, obstinate, or disobedient from an early age, or that they got into everything without any forethought (e.g., they were frequently moving, never finishing anything they started). Many of these children have no sense of danger and require close supervision. A low tolerance for frustration and dysregulation of emotional states are common. Some of these children have difficult temperaments and demand inordinate amounts of attention; they lack self-soothing regulatory mechanisms and are prone to intense and prolonged temper tantrums. These tantrums easily escalate into dyscontrol, and when this happens it takes these children a long time to regain self-control. In severe cases, biorhythm dysregulation may be present, as evidenced by sleep difficulties.

Symptoms of ADHD are conspicuous in the classroom: these children are distractible and disruptive. They are off-task and unable to remain seated. Commonly they have problems completing assignments, and they have problems taking turns and sharing with peers. Some children are intrusive and have limited social skills, whereas others have poor problem-solving abilities. Some children with ADHD develop early comorbidity. Children with the hyperactive-impulsive or combined types have problems with anger control and with affective modulation; these deficits contribute further to their limited social success.

According to Cantwell, the diagnostic evaluation of ADHD involves the following components (3, p. 982):

1. A comprehensive interview with all parental figures. This interview should be complemented by a developmental, medical, and school history of the child and a social, medical, and mental health history of family members.
2. A developmentally appropriate interview with the child to assess his or her view of the signs and symptoms and to screen for comorbidity.
3. An appropriate medical evaluation to screen for health status and neurological problems.
4. Appropriate cognitive assessment of ability and achievement.
5. The use of both broad-spectrum and more narrowly focused (i.e., ADHD-specific) parent and teacher rating scales.
6. Appropriate adjunct assessments such as speech and language assessment and evaluation of fine and gross motor function.

Because children with the combined type of ADHD need frequent corrective feedback (because of their impulsivity), they evolve a negative self-view that contributes to the early development of dysphoric affect. Frequently children with ADHD develop a defective self-concept and a poor sense of competence. According to O'Brien, self-esteem difficulties are the core psychological problems for these children (4, p. 117). The examiner needs to explore these complications to determine the extent of additional psychopathology in order to formulate a comprehensive treatment program. The examiner should ask the child to explain the reasons for the psychiatric examination and should help the child to explain, in his or her own words, the nature and extent of the problems.

Examiners should ask the following questions: Does the child display problems with hyperactivity-impulsivity in certain circumstances, or is this problem present all the time? Does it happen in most of the child's daily activities? Is the child able to concentrate in the classroom? Is the child able to stay on task? Does the child finish assignments? Does the child show task organization (see

"Behavioral Organization" section in Chapter 3). Are there are activities that grip the child's attention (e.g., playing certain games or watching television)? What television programs does the child watch? How are the child's social and problem-solving skills? This information has significant clinical relevance.

■ EVALUATION OF CHILDREN WHO HAVE ATTENTION-DEFICIT/HYPERACTIVITY DISORDER

As soon as the interviewer detects that the child is too hyperactive or impulsive and lacks means of self-regulation, self-structure, or self-control, he or she should structure both the physical space and the activities in which the child is permitted to engage. Space boundaries and a control of the quality, quantity, and modality of stimulation are mandatory to maintain a safe and productive interview. Such control will help the child to focus and concentrate on structured tasks (e.g., involving building blocks, Legos, puzzles, or table games).

If the child is too easily distracted, the examiner should reduce the amount of stimulation by limiting the number of items available at any given time. Limiting and structuring the elements for specific tasks is important: a box full of crayons and an unlimited amount of paper are too distracting for an inattentive and disorganized child. Such a child should receive one crayon or one pencil and one piece of paper at a time. Similarly, the examiner should limit the number of blocks, Legos pieces, or other items that the child can use at any given time.

If the child is too fidgety or has difficulty remaining seated, the examiner should pull the child's chair close to the interviewing table so that the chair and table form a physical boundary. The examiner should instruct (and encourage) the child to concentrate on only one task at a time. The examiner should encourage and help the child to complete the assigned task before moving on to a new one. Throughout the interview, the examiner should note the child's response to structure and limit setting; these observations have important diagnostic and therapeutic implications. Ongoing support should be given when the child meets the examiner's expectations and when he or she abides by the provided structure. The examiner should help the child concentrate on the project at hand and should give support and reinforcement each time the child finishes a task. Transitions from one activity to the next should be handled with care, because these children have problems with moving on to new tasks.

The length of the interview is an important factor; brevity is the goal. After 15 or 20 minutes of active interviewing, the child needs a break (e.g., for a trip to the bathroom). In an intensely structured setting, the patient and the clinician tire easily.

The amount of structure needed in subsequent sessions will indicate how well the child is responding to ongoing behavioral and psychopharmacological interventions. Observations made during structured interviewing, and changes observed in ratings on specific checklists completed by the examiner, teachers, or parents, are helpful in ascertaining whether changes at school, at home, or in any other setting have been made in response to treatment.

Social skill difficulties are significant problems for some children with ADHD. Cantwell described this comorbidity as an inability to pick up social cues, which leads to interpersonal difficulties (3, p. 981).

In assessing these children, nonverbal learning disabilities need to be ruled out. Issues related to the differential diagnosis of ADHD are presented in Chapter 7.

■ EVALUATION OF AGGRESSIVE, HOMICIDAL, AND SELF-ABUSIVE BEHAVIORS

Otnow Lewis's advice to clinicians working with children who have conduct disorder is particularly applicable to those dealing with aggressive and violent behaviors: "Clinicians are obliged to attempt to overcome the negative feelings toward the child that may be aroused by the child's frightening and obnoxious behaviors. One must embark on the evaluation of a behaviorally disturbed child with curiosity and an open mind" (5, p. 571). Negative responses toward the patient (i.e., countertransference) may interfere with the clinician's ability to thoroughly and systematically assess the child (see Chapter 11).

If the clinician knows in advance that the child is likely to be aggressive or self-abusive, he or she should make preparations beforehand to meet the child's special needs. No matter how syntonic a child's aggression seems to be, it is helpful to assume that the child is anxious, if not afraid, of the possibility of losing control. If the clinician senses that the child has this anxiety, he or she should reassure the child that every effort will be made to help him or her stay under control and that help will be provided to help him or her regain control, if needed. The examiner may need to consider psychopharmacological interventions, hospitalization, or other options. The diagnostic interview should be stopped whenever the examiner becomes concerned with his or her personal safety. If this happens, the examiner should take the steps needed to prevent the patient from injuring anyone (see Chapter 1).

During the evaluation of a volatile, labile, or aggressive adolescent, the examiner should try not to provoke the patient any further. The examiner should also be attentive to signs that the patient is about to lose control. Regardless of the etiology of the aggressive behavior, all communications and interventions need to take into account that the patient is struggling to maintain self-control and that there is an ongoing disturbance in the child's sense of self—a narcissistic injury that needs to be identified, abreacted, understood, and repaired. Something has threatened the patient's self-esteem and self-concept to the point that he or she resorts to aggressive behavior to restore self-esteem (i.e., to repair the perceived injury). If the examiner knows the nature of the injury, he or she should offer empathic comments regarding the perceived injury, evaluate the patient's response to such comments, and explore alternatives to deal with the perceived injury. The examiner will be more successful if he or she assesses aggression in this broader context and prudently assumes that the patient may lose control at perceived provocations.

Depending on the individual case, the patient may appear defensive, suspicious, fearful, or ashamed. If the patient feels humiliated or has been humiliated, he or she may anticipate further humiliation or even retaliation for aggressive, hateful, and vengeful feelings. Some adolescents who are struggling with aggressive feelings may experience shame or guilt secondary to intense anger and the fear of losing control.

The examiner's emphasis in dealing with aggressive adolescents is to determine their propensity for violence and to establish whether such adolescents are at imminent risk of losing control. If the examiner determines that the patient is on the verge of losing control, he or she needs to be extra cautious in his or her approach and demeanor and should be particularly judicious with his or her words.

Regardless of the nature of the aggression, the examiner's priority is to help the patient regain a sense of self-control. Lion expressed this principle in the following manner: "The evaluator's goal [when meeting belligerent and violent patients], whenever possible, is to convert physical agitation and belligerence into verbal catharsis. This principle holds true irrespective of the etiology of the patient's violence" (6, p. 3).

Because a history of violence is the best predictor of future violence, the examiner should make a comprehensive inquiry into this area. The following questions may be pertinent: Has the child ever lost control? What has been the nature of the child's dyscontrol? Has the child ever hurt someone? Does the child intend to harm someone? Has the child developed a plan to kill someone? The examiner should remember his or her duty to protect potential victims.

Many adolescents exhibit a facade of bravado or a bullish attitude. The examiner should take these surface behaviors seriously. An attempt to challenge these defenses carries a serious risk and is not recommended; the child might act out to prove to the examiner that he or she can do what he or she says. By stressing the dangerousness of threatened behaviors and highlighting the potential risks of what the adolescent is contemplating or the repercussions of the intended behaviors, the examiner may help the adolescent to take another look at his or her intentions and may also help the adolescent to better understand his or her potential for acting out.

Being honest, direct, and compassionate are indispensable qualities in building trust with aggressive children. When adolescents have grown up in deceptive and manipulative environments, they expect that everyone else (the examiner included) will try to put something over on them or to "con" them. If being honest and direct are indispensable qualities, they are of particular importance when dealing with hostile and assaultive adolescents. Issues need to be discussed plainly and directly.

It has been emphasized that when the examiner meets the adolescent, the examiner should make explicit what is already known about the adolescent and should encourage the adolescent to present his or her side of the problem. Consider the following case example:

> Todd, a 13-year-old Caucasian adolescent, came reluctantly for a psychiatric evaluation. He said to the examiner, "I don't have to see you. I don't need any help." He was evaluated because of physically abusive behavior toward his mother. He had also threatened to kill her. Recently Todd had brought a loaded gun into his house and had threatened to use it against his mother. Todd had beaten his mother many times before. He was unruly and at home did pretty much what he wanted. He was the only male in the household.
>
> The interview focused on Todd's homicidal intentions toward his mother:

> *Interviewer*: I understand you want to kill your mother.
> *Todd*: I don't like that bitch.
> *Interviewer*: You have threatened to kill her.
> *Todd*: She gets on my nerves. I hate her.
> *Interviewer*: You took a loaded gun and threatened to kill her.
> *Todd*: I was joking.
> *Interviewer*: You seem to be capable of killing her.

Todd: I just wanted to see what she was going to do.

Interviewer: Sounds like you are looking for reasons to kill her.

Todd: She makes me so mad!

Interviewer: You are looking for excuses to do it.

Todd began to seem anxious and smiled nervously. He said that he didn't want to live at home anymore. The examiner said, "There is a part of you that does not want to lose control."

At this point, Todd let his guard down, and his bullish facade faded. He acknowledged that he had problems controlling himself and was receptive to the examiner's recommendations. The interview proceeded in a more comfortable tone, and Todd's interest and participation in the diagnostic assessment improved.

Although psychiatric examiners pay attention to issues of aggressive behavior (e.g., physical and sexual abuse) perpetrated against children, they are less attentive to the aggressive and other abusive behaviors that children perpetrate against their parents and siblings. These aggressive behaviors need to be explored on a regular basis. Other behaviors that tend to be ignored are aggressive behaviors between boyfriends and girlfriends; violent interactions within these relationships are becoming more frequent.

The following case example illustrates an interview with a primitive, aggressive, and self-abusive female adolescent:

Sally, a 17-year-old Caucasian adolescent, had been admitted to the state hospital many times for severe episodes of explosive and assaultive outbursts accompanied by self-abusive behaviors. She had severe impairments in interpersonal relationships: she was markedly withdrawn and stayed away from people most of the time. Although endowed with normal intelligence, she had major problems in school because of her pervasive dysphoria and temper outbursts. As she grew older, her attendance at school became a regular problem because she had difficulties waking up in the mornings. She had an "awful" mood in the mornings, but her mood and attitude improved somewhat by noon every day. Her school schedule had been adjusted accordingly.

Sally's self-abusive behavior consisted of savage self-biting and self-cutting of the forearms and self-inflicted injuries to the hands and knuckles that resulted from hitting walls. She had been assaultive to many members of the hospital staff and to peers: she had been put in restraints and had received additional medications as needed on numerous occasions. Many psychopharmacological treatments had been tried unsuccessfully. Haloperidol was the only medication that seemed to be effective consistently.

The psychiatric consultant was asked to ascertain whether Sally exhibited evidence of an affective disorder. About a dozen clinical staff members attended this consultation. Upon arriving at the consultation, Sally refused to sit in the designated chair. She was a heavyset adolescent with ambiguous secondary sexual characteristics: her haircut, facial appearance, and demeanor lacked any femininity. Shortly after sitting down, she stood up and said, "Fuck you" to the group, began to suck her right thumb, and exited promptly from the room, grumbling on her way out. The consultant felt that the large audience had overwhelmed her and that a more private evaluation was needed.

The consultant found Sally sitting with a nurse in the hospital lobby area. She was sucking her thumb and rubbing her eyebrows, rituals she did regularly when she felt anxious or overwhelmed. The consultant attempted to engage her in a verbal exchange while allowing her to keep her distance (the consultant sat at least 15 feet away from her). Sally acknowledged that too many people made her nervous. The interaction continued at a distance, with Sally and the consultant speaking loudly to each other.

The consultant, sensing that Sally was not amenable to a variety of topics, chose to test the waters by bringing up the topic of discharge. Initially Sally said that she was never going to leave, but when the nurse said that she thought Sally had been working on this goal, Sally agreed to discuss what she needed to do to leave the hospital.

The consultant asked Sally if he could sit closer to her. She said it was fine with her. He sat one chair away from her and continued the psychiatric interview. She wanted to go home, although her family was not looking forward to her return. The consultant asked Sally what was expected of her before she could go home. She spoke about the need to control her anger and to be less self-abusive. He then asked what kind of progress she had made in those areas. She lifted the left sleeve of her shirt, showing him thick resolving scabs from recently inflicted self-injuries. Sally indicated that she was now less self-abusive than before. She also said that she was trying to control herself better and was doing so by staying away from people.

The consultant asked Sally if she could talk about her mood in the mornings. She nodded and said that she had a very bad mood in the mornings; she felt very angry and feared losing control and hurting someone at those times. To control these feelings, she would try to sleep until noon because by midday she felt in better control of herself. She denied feeling suicidal and said that she did not want to hurt anyone but acknowledged that she felt very nervous around people.

The consultant had observed by this time that any topic that raised Sally's level of anxiety would simultaneously elicit the self-regulatory behaviors of thumb sucking and eyebrow rubbing. The consultant asked Sally who her best friend was, and she said it was her 4-year-old cousin, who liked her and played with her. Her second best friend was her father. The consultant had learned that Sally's mother, who had abused drugs, abandoned Sally in early infancy. He did not ask her to discuss anything related to her mother.

Sally refused to say whether there were any other important persons in her life. When the consultant approached the issue of medications, she said that they did not help. When she was reminded about the haloperidol, she acknowledged reluctantly that it had helped. She denied experiencing any hallucinations. She even denied feeling paranoid. When asked what sort of activities she enjoyed, she said that she liked to take care of plants.

By this time she was smiling occasionally and even became playful by making fun of the consultant. After asking Sally about the presence of paranoid feelings, the consultant asked her if she had any unusual experiences. She said she had "EPS." The consultant thought she had said "ESP" and continued without catching his mistake. When the consultant realized that Sally had said EPS, Sally began to laugh. She said that she had fooled him. Both Sally and the consultant laughed. Sally then said that sometimes she knows what the other person is going to say. The consultant replied that ESP is important in dealing with people. As the interview proceeded, Sally agreed that she had a big problem with her mood and agreed to try some medications that might help her with this problem.

The consultant closed his contact with Sally on positive terms. When he was leaving the hospital building, he could see Sally at a distance. She waved at him, and he waved and smiled back at her.

This interview was carried out in unusual circumstances; Sally was a very uncooperative and volatile patient. Because of her unpredictability, the consultant made a special effort not to aggravate her more, and he took great care in forming and maintaining an alliance with her. The consultant was deliberate in the selection of areas or issues that he felt were appropriate and safe to discuss. Despite these difficulties, there was a genuine engagement, and the evaluation was helpful and productive. The information and observations gathered during the interview helped the consultant to conclude that Sally exhibited evidence of a mood disorder and an anxiety disorder.

The examiner should strive to determine the history and epigenesis of aggressive behaviors. Aggressive children frequently have a history of problematic temperament, persistent oppositional behaviors, impulsiveness or conduct problems, poor social cognitions, coercive discipline (i.e., involving physical punishment), and peer relationship problems. Self-abusive behavior is a common symptom in impulsive-aggressive children.

Loeber and Hay propose an epigenesis of aggressive behavior that starts with the infant's difficult temperament and an unsuitable caregiver (poor infant-caregiver matching) (7). This is followed by the persistence of oppositional behaviors, which produces a developmental arrest in the socialization process in a variety of ways. The parental figure then gives up, out of frustration over the child's lack of response. The parent begins to pay attention exclusively to the child's negative behavior and becomes unresponsive or stops giving positive feedback. This alters the child's social cognitions. The child begins to perceive bad intentions from others and to display aggression as a means to solve problems because he or she lacks adaptive problem-solving skills. This pattern of response creates rejection from the group. At this point, association with deviant peer groups is an expected step.

When assessing the presence of aggressive or assaultive behavior, the examiner should obtain the patient's passive and active histories of violence. The passive history relates to victimization (e.g., the patient's history of physical or sexual abuse); the active history refers to violence perpetrated against others, including physical or sexual violence (e.g., physical assault, rape).

The examiner should strive to link the aggressive behavior to specific psychiatric syndromes and other comorbid conditions (e.g., ADHD, conduct disorder, bipolar disorder, psychotic disorders, substance abuse disorders) that may contribute to aggressive dyscontrol. Aggressive children demonstrate serious deficits in problem-solving skills and peer relationships. These deficits should be addressed in a comprehensive treatment plan that focuses on aggressive behaviors and related problems.

Otnow Lewis describes evidence, in violent youth offenders, of psychosis (e.g., paranoid delusions), affective disorders, neuropsychological dysfunction (e.g., language and cognitive deficits), brain injury (e.g., psychomotor seizures associated with epilepsy), hyperactivity, impulsivity, and other signs of brain dysfunction (i.e., organicity) (8, pp. 564–565). The dyscontrol is an end-pathway deficit that results from brain injury related to a variety of causes. These violent persons have a history of head trauma as a consequence of physical abuse. Evaluation of the presence of brain injury and dysfunction in violent adolescents must be pursued systematically. Otnow Lewis has added dissociative disorders to a number of comorbid conditions the examiner should scrutinize methodically in children with behavioral dyscontrol (8, p. 567).

Biederman et al. have addressed the role of bipolar disorders as a cause of aggression and behavioral dyscontrol: "Since juvenile mania has high levels of irritability that can be associated with violence and antisocial behavior . . . this overlap between BPD [bipolar disorder] and conduct disorder is not surprising. . . . If this overlap continues to be confirmed, these findings may provide some new leads as to the possibility of subtypes of mood-based antisocial disorders not previously recognized" (10, p. 1006).

Children with so-called borderline disorder psychopathology display a broad spectrum of functional impairments, including overwhelming rage and violent fantasies (with extreme anxiety and loss of control); rapid regression in thinking and reality testing; affective control difficulties; extreme vulnerability to stress with psychotic decompensation; chronic regressive states; severe separation anxiety; generalized restricted development (in relationships, affect, cognition, and language); and schizoid retreat into preoccupations with fantasy life and withdrawal from relationships (11, p. 33).

■ EVALUATION OF BIPOLAR SYMPTOMS

The diagnosis of bipolar disorder in preadolescence is a major clinical challenge for child psychiatrists because the classical picture of this disorder is uncommon in patients of this age. The clinical features of bipolar disorder in childhood and adolescence are not similar to those described in adult patients. Bipolar disorder in its classical manifestations becomes more common as the child advances through adolescence. During adolescence, the clinical picture becomes more similar to that described in adults.

The controversy surrounding the diagnosis of mania in preadolescence is similar to the controversy surrounding the diagnosis of depression before it was recognized officially in the mid-1970s. Many clinicians do not accept that early latency age children or preschoolers might exhibit such a severe symptom complex. Klein et al. endorse Carlson's view that symptoms of mania represent a nonspecific index of severity rather than a specific indication of bipolar disorder. These authors believe that evidence for the validity of childhood mania is lacking (12, p. 1095). Hechtman explains that the overuse of the bipolar diagnosis in children is due to 1) modifications to DSM-IV diagnostic criteria (irritability for mania, chronic instead of episodic course) and 2) the overlap of diagnostic criteria between ADHD and bipolar disorder (13). Five of seven symptoms for the diagnosis of mania are shared with ADHD. Hechtman asserts that the bipolar diagnosis should not be made lightly and that it should require strong, sound evidence. She comments that there are no large epidemiological studies supporting the overinclusiveness of bipolar diagnosis. Pliszka supports the need for longitudinal studies and favors strict criteria for bipolar diagnosis (14). He points out diagnostic ambiguities between intermittent explosive disorder and bipolar disorder. Hechtman and Pliszka warn that psychopharmacological response should not be considered confirmatory of bipolar disorder. The controversy regarding the early presentation of bipolar disorder is not new. Kraepelin found that 0.4% of his patients had displayed manic features before age 10 years (15, p. 187). Skeptical clinicians believe that early bipolar disorder in children is nothing more than severe ADHD.

The critical factor in the differential diagnosis of early-onset bipolar disorder is not the ADHD symptomatology, because manic children and children with ADHD overlap significantly in this area. The difference is in the mood presentation and, more important, in the history of mood dysregulation. Unfortunately, many children exhibit both problems.

Findings by Geller and Luby seem to substantiate the existence of prepubertal mania (16). Their studies included a group of children with bipolar disorder who had a mean age of 11.0 ± 2.7 years at study entry and a mean age at onset of 8.1 ± 3.5 years. Manic symptoms that were significantly more frequent among children with bipolar disorder, in comparison with children with ADHD, included elated mood, grandiosity, decreased need for sleep, racing thoughts, and hypersexuality. Grandiose delusions occurred in 55% of the children with bipolar disorder, and cycles classified as rapid or ultrarapid (multiple episodes lasting a few days to a few weeks) or ultradian (multiple shifts daily) occurred in 83.3% of the children with bipolar disorder.

We believe that childhood mania does exist, that this clinical entity is uncommon, and that the diagnosis of bipolar disorder in preadolescence is overused.

The following case example involves a preadolescent child whose manic condition had not been identified:

> Tony, a 5-year-old Caucasian boy, had been admitted to an acute inpatient setting for evaluation of severe aggressive behaviors at home and at school. He also displayed overt and inappropriate sexual behavior, including attempts to have sex with a dog. Tony had a history of mood fluctuations, unpredictable temper, clear depressive trends, and even suicidal behaviors. He had been neglected and had been sexually abused by his 16-year-old brother. At the time of admission to the acute program, Tony had been living with his maternal great-grandmother, who allegedly infantilized him. Tony's natural parents were psychiatrically ill: his mother had a diagnosis of bipolar disorder, and his father had alcoholism. There was a family feud regarding Tony's most suitable rearing environment because other relatives felt that his great-grandmother was senile and mentally unstable.
>
> The therapist who sought the psychiatric evaluation had told the psychiatrist with amusement that Tony had the whole unit in stitches: he went around the unit cracking jokes and making everybody laugh. Tony's undeniable manic episode had not been recognized. He displayed euphoric mood and pressured speech and was driven and overly friendly, and his history of hypersexuality and family background of bipolar illness had been overlooked.
>
> *Postscript.* Tony is now a 15-year-old adolescent. He has displayed intermittent manic and psychotic behaviors over the years. From time to time he becomes paranoid and aggressive in response to delusional perceptions. Tony's comorbid anxiety and

somatoform symptoms are incapacitating. He lives with his maternal grandfather and is enrolled in special education. His great-grandmother has been in a nursing home for several years. Tony has continued to receive psychiatric treatment since the initial contact.

Bowring and Kovacs proposed four factors that make early identification of bipolar disorders difficult (17):

1. The low incidence of the disorder in clinical populations and the resulting low rate of exposure for clinicians. (However, bipolar disorder may be more common than was previously thought.)
2. Cross-sectional and longitudinal variability of symptoms. The symptoms of mania are probably intrinsically labile, and there are likely to be gradients of severity within a given episode. Labile, unstable, and changeable mood is unusual in children younger than age 10 years; in childhood, irritability and belligerence are more common than is euphoria.
3. The overlap between symptoms of mania and other disorders (e.g., ADHD, conduct disorders, and substance abuse). This overlap is a source of diagnostic confusion. Clinicians commonly dichotomize the diagnosis: the child has either bipolar disorder or ADHD, bipolar disorder or conduct disorder, bipolar disorder or substance abuse. These patients may have all of these disorders concomitantly.
4. The connection between developmental stage and symptom expression. Symptoms of a manic episode may be difficult to distinguish from developmentally appropriate behaviors. For example, symptoms such as grandiosity and inflated self-esteem need to be considered from a developmental perspective.

According to Bowring and Kovacs, "Particular attention must be paid to the age at which symptoms emerge, the vicissitudes of the symptoms, the temporal relationship between them, and the evolution of the syndrome. Historical information should be obtained from adult informants who are able to describe the young patient's behavior, mood, and functioning over time" (17, p. 614).

Wozniak et al. expressed the developmental aspects of bipolar disorder clearly and succinctly: "We found these children to have a developmentally different presentation from adults with BPD [bipolar disorder] such that the majority of these children presented with irritable rather than euphoric mood disturbance, a chronic rather than an episodic course, and a mixed presentation with simultaneous symptoms of depression and mania" (18, p. 1577). In other words, "it is developmentally possible for childhood-onset manic-depressive illness to be more severe; to have a chronic nonepisodic course; and to have mixed, rapid-cycling features similar to the clinical picture reported for severely ill, treatment resistant adults (19, pp. 1168–1169).

Hypomanic features are sometimes disregarded because they are mistaken for normative childhood behaviors. For example, silliness and clownlike behavior are often mistakenly considered as normal behaviors of childhood. Parents of hypomanic children often report that their children are unusually happy, are very silly, laugh without any apparent reason, or show an unusual degree of expansiveness, often out of character with their more subdued, if not depressed, demeanor. More often, though, a protracted course of irritable mood and prolonged dysphoria is the rule. The moods of these children shift unpredictably, and the children's negative moods are prolonged and intense despite efforts by sensitive caregivers to soothe them. Prolonged temper tantrums and bouts of violent, destructive, and uncontrollable behaviors are the norm rather than the exception in early-onset bipolar disorder. Parents report mood fluctuations even during the same day, and these mood changes often seem unmotivated. The clinician should suspect early-onset bipolar disorder when the following complaints are present: recurrent dejected states, prominent irritability, and proneness to angry outbursts in response to even minor provocations.

The examiner should assess bipolar symptoms in terms of the

child's developmental state. For example, a preadolescent with bipolar disorder explained his high energy level by saying that he felt like "I have 100 jet engines in my body." In Joe's case example (see later in this chapter), the adolescent exercised excessively for long periods of time without experiencing exhaustion.

Grandiosity may have age-related manifestations. Bipolar children frequently believe they are superheroes (e.g., Superman, Batman, Spiderman, Wonder Woman). These children believe they can perform incredible feats such as "defending the world from alien invaders" because they believe they have special strength or special abilities. Some bipolar children believe they can fly, have attempted to do so, and have been injured when they jumped from high places.

Most frequently bipolar children display or verbalize aggressive themes, for example, "I can beat anybody." One 7-year-old child felt so strong and invincible that he said, "I can beat even God." Another 7-year-old child expressed her grandiosity by boasting, "I have two thousand boyfriends." Yet another 7-year-old child claimed that he was a millionaire and kept making plans for all the money he expected to receive from his disability. Adolescents may be involved in schemes "to get rich fast" that are similar to the economic misjudgments made by manic and hypomanic adults. For example, a 16-year-old adolescent stole a number of checks from his grandfather and forged his signature with the idea of buying some stereo equipment at a cheap price. He was convinced that he could resell the equipment at a big profit.

Patients sometimes exhibit entrenched traits of arrogance and condescension (see Habib's case example later in this chapter). These individuals believe they know more than do their parents, teachers, or psychiatrists. Because of their boastfulness and their persistent devaluation of others, they frequently clash with peers (because they feel put down) and with authority figures (because they believe they know better than the authority figures). It is not surprising that these children lack friends and get into frequent conflict with authority figures, including the law. Parents and other significant figures in these children's lives are often impressed by the children's display of knowledge or by their use of sophisticated language. Parents may believe that these children have superior intellectual abilities and become incredulous only when faced with the reality of their children's abilities.

The expression of hypersexuality also needs to be assessed in reference to developmental norms. Several of the case examples in this chapter (see Tony, Kathy, and Joe) illustrate inappropriate sexual behavior or hypersexuality. Compulsive masturbation, promiscuity, and other forms of sexual preoccupation must be explored, and the examiner should exclude sexual abuse as the cause of these abnormal behaviors.

Because a mixed clinical picture seems to be the norm, the examiner must inquire about depressive feelings when the child exhibits hypomanic traits, and vice versa.

Consider the following case examples:

Kathy, an 11-year-old Caucasian girl, had been followed up for a bipolar disorder that had started about 1 year earlier. She appeared floridly manic. She was markedly euphoric (e.g., she laughed boisterously on an ongoing basis), was driven and restless (e.g., she was unable to sit still for a prolonged period of time), and was in need of continual redirection. She also had trouble sleeping at night. Kathy was sexually preoccupied, and the obsessional quality of her sexual thoughts was quite disturbing. At school she had boasted in front of the class that she was Lorena Bobbit. She took a razorblade to school and announced, "I am going to cut the penises from all the boys." This created a great amount of consternation among her classmates, and as a result, she experienced further rejection by her peers. Kathy also displayed conspicuous regressive behavior. When with her mother, Kathy would touch her repeatedly and often told her mother, in an endearing but childish manner, "You are so pretty" or "You are so beautiful!" Occasionally she would put her head on her mother's lap. When Kathy interacted with her mother, she would talk in a childish and regressive manner.

Kathy also exhibited significant depressive symptoms: she complained that she felt depressed; cried frequently; and was unhappy about her looks (she was overweight), her lack of friends, and her feeling that her peers had rejected her. Frequently she became withdrawn and said that she wanted to die.

Kathy's clinical presentation is not very different from Joe's:

Joe was a 14-year-old Hispanic adolescent, who 2 years earlier had been diagnosed with bipolar disorder with mixed features. He had been hospitalized multiple times in acute psychiatric units for suicidal, homicidal, and psychotic behaviors. At the time of the last hospitalization, Joe complained of being very depressed. He said that he wanted to kill himself and had heard commanding hallucinations ordering him to do so. He had problems concentrating and had no motivation to do his homework. He felt very guilty, ashamed, and remorseful about the sexual feelings he had experienced toward his 37-year-old aunt. These feelings had a compulsive quality. In the past Joe had complained about feeling like having sex with his dog, and he was also disturbed by this feeling. Joe reported feeling like Superman. He experienced a great deal of energy: on one occasion, he lifted weights for an entire day because he didn't experience any feeling of tiredness.

The following case example provides a dramatic illustration of mixed manic and depressive features:

Habib, a 12-year-old mixed-raced boy (his mother was Caucasian and his father Arabic), was admitted to an acute care psychiatric unit after he attempted to hang himself. He had tied his belt to a high bar in the bathroom, had put the belt around his neck, and was about to jump when he was found. This incident occurred at a psychiatric residential treatment facility.

Habib had been admitted to the residential program 2 months earlier, after his mother believed she could no longer handle his aggressive, explosive, oppositional, and defiant behaviors. He had been hospitalized 9 months before that for suicidal and homicidal behaviors. Before the residential placement, Habib had felt progressively depressed and hopeless, and he had trouble sleeping. He dreamed that his father was dying. In reality, his stepfather, who had been like a real father to him, was dying of terminal lung cancer. Since his first admission, Habib had been followed in outpatient therapy and had been tried on a number of psychotropic medications without significant benefits.

Habib was a very bright child and was an excellent student. He had very few friends because of his domineering, condescending demeanor and his low tolerance for frustration. He had particular problems with his 11-year-old sister, who apparently was afraid of him.

Habib's stepfather died 5 weeks before the most recent suicidal crisis. This was a major loss for Habib and his family. His mother was overwhelmed with her husband's death. Habib had been progressing satisfactorily in the residential program, and a discharge date had been set for him to return home, but his mother dreaded his return. Habib's mother, feeling incapable of handling him, told Habib over the phone that she was planning to put him in a shelter while he waited for a group home placement. It was at this point that Habib planned to commit suicide. He wrote the following suicide note:

To whom it may concern,

I have been torn to shreds emotionally, mentally, and spiritually. All the strings in my life have been cut. My mother, my own flesh and blood, has cut the last one today. Now I have no reason to live. There were many things I wanted to do that I will be able to do in heaven. I wanted to write the best book of all time. I wanted to play in the NFL and NBA. I wanted to be a star in the movies and a singer. I wanted to go to Harvard and Harvard Law to become a litigator. I wanted to be rich and not have to worry about money. I wanted to skydive and bungee jump and go river rafting. I wanted to improve the world with my inventions. I wanted to fly a fighter jet in combat for the marines.

I wanted to travel the world and beyond. But more than anything else I wanted a family, parents, children, and grandchildren. I wanted love. I refuse to live in this chaotic world. FUCK YOU, MAMA!

I love you Casey, Ebony, Meggy, Sleepy, Spike, Sugar, Fay, Thena, Precious, La'Britt, Goodwin, Matthew F., Troy, Ricky P., Brandon L., Scooter, Troy, and every one from the Center [Habib listed all of the residential placement staff members].

Sincerely,

Habib

P.S. I also wanted to be a big-time artist, design shoes, and create games.

The reader of this letter will recognize Habib's pressured speech, his marked verbosity, his depression, his sense of hopelessness, and his boundless grandiosity. When Habib mentioned his inventions at the residential program, and the therapist expressed curiosity about them, Habib asked the therapist to sign a letter in which the therapist would promise not to infringe on his patent inventions.

Constitutional and developmental affective dysregulation are implicated in early-onset bipolar disorder. According to Akiskal,

From a very young age, children of bipolar parents evidence difficulty modulating hostile impulses, extreme emotional responses to relatively minor provocations such that the responses greatly outlast the provocation, and heightened awareness of and distress for the suffering of parents and others. . . . by late childhood, they have significantly higher rates of comorbid depressive, anxious, and disruptive behavioral problems. . . . Such comorbidity might be interpreted as an indication of emerging dysregulation along irritable-cyclothymic temperamental lines. . . . these findings testify to the affective and behavioral liabilities, as well as the personal qualities of an emerging bipolar temperament." (20, p. 758)

To this, not surprisingly, the author adds: "Encounters [of children with a bipolar profile] with peers and adults, especially parents sharing the same temperamental dispositions, are bound to be intense, tempestuous and some times destructive" (20, p. 758). Akiskal concludes,

> The profile of the child at risk for bipolar illness emerging from the . . . literature review suggests that whatever emotion—negative or positive—these children experience, they seem to experience it intensely and passionately. Their behavior is likewise dysregulated and disinhibited, which leads to an excessive degree of people-seeking behavior with potential disruptive consequences. (20, p. 758)

The difficulties of ascertaining the diagnosis of bipolar disorder, as expressed by Carlson in 1990, are still valid today:

> While the distinctions between normality, hypomania and mania reflect differences of degree of disorder, differences between mania, psychotic mania, schizo-affective mania and schizophrenia raise questions of different disorders. Moreover, there is still no unequivocal way to make distinctions. Such time-honored criteria as degree of thought disorder, or presence of Schneiderian first rank symptoms and mood incongruent with psychotic symptoms, at least during the manic episode, have not been reliable in distinguishing a manic course from a schizophrenic course. (21, p. 332)

Carlson's point is also emphasized by Goodwin and Jamison: "Perhaps the major error in the differential diagnosis of manic-depressive illness in adolescents results from the over diagnosis of schizophrenia" (15, p. 190).

Examiners should exercise caution when diagnosing first psychotic breaks during adolescence because many presentations appear to be schizophreniform in nature. The clinical picture changes into a bipolar presentation as the clinical course unfolds.

Bipolar disorder diagnosis is also missed in children who abuse alcohol and other substances. Alcohol abuse in preadolescents is closely associated with affective disorders. Goodwin and Jamison quote Famularo, who asserted that "seven of their ten cases of preadolescent alcohol abuse or dependence were bipolar or cyclothymic, and the remaining three had closely related disorders (major depression with conduct disorder, atypical psychosis, and atypical affective disorder)" (15, p. 190).

Table 5–1 lists the constellation of history, signs, and symptoms that raise the index of suspicion of a bipolar diagnosis.

■ EVALUATION OF OPPOSITIONAL BEHAVIORS

Oppositional children pose the greatest challenge for the examining psychiatrist. The challenge is not so much in formulating a diagnosis but in establishing a diagnostic and treatment alliance. Oppositional children most often arrive at the psychiatric evaluation already disgruntled, refusing to speak, and with a defiant, uncooperative attitude. The examiner will know that the interview will be a trying affair if the child avoids eye contact and exhibits a downcast demeanor and a tense, if not angry, countenance.

Because oppositional children are hypersensitive to authority figures and are prone to active oppositional or defiant behaviors at the slightest perception of provocation, the examiner needs to avoid stimulating the child's oppositional and provocative defenses. Simply, the examiner needs to avoid falling into the provocative trap enacted by the patient. Refusal to talk or defiant mutism could stimulate angry counterresponses in the examiner; this is in part because the child wants to enact a power struggle and wants to be the victor. The examiner should be aware that the oppositional behavior may be related to a dysphoric state, an affective disorder, or other psychiatric or neuropsychiatric conditions.

The examiner should attempt to soften the child's provocative facade by relating to the patient in a straightforward but caring and concerned manner. The child becomes a victor if the examiner falls into the child's trap or if the examiner gives up the interviewing effort out of frustration over the child's lack of cooperation. Facing

---

TABLE 5–1. **History, signs, and symptoms associated with bipolar disorder**

Comorbidity. ADHD, conduct disorder, substance abuse disorder, borderline personality disorder, and anxiety disorders are common.

Evidence of elation during the AMSIT. The euphoria is usually infectious. Mixed mood, including depressive and hypomanic (or manic) trends, may be present.

Evidence of grandiosity. Some children feel that they have special powers; they want to perform the feats of superheroes (e.g., Superman, Batman). Some have made attempts to fly. Other children are hard to teach because they "know it all." Many are condescending toward peers. Frequently, these children have no friends because they have alienated peers with their devaluating and condescending attitude. Thus, delusions of grandeur, primary identification with superheroes, and paranoid symptomatology may be prominent.

Judgment impairment. Hypomanic and manic states always involve impaired judgment. Hypersexuality, perverse sexual activity, participation in ill-conceived financial schemes, frequent "joyriding," and other impulsive actions are commonly reported.

Mood dysregulation. Commonly, these children have a background of chronic mood disorder with mostly depressive symptomatology. Moodiness and, particularly, irritability are commonly present. These children have histories of intense and prolonged temper tantrums and difficulties with anger control. Frequently they have been violent, assaultive, suicidal, or self-abusive. Severe preadolescent depression with psychomotor retardation may be a forerunner of bipolar disorder.

Positive family history. A family history of mood disorders—in particular, bipolar disorder (more so when a three-generation history of the disorder is present)—makes the diagnosis probable.

Presence of homicidal or suicidal behavior.

Pressured speech and rushing thoughts.

Psychomotor activation. These children are hyperactive if not driven and are restless and very impulsive. They may be distractible (many patients have been diagnosed with ADHD or may have comorbid ADHD). Other related symptoms are the lack of a need for sleep (i.e., insomnia) and a high level of energy.

(continued)

TABLE 5–1. **History, signs, and symptoms associated with bipolar disorder** *(continued)*

Psychotic symptomatology. Psychotic features are common. Auditory hallucinations, often of a commanding nature, are present. Depressive delusional manifestations have been considered to be predictive of a bipolar diathesis. Psychotic depressions are common: the earlier the presentation of depression the greater the likelihood of psychotic symptomatology.

an overtly uncooperative and defiant child, the examiner may feel great temptation to plead for cooperation, to give advice, or to become patronizing. These strategies must be avoided at all times. The following case example illustrates some of these issues:

Raul, a 12-year-old Hispanic boy, was evaluated for progressively aggressive behavior at home and at school. He had been involved in fights at school and had been suspended a number of times. He had been suspended recently for physically assaulting a third grader. After assaulting the boy, he threatened to kill anyone who reported the incident. At home, Raul got into frequent fights with his younger brother and argued with, talked back to, disobeyed, and provoked his mother on a regular basis. The night before the evaluation, Raul threatened to run away and also threatened to kill himself. A short time before the evaluation, Raul's 8-year-old sister had been removed from the home after it was found that their 14-year-old brother had sexually abused her.

During the preceding 6 months, Raul's mother had noticed that he was becoming progressively more irritable. She also reported that he had daily angry outbursts toward her and his siblings. Raul had been in a psychiatric hospital for treatment of a major depressive episode with psychotic features 4 years earlier. He had been followed up in outpatient therapy on a weekly basis. At the time of the current evaluation, Raul was taking antidepressants.

Since Raul was 8 years old, his father had been in prison for dealing drugs. Raul was in the sixth grade in a special education program, but because of the recent episode of dyscontrol, he was supposed to attend an alternative school. He had no significant medical or surgical history. According to Raul's mother, he had reached his developmental milestones in a timely manner. Raul's mother was afraid that her son had used drugs, and she suspected him of associating with gangs.

Raul was in a dysphoric mood when he entered the interview room. He wore casual clothes, and his hair was shaved on both sides of his head. He gave the examiner a defiant look. The interview proceeded as follows:

Interviewer: Why were you brought for this evaluation?
Raul (responding in an irritated manner): Go and ask my mother.
Interviewer: Do you know why you were brought to see a psychiatrist?
(Raul shrugged his shoulders and didn't say anything.)
Interviewer: What problems do you have at home?
(Raul shook his head, made a gesture of displeasure, and shrugged his shoulders again.)
Interviewer: What problems do you have at school?
Raul: Fighting.
Interviewer: Have you ever been suspended?
Raul: Two times.
Interviewer: I wonder if you have been expelled.
Raul: No.
Interviewer: What kind of fights were those?
Raul (shouting defiantly): That is something private. That stupid teacher.
Interviewer: Have you ever been in a gang?
Raul: That's personal.

Because Raul had begun to answer some questions, the examiner repeated some of the earlier questions.

Interviewer: What problems do you have at home?
Raul: Fighting with my brother and arguing with my mother.
Interviewer: Who lives at home?

Raul: My mother and two brothers.

Interviewer: Do you have a father?

Raul: He is in prison. (Raul looked down at his lap.)

Interviewer: Why is he in prison?

Raul: That's personal. (Raul gave the examiner a defiant look.)

Interviewer: Have you ever gone to see him?

Raul: No. (Raul became less confrontational.)

Interviewer: Does he ever write to you? Do you ever write back?

Raul (with sadness): I can't read. (Raul's face appeared downcast, and he rested his head on the table.)

Interviewer: You are sad.

(Raul nodded but didn't say anything. His head was resting on the table at this time.)

Interviewer: Do you ever cry?

(Raul nodded again.)

By this time, Raul's demeanor had softened, and he was more amenable to an extended interview. By the end of the psychiatric examination, Raul was more animated and appeared less defiant. The interview was difficult and filled with tension, but as the engagement increased, the tension and pressure decreased. By the end of the interview, the examiner had empathic and positive feelings toward Raul. The examiner persisted in the goal of completing the psychiatric examination in spite of Raul's persistent defiance and obstructionism. The examiner was firm but related to Raul in a caring manner and avoided responding to his provocations.

Table 5–2 offers some suggestions on how to deal with and respond to a child's oppositional behaviors.

Oppositional behavior coexists with a variety of comorbid conditions such as depressive and psychotic disorders and ADHD. Oppositional behaviors are prominent in children with conduct disorders. Severe oppositional behavior is common in children with language disorders (receptive disorders in particular), cognitive deficits, limited problem-solving skills, and other neuro-

---

TABLE 5–2. **Productive and counterproductive approaches in dealing with oppositional children**

Productive approaches

Use these helpful interventions

Approach the child in a matter-of-fact manner

Display warmth and benevolence

Exercise self-control and become aware of your tone of voice

Use a positive and assertive tone of voice

Model problem-solving

Focus on the problem at hand, not on the child

Foster the child's cooperation

Engage the child in the solution of the problem

Praise the child's steps toward resolving the problem

Try playfulness and humor

Do not miss any opportunity to praise or reward the child's prosocial behavior

Be empathic toward the child's plight

Pinpoint your awareness that the child is hurting

Attempt to identify with the child's problems

Help the child to verbalize sources of distress

Assist the child in regaining control

Give the child opportunities to save face

Use sensitive redirection

Keep behavioral expectations

Emphasize the child's strengths and positive expectations

Make child aware of behavioral consequences

Exercise consistent limit setting

Focus on the here and now

Reverse roles (help the child to verbalize the experience)

Counterproductive approaches

Use overt confrontation

Engage in power struggles

Take a threatening or intimidating stance

Ignore the child

(continued)

TABLE 5–2. **Productive and counterproductive approaches in dealing with oppositional children** *(continued)*

Counterproductive approaches *(continued)*

Dramatize or patronize

Personalize the problem

Remind the child of previous mistakes

Humiliate the child

Be concise and to the point when you address the child

Do not give up. Do not give in!

psychological deficits and in children with narcissistic features. Many oppositional children have a history of abuse, significant parental inconsistency, and exposure to parental discord or family violence.

■ REFERENCES

1. Barkley RA: ADHD and the Nature of Self-Control. New York, Guilford, 1997

2. Faraone SV, Biederman J, Weber W, et al: Psychiatric, neuropsychological, and psychosocial features of DSM-IV subtypes of attention deficit hyperactivity disorder: results from a clinically referred sample. J Am Acad Child Adolesc Psychiatry 37:185–193, 1998

3. Cantwell DP: Attention deficit disorder: a review of the past 10 years. J Am Acad Child Adolesc Psychiatry 35:978–987, 1996

4. O'Brien JD: Children with attention-deficit hyperactivity disorder and their parents, in Psychotherapies With Children and Adolescents. Edited by O'Brien JD, Pilowsky DJ, Lewis OW. Washington, DC, American Psychiatric Press, 1992, pp 109–124

5. Otnow Lewis D: Conduct disorder, in Child and Adolescent Psychiatry: A Comprehensive Textbook, 2nd Edition. Edited by Lewis M. Baltimore, MD, Williams & Wilkins, 1996, pp 564–577

6. Lion JR: Clinical assessment of violent patients, in Clinical Treatment of the Violent Person. Edited by Roth LH. New York, Guilford, 1987, pp 1–19

7. Loeber R, Hay DF: Developmental approaches to aggression and con-

duct problems; development through life. Edited by Rutter M, Hay DF. Oxford, England, Blackwell Scientific, 1994, pp 488–516

8. Otnow Lewis D: Conduct disorder, in Child and Adolescent Psychiatry: A Comprehensive Textbook. Edited by Lewis M. Baltimore, MD, Williams & Wilkins, 1991, pp 561–573

9. Otnow Lewis D: Diagnostic evaluation of the child with dissociative identity disorder/multiple personality disorder. Child Adolesc Psychiatr Clin North Am 5:303–331, 1996

10. Biederman J, Faraone S, Mick E, et al: Attention-deficit hyperactivity disorder and juvenile mania: an overlooked comorbidity? J Am Acad Child Adolesc Psychiatry 35:997–1008, 1996

11. Lewis M: Borderline disorders in children. Child Adolesc Psychiatr Clin North Am 3:31–42, 1994

12. Klein R, Pine DS, Klein DF: Resolved: mania is mistaken for ADHD in prepubertal children. Debate forum. Negative. J Am Acad Child Adolesc Psychiatry 37:1093–1096, 1998

13. Hechtman L: ADHD and bipolar disorder. The ADHD Report 7:1–3, 1999

14. Pliszka S: Bipolar disorder and ADHD; comments on current controversy. The ADHD Report 7:9–11, 1999

15. Goodwin FK, Jamison KR: Childhood and adolescence, in Manic-Depressive Illness. Edited by Goodwin FK, Jamison KR. Oxford, England, Oxford University Press, 1990, pp 186–209

16. Geller B, Luby J: Mania in young children (letter). J Am Acad Child Adolesc Psychiatry 37:1005, 1998

17. Bowring MA, Kovacs M: Difficulties in diagnosing manic disorders among children and adolescents. J Am Acad Child Adolesc Psychiatry 31:611–614, 1992

18. Wozniak J, Biederman J, Mundy E, et al: A pilot study of childhood-onset mania. J Am Acad Child Adolesc Psychiatry 34:1577–1583, 1995

19. Geller B, Luby J: Child and adolescent bipolar disorder: a review of the past 10 years. J Am Acad Child Adolesc Psychiatry 36:1168–1176, 1997.

20. Akiskal HS: Developmental pathways to bipolarity: are juvenile-onset depressions pre-bipolar? J Am Acad Child Adolesc Psychiatry 34:754–763, 1995

21. Carlson G: Annotation: child and adolescent mania; diagnostic considerations. J Child Psychol Psychiatry 31:331–341, 1990

6

EVALUATION OF OTHER SYMPTOMS

We discuss in this chapter a number of symptoms that do not fit well into the categories of either internalizing or externalizing symptoms. The assessment of these symptoms may involve agencies such as the legal system.

■ EVALUATION OF SYMPTOMS OF ABUSE

The clinical evaluation of abused children deals predominantly with the psychological consequences of the abuse. Its major goal is to evaluate the effect of the abuse, that is, the psychological consequences of the abuse on the child's developmental process and on the psychological functioning of the child and his or her family. Such an evaluation aims to develop a comprehensive assessment of the child and the family and to elaborate an accurate psychiatric diagnosis and a comprehensive treatment plan.

The examiner's first step in evaluating abused children is to clarify his or her role in the overall assessment process. The purpose of the evaluation will determine the examiner's approach and the information he or she will gather. The approach taken depends on whether the examiner is performing a forensic or a clinical examination. Because of the legal implications, the examiner must pay particularly careful attention to the facts in a forensic assessment. Ascertaining the facts in allegations of sexual abuse is a delicate, difficult, and uncertain enterprise (1, 2). Even the pelvic examination is fraught with uncertainties and controversy (3). Ascertaining facts in child abuse investigations is very difficult. One would think that the medical pelvic examination would be more effective as a fact finding examination. That is not the case. These findings are controversial.

The use of anatomically correct dolls to elicit information regarding possible sexual abuse is a controversial practice. Anatomically correct dolls should be considered as part of a set of stimuli that can function as communication and memory aids for children and other individuals who have immature language, cognitive, or emotional development or impaired communication skills (4, p. 375). Support seems to be gathering for the use of anatomically correct dolls in sexual abuse evaluations (5). Table 6–1 lists the benefits of using these dolls. Britton and O'Keefe found that, in comparison with nonanatomically detailed dolls, the use of anatomically detailed dolls had no effect on the outcome of the assessment of children who were thought to be victims of sexual abuse (6).

Benedek and Schetky warn that sexual abuse treatment should not be initiated without confirming that such abuse happened in the first place (2, p. 916). These authors consider comprehensive psychological evaluation an important part of the total assessment and emphasize the need for a comprehensive psychiatric evaluation of the child and the family and for extensive collateral corroboration from school, other families, and other relevant sources.

TABLE 6–1.   **Benefits of using anatomically correct dolls**

They do not distress or overstimulate the child.

They assist in the identification of idiosyncratic naming of body parts.

They increase verbal productivity during the examination.

They may be useful as communication and memory props.

They are helpful in working with immature children and with children who have cognitive deficits or impaired language.

Source.   Adapted from American Psychological Association 1991 (5).

The clinician needs to focus his or her attention equally on the child's narrative and on historical truths: "Clinicians should not attempt to be detectives in search of historical truth, but neither should they blur narrative and historical truth" (7, p. 90).

Special Considerations in Interviewing Abused Children

Clinicians should always keep in mind their legal responsibilities when dealing with abusive situations: they are obligated to report abuse (even suspected abuse) to child protection agencies.

When interviewing children who may have been abused, the examiner must be particularly careful to avoid asking leading questions (8). Because leading questions sometimes are unavoidable, the examiner must assess carefully how such questions may have biased the information gathered.

Rapport is particularly important in assessments of this nature. Rapport helps to improve the child's sense of trust and comfort and decreases the degree of defensiveness and apprehensiveness the child may exhibit in communicating these sensitive, often secretive, issues. The examiner should use the same vocabulary that the child uses, no matter how incorrect such terms may seem to the examiner. This is not the time to instruct the child on correct anatomical terms.

Questions like "Have you ever been physically or sexually abused?" are of uncertain value because the child may have been told not to tell or the child may feel a duty to protect his or her family. The examiner should begin the evaluation by exploring how the child is disciplined. The following questions are helpful: When you have done something wrong, how do your parents discipline you? Have you ever been spanked? Have you ever been punished? Has your father or your mother ever lost control in disciplining you? Has anyone ever used a belt on you? Have you ever been whipped? When asking these questions, the examiner needs to be sensitive to different cultural attitudes toward physical discipline.

The sensitive exploration of the topic of sexual abuse may begin with the following questions: Has anyone ever touched you where they shouldn't? Where? When did that happen? Did you tell anyone? Did you tell your mom? If the child answers "no" to this question, the examiner should ask whether there was a reason why the child couldn't tell the parent. If the child reports that "nasty" acts were done to him or her, the examiner should encourage the child to provide details of what happened, but the examiner must be particularly careful not to suggest answers nor to present leading questions.

The examiner must note the events narrated by the child in the child's own words (i.e., using the child's own language and expressions).

Most sexually abused children have been threatened by the perpetrators of the abuse and have been told not to talk about it. Often these children have been told that horrible things, including death, will happen to them or their family if they disclose the abuse. The examiner should remember that the child is aware at all times of the possible repercussions of disclosure. The examiner's empathic understanding of the child's fear should reassure the child. When a child reveals sexual abuse, the examiner may tell the child that he or she knows that when things like that happen to children they are often told not to say anything to anyone. The examiner can then ask the child to tell him or her about any threats the perpetrator may have made. The examiner should explore the nature of the threats and reassure the child about his or her fears and about any retaliation he or she anticipates. If the child has active symptoms of posttraumatic stress disorder, the fear of retaliation may reach psychotic proportions. When needed, the examiner should reassure the child that he or she will be safe and protected and that the examiner will make every possible effort to avoid any negative consequences for making the disclosure. If the examiner concludes that the child's safety cannot be guaranteed or that the traumatization is likely to continue, he or she should arrange with child protective services to place the child temporarily in a safe environment until the concerns with safety are resolved.

All forms of psychological manipulation on the child and any form of cajoling or pressuring of the child are absolutely proscribed. Pressure from the examiner to remember traumatic events may promote confabulation (7, p. 86). Confabulation is discussed in more detail in the last section of this chapter.

A child's ability to remember traumatic events may vary. Some memories may be clear, and some may be clouded; some memories may be corroborated and others may not. Four of the categories in Allen's classification of memories regarding sexual abuse are of particular clinical and legal relevance. Category 4 includes clouded memories for which corroborating evidence is lacking, category 5 includes memories of trauma that are highly exaggerated or distorted, and categories 6 and 7 include memories of trauma that may or may not have occurred in individuals who believe they were abused (7, p. 89). Memory distortion may occur if the patient has been exposed to suggestive techniques or has experience with therapists who erroneously believed that the patient's symptoms were the result of childhood sexual abuse (7, p. 89).

Examiners should remember the moral and legal implications of accepting the patient's disclosures at face value. They must exercise caution and attempt to substantiate the truthfulness of the patient's revelations. Frankel asserts this point: "Those therapists who emphasize that what is recalled is a previously disconnected and accurate memory of a childhood event that has never before been recognized might be correct in some instances; however, these therapists should not underestimate the consequences of such material, which has been regarded as truth but is actually the product of imagination, becoming the basis of either accusations within the family or litigation" (9, p. 69). Children may "remember" things that they have not experienced. In a discussion of Ceci's research on memory retrieval in small children, Terr et al. commented, "If children are coached . . . the incorrect suggestion that they have heard may turn up as memories. Using strong and repeated suggestions, Ceci's group was able to impart episodes that never took place into some preschoolers' minds" (10, p. 619). The examiner should also be aware that the act of reporting previous experiences modifies the nature of the child's narrative memory (7, 11; see also the "Memory Impairments" section in Chapter 7). These issues are described in further detail in the last section of this chapter.

Abused children are prone to future psychopathology, and they are prone to repeat abusive behavior with peers and, later, with spouses and their own children. The idea that physical abuse may be repeated is commonly accepted, but the tendency of abused children to act out the experience of sexual abuse with other children should also be explored (see Carlos's case example in Chapter 10). Children who have experienced sexual abuse should be asked whether they have done or have attempted to do the same thing to other children.

Developmental Consequences of Abuse

The examiner should attempt to identify any developmental deviations created by physical and sexual abuse. Cicchetti and Toth described specific mechanisms by which abusive experiences disrupt or interfere with the formation of fundamental functions or psychological structures (12, pp. 546–554; see also Chapter 8). These developmental deviations create or contribute to the development and maintenance of psychopathology (Table 6–2).

Examiners will encounter a variety of psychopathological syndromes in abused children. For example, van der Kolk et al. suggests that posttraumatic stress disorder does not occur in isolation (13, p. 89). Frequently it is associated with dissociation, somatization, and dysregulation of affect, including difficulties with anger modulation, sexual involvement, and aggression against the self and others. These symptoms are found together in the same in-

TABLE 6–2.	Developmental disruptions fostered by physical and sexual abuse experiences

Affect regulation (by promoting affect dysregulation—e.g., low tolerance for frustration, anger dyscontrol)

Normative attachment (by promoting atypical attachments—e.g., avoidant, resistant, and disorganized types)

Self-system (by promoting a defective self-concept and lower self-esteem, deficits in internal state language, and lower capacity for symbolic play)

Supportive peer relationships (by disrupting social competence and promoting a tendency to physical and verbal aggression in peer interactions)

Positive adaptation to school (by contributing to school maladaptation secondary to deficits in social cognitions and limited academic achievement)

dividuals and their cooccurrence is at least in part a function of the age at which the trauma occurred and the nature of the traumatic experience. Table 6–3 lists psychiatric disturbances commonly found in sexually abused children and adults. According to Green (14), these disturbances may represent sequelae of the abusive experiences.

Dissociative Symptoms

Dissociative disorders, including dissociative psychoses, are frequent complications of severe childhood abuse; unfortunately, these disorders often are not diagnosed correctly. Dissociative psychoses are frequently misdiagnosed as schizophrenia (15, 16). Otnow Lewis corroborates this point: "[T]he command auditory hallucinations, the experience of hearing voices speaking to each other in one's head, the sense of being controlled by these voices, the delusional system of hierarchies of imaginary companions, the blocking, and the illogical thinking of children with DID/MPD [dissociative identity disorder/multiple personality disorder] often

TABLE 6–3.	Psychiatric disturbances commonly observed in sexually abused individuals

Disturbances in children

 Anxiety disorders, including posttraumatic stress disorder (see Glenn's case example in Chapter 3)

 Depression and suicidal behaviors

 Dissociative and hysterical symptoms

 Disturbances in sexual behavior

Disturbances in adults

 Anxiety disorders, including posttraumatic stress disorder

 Substance abuse

 Borderline personality disorder

 Multiple personality disorder

 Revictimization

 Sexual dysfunction

 Sexual offending

Source. Based on Green 1993 (14, pp. 892–896).

lead to a misdiagnosis of schizophrenia" (17, p. 307). Otnow Lewis reviewed complex dissociative symptomatology (DID/MPD) and the difficulties of differentiating it from normal fantasy life, schizophrenia, mood disorder, seizure disorder or narcolepsy, borderline personality disorder, conduct disorder, or antisocial personality disorder (17, pp. 304–309).

 In the evaluation of children suspected of having dissociative disorders, it is important to recognize that a number of symptoms are secretive and that children invariably are unaware of these disorders or of the switches from one state of mind to another that occur in association with them. The examiner should explore the presence of behaviors such as getting lost in fantasy, spacing out, losing track of time, or disconnecting from what is going on in the real world. The examiner may ask the child the following questions: Are you able to go into a world of your own? Is there any special place in your head or in your imagination where you go when things get too painful, or a place where you go to seek comfort? The examiner should ask about the presence of depersonalization, out-of-body experiences, premonitions, or feelings of being controlled from outside.

Another important part of the evaluation of dissociation is the examination of memory disturbances, gaps in time, lack of recollection of important personal or family events, and fugue state experiences. Recurrent somatization, pseudoseizures, and self-abusive or self-mutilating behaviors may be indicators of dissociative states. The same could be said about precocious sexual behaviors. More obvious and more suggestive of the presence of these states are behaviors indicating that the child uses different names; that he or she has subjective experiences of being like two or more people; or that he or she experiences a sense of being possessed or a sense of unfamiliarity with the self.

Other issues that need to be explored in abused children with dissociative symptoms are the presence of imaginary companions and the presence of auditory hallucinations. In these hallucinations the voices are of a variable nature: some console, some counsel, some give orders, and some intimidate. The differentiation of these perceptual experiences from other psychotic states, from fantasy play, or from malingering may be a great challenge for the examiner. The only way the examiner can differentiate these experiences is through extended and sensitive questioning, the gathering of collateral information, and the use of other techniques (e.g., writing and drawing) or procedures such as psychological testing.

Other Symptoms of Abuse

Pervasive refusal. Lask et al. described a potentially life-threatening, extreme form of posttraumatic stress disorder, which they named *pervasive refusal* (18, pp. 868–869). This avoidance variant is characterized by a refusal to eat, drink, walk, talk, or care for oneself. Children with this disorder demonstrate willfulness in their symptoms and great fear of disclosing the nature and extent of their trauma. Children adopt this behavior as a way of escaping an intolerable situation.

Self-abusive behavior. Calof described chronic self-injury in adult survivors of childhood abuse (19, 20). Similar symptomatology is often observed in children and adolescents with abusive backgrounds. When a child exhibits self-abusive behavior, the examiner should ask about prior sexual or physical trauma.

■ EVALUATION OF REGRESSIVE BEHAVIOR

During the initial psychiatric examination, the examiner may be confronted with the emergence of regressive behaviors in a patient. In general, regressive behavior denotes a behavior or demeanor that would be more appropriate for a child who is younger than the patient's chronological age. Regressive behaviors may take a variety of forms: the child may resort to baby talk, decide not to talk at all, curl up into the fetal position, or become deliberately provocative. These behaviors may become major obstacles in the diagnostic assessment, and unless they are overcome the diagnostic interview may come to a standstill.

If a child begins to act younger than his or her age, the examiner can try a simple technique to motivate the child to behave more adaptively. The technique consists of contrasting the child's behavioral age with his or her chronological age. The examiner calls the child's attention to the way he or she is behaving and attempts to engage the child by asking, "How old do you think you were when you used to do that?" Usually, the child responds with an age that is quite a bit younger than his or her actual age. After this age has been agreed upon, the examiner asks the child how old he or she is. The child immediately states his or her chronological age. The examiner then asks the child how old he or she would like to behave. Most children readily favor their chronological age. The examiner then indicates to the child that from then on, he or she will help the child to behave that age by reminding the child every time he or she begins to act younger.

This simple technique works when it is done with equanimity and humor. The playfulness of this technique belies its power. The technique works because it promotes a therapeutic ego split; it puts the regressive ego in opposition with the most adaptive ego functioning part. The technique creates or, more properly, activates a conflict between the more adaptive ego and the more immature or regressive part. This technique appeals to the child's internal controls because it puts the child in conflict with himself or herself. Further therapeutic alliance may be built around the goal of controlling or decreasing the influence of the regressive part. The examiner may explain to the child that sometimes the immature part takes control and gets the child in trouble. The child may be challenged to come up with ideas on how to manage the immature part.

Regressive behavior is common in patients undergoing malignant decompensations (e.g., in acute psychotic episodes and schizophrenia). Serious and stable regressions are also present in severe bipolar disorder. Less severe forms of regression are common in children going through developmental transitions (e.g., from preschool to elementary school and during adolescence), in children undergoing stress (e.g., related to family, school, or friends), in children who are deprived or abused, and in children who have severe psychiatric disorders (e.g., mood, anxiety, or psychotic disorders). Regressive behaviors are not always associated with functional disorders. Regressive behaviors may be associated with delirium and other organic conditions (see Chapter 7).

■ ASSESSMENT OF TRUTHFULNESS IN ABUSED CHILDREN

When there are concerns about the patient's truthfulness, the examiner should be particularly careful about the types of questions he or she asks. Leading questions must be avoided at all times. As discussed earlier in this chapter, the examiner should use the same language that the patient uses: the examiner must use the patient's words and expressions, no matter how incorrect or inappropriate they may sound. The introduction of different words or expressions may change the patient's intended meaning. These recommendations are even more important in forensic interviews, regarding allegations of physical or sexual abuse. The following case example illustrates a situation in which the examiner respected these principles:

> Mary, a 14-year-old Caucasian adolescent, claimed that she had been raped by a 21-year-old man. When describing what the man had done to her, she said that the man had "perpetrated" her. When Mary was asked to explain, she said that the man had "gone all the way." She added that he had put his "thing" inside of her. Mary reported her story consistently when she was asked about the incident. This was compatible with a truthful story. The examiner understood that Mary wanted to say "penetrated" but did not correct her. The examiner also understood that "thing" meant "penis," but he did not correct her then either. Instead the examiner asked Mary to explain what "perpetrated" and "thing" meant.

Bernet (21) has clarified many important concepts in the identification of false statements of sexual abuse. Allegations of sexual abuse are true in about 90% of the complaints. As a result, the first assumption should be that the allegations may be true. Bernet organizes the mechanisms of false statements of sexual abuse into three groups:

1. The false statement arises in the mind of the parent or other adults and is imposed on the mind of the child. This may be due to
   a. *Parental misinterpretation and suggestion.* The parent takes an innocent remark or a neutral piece of behavior and inflates it into something worse and inadvertently induces the child to endorse his or her interpretation.
   b. *Misinterpreted physical condition.* A vindictive or anxious parent or a health professional may jump to the conclusion that the child's injury or illness is due to sexual abuse rather than accepting a more benign explanation.

c. *Parental delusion.* The parent is paranoid, very disturbed, and shares the distorted view of the world with the child, who comes to share the same delusion. There may be a folie à deux (shared delusion), or the child may give in to the parent's contention that abuse occurred.

d. *Parental indoctrination.* This occurs when the parent fabricates the allegation and instructs the child in what to say.

e. *Interviewer suggestion.* Previous interviewers may have contaminated the evidence by asking leading or suggestive questions.

f. *Overstimulation.* The parent lacks modesty or discretion and exposes the child to nudity or sexual activity.

g. *Group contagion.* The child and parents fall victim to epidemic hysteria.

2. The false statement is caused primarily by mental mechanisms in the child that are not conscious or not purposeful.

a. *Fantasy.* The child may confuse fantasy with reality.

b. *Delusion.* Delusions about sexual activities may occur in children and adolescents in the context of psychotic illness.

c. *Misinterpretation.* The false belief is based on an actual happening.

d. *Miscommunication.* The false allegation arises out of simple verbal misunderstanding.

e. *Confabulation.* The person fabricates statements or stories in response to questions about events that the person does not actually recall.

3. The false statement is caused primarily by mental mechanisms in the child that are usually considered conscious and purposeful.

a. *Pseudologia phantastica,* also called *fantasy lying* and *pathological lying.* The person tells stories without discernible motive and with such a zeal that the subject may become convinced of their truth.

b. *Innocent lying.* Young children frequently make false statement because that seems to be the best way to handle the situation they are in.

c. *Deliberate lying.* This refers to self-serving, intentional fab-
rications that are common among children and adolescents.

Bernet makes clear the distinction between confabulation and
pseudologia phantastica:

1. The social context is different: Confabulation is evoked by
questions raised by another person. Pseudologia phantastica is
created to impress and influence others.
2. The form of the statement is different: Whereas confabulation
is usually a short statement in response to a specific question
when the person has no real memory for the answer, in
pseudologia [phantastica] there is a lengthy, complex story
that goes beyond the question raised and is delivered with zest
and in an engaging manner.
3. Confabulation and pseudologia [phantastica] differ in the way
the person responds when confronted with contradictory evidence: The confabulator sticks to his or her story, whereas the
individual with pseudologia [phantastica] drops the story and
moves on to another one (21, p. 908).

Bernet also distinguishes confabulation from misinterpretation:

A misinterpretation may cause a false belief but is derived from
something that actually happened. A child with a misinterpretation may say that two people were fighting when in reality they
were having sexual intercourse. A confabulating child may say
that two people were fighting when they were having an unremarkable conversation. Confabulation is also different from deliberate lying in that the child who is lying knows that he or she
is trying to deceive. The confabulator does not realize what he or
she is doing. Pseudologia is different from deliberate lying in
that the delinquent liar intends to deceive and knows exactly
what he or she is doing. In pseudologia phantastica, the fabulist,

intending to enhance an interpersonal relationship or influence
another person, does so by embellishing the stories and may be
so involved in the deception that he or she comes to believe it.
(21, p. 908)

The following case example is an intriguing illustration of
pseudologia phantastica in a very disturbed adolescent:

Victor, a 15-year-old Caucasian adolescent, presented with a
prolonged history of psychiatric problems including a profound
inability to establish and to maintain interpersonal relationships,
lying, stealing, destructiveness with lack of remorse, severe
enuresis, difficulties at school, sexually inappropriate behaviors,
aggression toward his peers, and a lack of interest in participating in treatment. He had been in state custody for 8 years because his family had abandoned him. His natural mother had a
history of a neurological disease and polysubstance abuse. Victor had a history of multiple placements and multiple psychiatric
hospitalizations. At birth, Victor was thought to have fetal alcohol syndrome. On earlier testing, Victor was found to have a
borderline level of intelligence.

Victor had been evaluated when he was readmitted to an
acute psychiatric program for aggressive and inappropriate behaviors including the difficulties already mentioned. Victor exhibited involuntary movements of the mouth and jaw. These
dystonic signs had been erroneously considered as the "bizarre
mannerisms of an elderly man." When Victor was asked his
name, he said, "I'm a third degree Nijitsu." The examiner asked
Victor what a Nijitsu was. He replied, "We're licensed to carry
weapons. Nobody else carries weapons in America." The examiner asked, "What kinds of weapons?" Victor replied, "Swords,
knives, stars, nunchakus, sticks, slingshots." He reported that his
father was a Ninja and asserted that he was not an American.
"I'm Japanese-Indian, second generation of Americans," he
said. He stated that he had studied with a samurai who had been
stabbed to death with a sword. He claimed that his father had
died in combat, and he repeated that he was not an American.

Victor's verbalizations could be considered megalomanic
delusions. He did not strongly uphold any of his beliefs: when

the examiner would challenge one confabulated idea, he would create a new one. What was intriguing was the lack of emotion he displayed when he presented his fantastic background. A pediatric neurologist determined that Victor had tardive dystonia and other neurological problems. Neuropsychological testing was positive for multiple neuropsychological deficits, including bilateral fine motor deficits, receptive and expressive language disorder, poor verbal learning, memory and attention difficulties, and executive dysfunction. Multiple factors, then, contributed to Victor's pseudologia phantastica.

■ REFERENCES

1. Benedek EP, Schetky D: Problems in validating allegations of sexual abuse; part 1: factors affecting perception and recall of events. J Am Acad Child Adolesc Psychiatry 26:912–915, 1987

2. Benedek EP, Schetky D: Problems in validating allegations of sexual abuse; part 2: clinical evaluation. J Am Acad Child Adolesc Psychiatry 26:916–921, 1987

3. Coleman L: Medical examination for sexual abuse: have we been misled? The Champion, November 1989, pp 5–12

4. Koocher GP, Goodman GS, White CS, et al: Psychological science and the use of anatomically detailed dolls in child sexual-abuse assessments. Psychol Bull 118:199–222, 1995 [Reprinted in Hertzig M, Farber E (eds): Annual Progress in Child Psychiatry and Child Development. New York, Brunner/Mazel, 1996, pp 367–425]

5. American Psychological Association: Minutes of the council of representatives. Am Psychol 46:722, 1991

6. Britton HL, O'Keefe MA: Use of nonanatomical dolls in the sexual abuse interview. Child Abuse Neglect 15:567–573, 1991

7. Allen J: The spectrum of accuracy of childhood trauma. Harvard Rev Psychiatry 3:84–95, 1995

8. Goodman GS, Saywitz KJ: Memories of abuse: interviewing children when sexual victimization is suspected. Child Adolesc Psychiatr Clin 3:645–661, 1994

9. Frankel FH: Dissociation: the clinical realities. Am J Psychiatry 153(Festschrift suppl):64–70, 1996

10. Terr LC, Bloch DA, Michel BA, et al: Children's memories in the wake of *Challenger*. Am J Psychiatry 153:618–625, 1996

11. Lewis M: Memory and psychoanalysis: a new look at infantile amnesia and transference. J Am Acad Child Adolesc Psychiatry 34:405–417, 1995

12. Cicchetti D, Toth SL: A developmental psychopathology perspective on child abuse and neglect. J Am Acad Child Adolesc Psychiatry 34:541–565, 1995

13. van der Kolk BA, Pelcovitz D, Roth S, et al: Dissociation, somatization, and affect dysregulation: the complexity of adaptation to trauma. Am J Psychiatry 153(Festschrift suppl):83–93, 1996

14. Green A: Child sexual abuse: immediate and long-term effects and interventions. J Am Acad Child Adolesc Psychiatry 32:890–902, 1993

15. Putnam F: Dissociative disorders in children and adolescents; a developmental perspective. Psychiatr Clin North Am 14:519–531, 1991

16. Hornstein NL, Putnam F: Clinical phenomenology of child and adolescent dissociative disorders. J Am Acad Child Adolesc Psychiatry 31:1077–1085, 1992

17. Otnow Lewis D: Diagnostic evaluation of the child with dissociative identity disorder/multiple personality disorder. Child Adolesc Psychiatr Clin North Am 5:303–331, 1996

18. Lask B, Britten C, Kroll L, et al: Children with pervasive refusal. Arch Dis Child 66:866–869, 1991

19. Calof D: Chronic self-injury in adult survivors of childhood abuse; sources, motivations, and functions of self-injury (part I). Treating Abuse Today 5:11–17, 1995

20. Calof D: Chronic self-injury in adult survivors of childhood abuse; sources, motivations, and functions of self-injury (part II). Treating Abuse Today 5:31–36, 1995.

21. Bernet W: False statements and the differential diagnosis of abuse allegations. J Am Acad Child Adolesc Psychiatry 32:903–910, 1993

7

THE NEUROPSYCHIATRIC INTERVIEW AND EXAMINATION

In this chapter, we offer a practical and clinically oriented approach to the neuropsychiatric interview and examination of children and adolescents, including descriptions of the most common neuropsychiatric symptoms found in children and adolescents.

In most of the neuropsychiatric disorders of childhood the diagnosis of "brain damage" is incorrect. It is more appropriate to speak of "brain dysfunction" or "brain impairment." The concept of brain damage is associated with two erroneous assumptions: 1) that the brain was developing well until something damaged it and 2) that brain damage is irreversible. The first assumption is true in certain situations, for example, when hydrocephalus follows tuberculous meningitis or when epilepsy follows a penetrating head injury. Most commonly, however, brain development may have been abnormal from the very beginning, perhaps as a result of an inherited disorder, chromosomal abnormality, or chromosomal mutation. In terms of the second assumption, children do grow out of disorders such as epilepsy and even cerebral palsy (1, p. 172).

The neuropsychiatric evaluation is a specialized, structured, and orderly examination of a number of specific functions and is aimed at determining assumed brain dysfunction or impairment that underlies behavioral, emotional, cognitive, or interpersonal disturbances. The field of neuropsychiatry correlates performance on specific tasks with certain neuroanatomical areas or with certain neurophysiological and neuropsychological events. The neuropsychiatric evaluation probes the integrity of neuropsychological functioning of many cortical association areas and of certain subcortical functions. It includes the assessment of attention; language; cognition; memory; visuospatial, motor, and sensory functioning; and executive functions. More specifically, the neuropsychiatric examination assesses functioning of the frontal, temporal, parietal, and occipital lobes and of subcortical regions. It also explores so-called soft neurological signs.

Cummings classifies the behavioral disturbances associated with neurological disorders in adults in two groups (2, p. 180). The first group, called the *neurobehavioral syndromes* (or deficit disorders), includes dysfunctions such as aphasia, amnesia, apraxia, agraphia, aprosody, acalculia, frontal lobe disorders, neglect, and anosognosia. These dysfunctions are correlated with injury to the cerebral cortex, deep hemispheric nuclei, or white matter tracts. The second group, called the *neuropsychiatric syndromes* (or productive disorders), encompasses idiopathic psychiatric symptom complexes such as delusions, hallucinations, depression, mania, personality alterations, anxiety, obsessive-compulsive disorders, and paraphilias.

In general, productive disorders are not associated with focal, or precise, anatomical lesions. In the productive disorders, the lesion must be present in the appropriate location for the disorder to occur; that is, the existence of the lesion by itself is often insufficient to produce the disorder. Other factors contribute to the expression of these disorders, such as age, unilateral or bilateral lesions, genetic factors, comorbidity, gender, premorbid personality, environmental stress, coping skills, and social supports (2, p. 180).

In contrast to such conditions in adults, in children and adolescents, neurodevelopmental disorders encompass a group of complex disorders that result from abnormal development of the central nervous system (CNS). This abnormal development results in delays, deviations, or a lack of emergence or progression in expected skill acquisitions.

The field of pediatric neuropsychiatry is in its infancy. This emerging field has borrowed a significant body of knowledge from the field of adult neuropsychiatry, but extensions and generalizations from one field to the other may not be appropriate. Pediatric neuropsychiatry is beginning to rely on its own experience, knowledge, and research methodology with pediatric subjects. Longitudinal developmental observations are needed to elucidate the nature of skill emergence and to determine atypical developmental pathways. These studies are needed in order to make adequate outcome prognostications regarding a variety of neurodevelopmental disorders.

Broadly conceived, the pediatric neuropsychiatric examination is based on a multidisciplinary approach that involves developmental pediatricians, pediatric neurologists, speech pathologists, developmental psychologists, geneticists, neuropsychologists, neuroradiologists, electrophysiologists, neurosurgeons, educators, and other specialists. The field deals with the assessment and treatment of congenital or acquired neurodevelopmental disorders.

In general, adult clinical neuropsychiatry focuses on the loss of neurological function and the process of its recovery *(rehabilitation)*. In contrast, pediatric clinical neuropsychiatry focuses on the emergence and developmental deviations of function *(skill acquisition)* and the process of functional habilitation. Pediatric neuropsychiatry also looks at the psychological and psychosocial consequences of neurodevelopmental disorders.

According to some authors, the neuropsychiatric examination of adults should be fairly broad, including an assessment of systemic and neurological functions, an examination for soft neurological signs, a detailed mental status examination and cognitive assessment, ancillary clinical tests (e.g., the Mini-Mental State

Exam, the Aphasia Screening Test), and laboratory tests (e.g., neuropsychological assessment, electrophysiological studies, brain imaging, spinal fluid studies, cerebral angiography, skull X rays, blood chemistries, urinalysis, VDRL, electrocardiograms, chest X rays, and endocrine and nutritional studies) (3, p. 4). These examinations should also be considered in the neuropsychiatric evaluation of children. The authors cited also feel that a valid cognitive examination should be thorough and systematic and should include assessments of motor behavior; language; memory; temporal, frontal, parietal, and occipital lobe function; and soft neurological signs. Furthermore, these examinations should be intercorrelated. Most tasks focus on specific higher cortical functions and cortical-associational regions and systems (3, p. 5). The same considerations apply in the field of pediatric neuropsychiatry.

■ ELEMENTS OF THE NEUROPSYCHIATRIC HISTORY

Gold asserted that the history is the cornerstone of neurological (or neuropsychiatric) diagnosis, much as it is in psychiatry (4, p. 1). The history often suggests whether the condition is static or progressive and whether it has an organic cause. The neuropsychiatric assessment involves a comprehensive maturational and developmental history, and the emphasis is on systematic data gathering. If at all possible, the history should be obtained from the child, even from young children, before historical data are obtained from the parents. This approach may generate information that is free of parental bias, which is often invaluable in making a diagnosis and in determining how the condition affects the child. A comprehensive neuropsychiatric history includes a systematic exploration and evaluation of the areas listed in Table 7–1.

Neuropsychiatric factors should be suspected in children who exhibit developmental delays (e.g., in achieving milestones), language delays (e.g., language acquisition, production, or comprehension delays), or learning problems; in children who have a

TABLE 7–1.   **Areas to explore in every comprehensive neuropsychiatric evaluation**

Family history of neurological or psychiatric illnesses

Gestational history

  History of mother's alcohol or drug consumption (including tobacco use) during pregnancy

  History of viral infections or other illnesses during early pregnancy

Prenatal, neonatal, and perinatal histories

History of exposure to heavy metals and other toxins

History of medical or surgical conditions

History of neurological disorders: seizures, loss of consciousness, and head trauma

Maturational history

  Developmental milestones

  Attachment history

History of language acquisition

History of motor coordination competence

History of attention-concentration development

History of consistent impulse control

History of control of aggressive behavior

History of control of sexual behavior

History of observance of rules and expectations

History of academic performance and learning competence

History of social and interpersonal functioning

History of psychiatric behavioral problems

History of drug abuse and intravenous drug use

History of practice of protected sex (sexual contact with HIV-positive individuals or with individuals who have sexually transmitted diseases)

history of cerebral palsy, movement disorders, perinatal insult, meningitis or meningoencephalitis, seizures, dementing conditions, or head trauma accompanied with prolonged loss of consciousness; and in children with sensorium impairment, recent onset of neurological signs, loss of intellectual capacity or acquired skills, sudden onset of regressive behavior, developmental arrests, or worse, developmental regression. This is not an exhaustive list of conditions in which neuropsychiatric factors need to be investigated.

Neuropsychiatric factors also should be investigated in the following psychiatric conditions: when a progressive loss of adaptive capacity or intellectual functioning has occurred; when delirium or other disturbances of the sensorium are present; when psychotic conditions or visual, olfactory, or other perceptual disorders are present; when catatonic or recurrent impulsive behavior exists; when children display chronic interpersonal difficulties; or when psychiatric symptomatology does not fit into other categories. Neuropsychiatric factors should be considered when psychiatric treatments seem to be ineffective, when there is no progress in the clinical course of a disorder, or when the patient's clinical condition deteriorates.

Beyond the so-called hard neurological signs, such as seizures and paralysis, the most frequent complaints of neuropsychiatric patients are attention-concentration difficulties, cognitive impairments, impulse-control problems, impairments of judgment, affect dysregulation, language disorders, learning difficulties, memory impairments, interpersonal difficulties, and regressive behavior.

Many neuropsychiatric syndromes that occur in childhood or in adolescence require timely diagnosis and treatment. Examples include phenylketonuria and other congenital or genetic metabolic diseases of the CNS; mental retardation syndromes such as Down syndrome, fetal alcohol syndrome, fragile X syndrome, and Williams syndrome; seizure disorders (e.g., petit mal seizures, psychomotor epilepsy, and other neuropsychiatric disturbances secondary to seizures or phenomena that occur either after or between seizures); aphasia; cerebral palsy; movement disorders such as chorea; and conditions such as Rett syndrome, Prader-Willi syndrome, Angelman's syndrome, Asperger's syndrome, and autistic disorder. Many severe adult neurological illnesses (e.g., Huntington's disease, Wilson's disease) have their onset in childhood, and child psychiatrists must be aware of their early presentation (5, p. 143).

■ NEUROPSYCHIATRY AND PSYCHOSOCIAL FACTORS

Neuropsychiatric conditions are susceptible to environmental influence. Favorable conditions facilitate early detection and prompt habilitation or rehabilitation of emerging deviations or developmental arrests. In contrast, symptoms may unfold unaltered or they may be maintained or worsened by adverse psychosocial circumstances (e.g., infantilism, inappropriate parenting).

Cook and Leventhal described two key findings related to the increased morbidity associated with neuropsychiatric disorders in childhood and adolescence (6, p. 639). First, children with neuropsychiatric disorders substantially affect their parents and siblings. Second, children with these disorders are often disabled for a long time. Frequently, the parents' response to a neurological problem creates additional handicaps for the child. Williams et al. articulated this concern in the following manner:

> Another common and more clearly psychological theme occurring throughout the spectrum of neuropsychiatric disorders in childhood and adolescence is the problem of dependency and its many permutations. While some degree of augmented parental solicitude and support is a natural and, indeed, healthy response to the sequelae of a chronic neurological dysfunction in a child, frequently this pattern becomes exaggerated as a by-product of features of anxiety, guilt, or demoralization in the patient, the parents or both. (7, p. 366)

Individuals with mental retardation and other developmental disorders are at greater risk for psychiatric disorders due to CNS dysfunction, peer rejection, and decreased coping strategies (6, p. 643). The psychological disability associated with a neuropsychiatric condition can be worse than the handicap itself: "In effect, the patient can be tempted, either unconsciously or consciously, to exploit the sick role with its associated dependency gratifications when feeling overwhelmed by ongoing life stresses" (7, p. 366). In general, the secondary gain from the illness occurs because the parents become inconsistent with limit setting. This is usually the result of parental guilt that interferes with appropriate and consistent discipline and limit setting. The parents feel somehow responsible for the child's neuropsychiatric condition and, as a consequence, become inconsistent in discipline and in boundary enforcement.

■ PERFORMING THE AMSIT ON A CHILD WHO HAS A NEUROPSYCHIATRIC DISORDER

The neuropsychiatric examination starts as soon as the examiner greets the child in the waiting area. The following observations are relevant in this regard: What is the child's appearance and overall complexion? What is the preliminary gestalt or impression? Are any dysmorphic features present?

As the examiner guides and follows the child toward the office, he or she should observe the child's gait, movement of upper and lower extremities, balance, and coordination and the child's sense of space orientation. After the child enters the office, the examiner should complete the mental status examination—including a neurodevelopmental evaluation (described in the next section)— and physical and neurological examinations.

We agree with Gold regarding the importance of inspection: "Observations may be more rewarding than examination, encouraging the clinician to acquire and use observational skills that may result in a diagnosis by inspection. This is obviously preferred to the performance of diagnostic studies that can be anxiety producing, painful, invasive and expensive" (4, p. 4).

■ ELEMENTS OF THE NEURODEVELOPMENTAL EVALUATION

Areas that need to be assessed in the neurodevelopmental evaluation are listed in Table 7–2 and are described in more detail in this section.

TABLE 7–2. **Elements of the neurodevelopmental evaluation**

1. Dysmorphic features
2. Abnormal posture and involuntary movements
3. Gross motor skills
4. Fine motor skills
5. Sensory functioning
6. Midline behaviors
7. Laterality and dominance
8. Cerebellar functions
9. Praxis
10. Receptive and expressive language functions
11. Information
12. Orientation to time and place
13. Abstraction ability
14. Writing and reading
15. Calculation ability
16. Immediate, short-term, and long-term memory
17. Executive functions

Assessment of Dysmorphic Features

The examiner should describe the child's stature (e.g., small or large), head size (e.g., microcephaly, macrocephaly), and any abnormalities of the skull structure. Young et al. highlighted the importance of the identification of dysmorphic features:

> The detection of minor congenital anomalies during the physical and neurologic examination may be more clinically pertinent. These stigmata are correlated with a variety of behavioral and intellectual deviations, even in children with no major physical pathology who do not fall into the conventional diagnostic categories. They also may have value in suggesting a chromosomal abnormality or an insult to the fetus during the first trimester of pregnancy. (8, p. 455)

The examiner should note whether any signs of readily identifiable syndromes are present, for example, Down syndrome, fragile X syndrome, fetal alcohol syndrome, Prader-Willi syndrome, or neurocutaneous disorders (e.g., ataxia-telangiectasia, neurofibromatosis, tuberous sclerosis, or Sturge-Weber-Dimitri's syndrome).

Assessment of Abnormal Posture and Involuntary Movements

The examiner should note the presence of tics, chorea, athetosis, or any other involuntary movements. He or she should also note whether the child stands or sits erect and whether the child displays stiffness, hypotonia, dystonia, or other unusual movements or abnormal postures. The examiner should look for acute extrapyramidal symptoms in children recently exposed to neuroleptic medications and for chronic extrapyramidal symptoms—such as chronic akathisia or chronic dystonia (tardive dyskinesia)—in children with extended exposure to these medications.

Assessment of Gross Motor Skills

The examiner should pay attention to child's motor function. Is it smooth? Spastic? Choreic? Dystonic? Athetoid? As the child walks, the examiner should observe his or her stance and gait. Is the child's standing base broad or variable? The examiner should note associated involuntary movements. Does the child display a normal steppage? Does the child limp? Waddle? Tiptoe? Is the child's gait stiff? When the examiner throws a ball to the child, is the child able to catch it? Is the child able to throw or roll back the ball?

In children with a history of cerebral palsy, the examiner should explore for signs of spasticity, rigidity, paralysis, dystonia, athetosis, chorea, or tremor. Spasticity and athetosis are the most frequent neurological sequelae of cerebral palsy, followed by rigidity and ataxia.

Assessment of Fine Motor Skills

The examiner should observe how the child grasps an object and how he or she manipulates toys. When the child is given a pencil or a crayon, the examiner should observe how the child picks it up and note the quality of the child's grasp. Is it normal? Is it unusual? Pencil grasp is an important indicator of motor control: it is a hard-to-change motor habit and is acquired early; it may represent a residual indicator of the maturation of the child's motor system at the time the child began to use a pencil. The quality of the grasp does not "stigmatize" the current motor repertoire but may be an early snapshot of past status during the period of motor skill learning (9, p. 726). The examiner should ask the child to copy a circle, a cross, a square, a triangle, and a diamond. A 2-year-old child will be able to copy the circle, a 3-year-old child the cross, a 5-year-old child the square, and a 6-year-old child the triangle. A 7-year-old child will be able to copy the diamond.

Assessment of Sensory Functioning

The examiner first asks the child to close his or her eyes. Then the examiner touches the child first on one limb and then another, each time asking the child to identify the body part. After this, the examiner simultaneously touches either ipsilateral or contralateral limbs and again asks the child to identify where he or she has been touched. The examiner can test the child for *graphesthesia* (ability to recognize symbols drawn onto parts of the body) by tracing numbers or letters onto the back of each of the child's hands and asking the child to identify them. To test for *stereognosis* (ability to recognize objects by touch), the examiner can ask the child to identify, without looking, items such as a coin, a paper clip, a key, or a stamp. The examiner should first ensure the child has these items in his or her vocabulary. The child needs to identify these items with each hand. These tests explore parietal lobe functioning. Stereognosis is well developed in early childhood, whereas graphesthesia is not well developed until age 6 or 7 years.

Denckla has reservations about the diagnostic validity of graphesthesia in children. She thinks this may be an inefficient test because little is known about the firmness of the association between mental image or visual memory of a letter, the name of the letter, and the dynamic-tactile experience of graphesthesia (9, pp. 724–725). The implication is that for these tests to be valid, a certain cognitive developmental level is required. Tactile sensory loss is common in children with cerebral palsy. Astereognosis and dysgraphesthesia are specific agnosia deficits observed in cerebral palsy. Denckla's reservations about the validity of graphesthesia in children may be also applicable to these tests.

Assessment of Midline Behaviors

The examiner should observe whether the child uses both hands coordinately and supportively and whether the child transfers any given item from one hand to the other. The examiner should also note whether the child is able to cross the body's midline (the examiner should note the extent to which the child's right hand, for instance, is able to cross the midline and operate on the left side of the body or vice versa). These behaviors reflect the functional integrity of the corpus callosum (10, p. 162). For example, one mother reported that her 8-year-old child, who had no evidence of motor difficulties, used only one hand even when he combed his hair or when he put on his belt. He also had attention problems, difficulties with learning, and problems with impulse control.

Assessment of Laterality and Dominance

Lewis clarified the concepts of laterality, preference, and dominance: *Laterality* is a measurable, specialized, central function of a paired faculty, such as eyes, ears, hands, and feet; *preference* is the subjective, self-reported experience of an individual, as opposed to laterality, which may be objectively measured; and *dominance* is a term used for the concept of cerebral hemisphere specialization, such as language and speech. Clinically, the examiner may merely be testing preference, which depends more on a peripheral organ than on a central mechanism (11, p. 445). Handedness is consolidated by age 5 years, footedness by about 7 years, eye lateralization by 7 or 8 years, and ear lateralization by about 9 years.

The examiner should observe which hand the child uses predominantly when manipulating objects and when asked to write or to draw. The examiner should also observe which foot the child uses when asked to kick a ball. The child's eye preference is tested by asking the child to look into a particular item in the office using a "telescope" (a rolled-up piece of paper).

A useful test to assess right-left discrimination consists of asking the child to follow some ipsilateral and contralateral commands. For example, for ipsilateral discrimination, the examiner asks the child, "With your right hand touch your right ear" or "With your left hand touch your left knee." For contralateral discrimination, the examiner asks, "With your right hand touch your left ear" or "With your left hand touch your right knee." A child can identify right and left hands by age 5 years; ipsilateral double orientation (e.g., left hand on left ear) should be possible by age 6 years and contralateral orientation by age 7 years. Problems in these areas are common in children who have learning disorders. Confusion of laterality should be suspected when the examiner extends a hand for a handshake and the child does not seem to know which hand to respond with.

Assessment of Cerebellar Functions

To assess cerebellar functions, the examiner should ask the child to stand up, put both hands out in front, and close both eyes; the examiner should then observe whether the child sways to the sides (Romberg's sign). The child should be asked to walk in a straight line, and the examiner should observe the child's balance and coordination. Next, the child should be asked to stand on one foot and then on the other and then to hop on one foot and then on the other. The examiner should observe the child's sense of equilibrium and the smoothness and proficiency with which the child accomplishes these tasks. The examiner also should assess the child's muscle tone and determine whether the child is hypotonic, normal, or hypertonic.

The role of the cerebellum in higher cortical functions, including language, has been recognized. A syndrome of mutism and subsequent dysarthria (imperfect articulation of speech) has been identified. This syndrome is not related to cerebellar ataxia and is characterized by a complete loss of speech that resolves into dysarthria (12, p. 746).

Assessment of Praxis

Ideokinetic, or ideomotor, praxis is the ability to perform an action from memory on request without props or cues. The child should be asked to demonstrate how he or she would use a key, a toothbrush, and a comb. The child's nonpreferred hand should be tested first. The child's kinesthetic praxis can be tested by asking the child to mimic the examiners' finger and hand movements. Difficulties with finger sequencing correlate with graphomotor dyspraxia and with poor handwriting (9, p. 725).

The examiner may ask the child to perform more complex tasks such as unbuttoning and buttoning his or her own shirt and untying and then retying his or her own shoelaces. The latter task involves complex functions, out of reach of children who have impairments in interhemispheric integration.

Assessment of Receptive and Expressive Language Functions

The examiner should attempt to differentiate among speech, language, and communication disorders. *Speech disorders* relate to difficulties in the production of speech. They relate to output problems and the utterance of meaningful and communicable sounds. *Language* is the organized and retrievable view of the self and the world; phonemics, morphemics, syntactics, and semantics relate to different aspects of integrated language. *Communication* relates to the social use of language, to the transmission of meanings between and among persons. The process of communication is regulated by a number of norms, so-called communication pragmatics (e.g., eye contact, turn taking, topic continuity). Delays in language acquisition could be global or could appear in only selected aspects of language acquisition. The latter are the most common language disorders.

When evaluating the child's language, the examiner should first observe the child's capacity to understand verbal communication. When the examiner interviews the child, he or she will have multiple opportunities to observe the child's understanding of verbalizations. The examiner should note whether he or she has to repeat questions frequently, use redundant and simple language, or supplement utterances with gestures or with deliberate nonverbal language. The examiner should also observe whether the child is unable to understand even simple expressions. As the child speaks, the examiner should note the child's fluency and pronunciation; prosody and gesturing; vocabulary, grammar, and syntax; and capacity for abstract thinking (see Chapter 3).

The capacity to name objects (*anomia*, or *dysnomia*, is the term used to describe disturbances in this capacity) may be tested by asking the child to name a number of body parts. The examiner should point to his or her own eyebrow, chin, wrist, or other body areas and ask the child to name the part. The examiner may also point to his or her own jacket, belt, wristwatch, collar, shoe, or tie, and ask the child to name those items. In adults, dysnomia may result from dominant temporal or parietal lesions. In children, the disturbance is related to significant developmental delays in language. For example, a 6-year-old child with significant developmental delays in language was retained in kindergarten. The examiner asked the child to name some body parts. When the examiner pointed to his ear, the child said "head"; when the examiner pointed to the child's foot, she said "leg."

In adults, disturbances of prosody and gesturing in which spontaneous gesturing and emotionality of speech are lacking could be related to frontal lesions; disturbances in the understanding of the prosody and gesturing of others could be related to temporal lesions (3, p. 8). Similar localization of functions has not been confirmed in children.

Assessment of Information

The child should be asked to narrate recent events. If the child demonstrates no awareness of or interest in recent news, he or she could be asked to talk about a favorite sport, favorite team, or favorite players. The following questions are commonly used in this part of the assessment: What town do you live in? What state do you live in? What is the state capital? Name the biggest cities in your state. Name the states that border your state. What is the capital of the United States? Who was the first president of the United States? Who is the current president? Do you know the vice president's name? Other factors to be considered when assessing this area are the child's level of intelligence and the child's cultural and socioeconomic background.

Assessment of Orientation to Time and Place

The child should be asked to identify where he or she is, including the name of the place, the floor, and so on. The examiner should ask the child to indicate, on a map, where north or south is. He or she may also ask the child to point to directions on a wall picture, for example, "In this picture, where is north?" The examiner should ask the child to indicate the day of the week and the date, including the month and the year. The child may also be asked to identify the season and the most recent holiday.

Assessment of Abstraction Ability

The examiner should note the child's complexity of thought as he or she responds to the examiners' questions during the interview. In adolescents and intelligent children, the examiner can test for abstraction ability by testing for similarities or by asking the individual to interpret proverbs.

Assessment of Writing and Reading

The child should be asked to write his or her name and the date. If the child is old enough, he or she should be asked to use cursive script because this type of writing is the most sensitive for detecting dysgraphia (difficulty in writing). The child should be asked to read and to carry out a written command, for example, "Go to the table, pick up the pencil, and bring it back to me."

Assessment of Calculating Ability

For the assessment of calculating ability, see the corresponding AMSIT section (see Chapter 3). Acalculia is a common developmental disorder and is a frequent concomitant of acute and progressive left posterior hemispheric lesions in children and adults (13).

Assessment of Immediate, Short-Term, and Long-Term Memory

As the examiner asks questions, he or she should observe the child's recall. Children who ask their parent (or other caregiver) either for assistance or to respond for them may have memory problems. Immediate memory can be tested by asking the child to repeat a number of digits forward and backward. By age 8 years, a normal child is expected to recall five digits forward and two or three digits backward; at age 10 years, the child should be able to recall six digits forward and four digits backward (11, p. 448). Short-term memory can be tested by giving the child three words and asking the child 5 minutes later to recall the words.

Assessment of Executive Functions

Executive functions could be defined as a number of higher cognitive activities (in an information-processing model), such as strategic planning, impulse control, organized search, flexibility of thought and action, and self-monitoring of one's behavior and activities; these functions help the child to maintain an appropriate mental set in order to achieve a future goal (10, p. 66). Such functions are thought to be localized in the prefrontal cortex. This area is not functionally mature until young adulthood (10, p. 69).

To assess executive functions, the examiner could ask the child to do a puzzle, for instance. The examiner should observe the child's behavioral organization and his or her capacity to maintain and to shift attention while performing the task. The examiner also should observe the child's degree of planning for and persistence with the given task and his or her approach to problem solving. The examiner should note the presence of impulsiveness, disinhibition, or perseverance.

■ INDICATIONS FOR CONSULTATION AND TESTING

Pediatric neurological consultation may be requested to ascertain the presence of neurological deficits and to pursue, when indicated, further neurological workup, including neuroimaging studies (e.g., computed tomography [CT] scan, magnetic resonance imaging [MRI]) (see Note 1) or electrophysiological studies (e.g., electroencephalogram [EEG], evoked potentials). Consultation with a speech and language pathologist is indicated when language and communication deficits are present. Speech and language assessment are currently underutilized. This evaluation helps the clinician to diagnose the nature of the language pathology and to determine an appropriate treatment approach. A geneticist should be consulted when chromosomal or genetic factors are suspected.

Assistance from psychologists and neuropsychologists is indispensable for both the evaluation and the treatment of neuropsychiatric conditions. The psychologist provides invaluable assistance in determining the child's intellectual abilities and achievement levels. Intellectual assessment scales, such as the Wechsler Intelligence Scale for Children Revised (WISC-R), indicate the child's verbal IQ (VIQ), which measures language-based, reasoning abilities, and the child's nonverbal performance IQ (PIQ), which measures visuospatial abilities. Test results may also suggest deficits that need further exploration through neuropsychological testing or language and speech assessment. When a discrepancy exists between the child's achievement level (i.e., grade placement in reading, spelling, or math) and the child's level of intelligence, the determination of learning disabilities, for purposes of psycho-educational programming, should be made. This general determination does not address the specific factors that contribute to the child's underachievement; elucidation of such factors may require neuropsychological testing.

The psychologist assists in the determination of subjective and interpersonal issues that are associated with neuropsychiatric disorders. These issues may precede, follow, or be concomitant with the evolution of neuropsychiatric pathology. Projective testing (e.g., Thematic Apperception Test, Rorschach Inkblot Test, Sentence Completion Test) helps the examiner to understand the child's ongoing psychological conflicts; to determine whether reality testing is intact; to establish the presence of thought disorder; to evaluate the child's relatedness (object relations), coping mechanisms, and psychological resources; and to establish the degree of depression or anxiety that may be present and the nature of the child's impulse control. The psychologist also helps the examiner to determine whether secondary gain is present.

Neuropsychological testing has a unique importance and relevance in the diagnosis and treatment of neuropsychiatric disorders. According to Harris, neuropsychological testing is

> particularly helpful in appreciating those mental status items that deal with speech/linguistic functions, memory, attention, executive functions (vigilance, set maintenance, planning, and inhibitory motor control), praxis (learned motor behavior), and visuomotor and visuospatial functions. In addition, the processing/production of social-emotional signals (including vocal tone, facial expression, and "body language," or gesture) is tested, although this is an area of ongoing research and new approaches are needed. (14, p. 20)

Harris emphasizes that "[t]he linking of test findings to adaptive function is crucial because children may compensate for the brain dysfunction in a way that the overall functioning is 'better than they look' on the tests applied" (14, p. 20).

Neuropsychological findings assist psychiatrists in the process of devising optimal rehabilitation programs for children who are recovering from brain injury or brain disease. Such findings also help child psychiatrists to construct—with the assistance of experts in special education, language pathology, and other specialties—optimal psychoeducational and remediation programs for children who have neuropsychological deficits.

■ INDICATIONS FOR NEUROPSYCHOLOGICAL TESTING

Neuropsychological testing is not a uniform examination: testing varies in scope and depth, and there are many schools and methods of neuropsychological assessment. Pendleton Jones and Butters explain:

> A major dichotomy in the field of neuropsychological assessment is characterized by the use of either a uniform battery for all patients or an individualized approach. Practitioners of an individualized approach usually administer a small, core group of tests to all patients, and then select further tests for the optimal elucidation of the referral questions or issues that may have been arisen during testing. Batteries undoubtedly have some advantages. These include comprehensiveness in the range of functions they sample. They greatly facilitate the combination of research with clinical objectives in that the same data-base will automatically be compiled for all patients. . . . A serious disadvantage of batteries is that they may be providing redundancy of information in some areas of functioning while achieving insufficient exploration of other areas. (15, p. 413)

Tranel, quoted by Harris (14), suggests a number of indications for neuropsychological testing (Table 7–3). In general, neuro-

TABLE 7–3. **Uses of neuropsychological testing**

Conducting diagnostic evaluation of developmental disorders

Identifying dysfunctional domains related to cognitive or behavioral disorders (nonverbal disabilities are the most challenging)

Detecting conditions not demonstrated on standard neurodiagnostic testing

Defining specific learning disorders (may also objectify subtle brain trauma)

Monitoring neuropsychological status

Assessing baseline and measuring recovery associated with therapies

Characterizing patient strengths for planning rehabilitation programs

Determining suitability for educational or vocational programs

Assisting in medico-legal situations

Determining responsibility in forensic examinations

Assisting in research

Source.   Based on Harris 1995 (14).

psychological batteries are reliable for children age 6 years and older. For younger children, neuropsychological testing involves combining a variety of age-appropriate motor, language, and cognitive tasks with various standardized assessments somewhat similar to those used in neuropsychological batteries administered to older individuals (16).

Table 7–4 summarizes the advantages and disadvantages of commonly used neuropsychological batteries and individualized approaches. One of the shortcomings of neuropsychological testing is the lack of ecological validity, meaning that testing results do not predict how the patient will perform in the real world (16). Table 7–5 summarizes the most common misconceptions about neuropsychological testing (regarding the testing process or its interpretation) that may lead to inaccurate expectations of the testing results in real-world settings (17). These misconceptions are equally applicable to neuropsychological testing and its interpretation in children and adolescents.

TABLE 7-4. **Advantages and disadvantages of the most commonly used neuropsychological batteries and individualized approaches**

Batteries	Advantages	Disadvantages
Halstead-Reitan Neuropsychological Battery (HRB)	Has been adapted for use with children: the Reitan-Indiana Test Battery for Children may be used with children ages 5–8 years; the Halstead-Neuropsychological Test Battery for Children is used with children ages 9–15 years.	As with other batteries, the accuracy of detecting structural brain damage declines when applied to psychiatric patients.
	Samples a wide range of functions.	Lacks measures of memory assessment.
	Trained clinicians can make inferences as to lesion localization and chronicity.	Lengthy and costly.
		Contains a large element of subjective evaluation.
		Does not reflect progress in neuropsychological assessment during the past 40+ years.
Luria-Nebraska Neuropsychological Battery (LNNB)	Brief and comprehensive.	Serious questions exist regarding standardization, validity, and reliability.
	Complex functions are divided into simple components so that more information is gleaned about the precise nature of the deficits.	It has been questioned whether the assessment method developed by Luria can be operationalized as a fixed battery.
	Can discriminate between brain-injured and control subjects and between brain-damaged patients and schizophrenic patients.	

Individualized approaches		
Boston Process Approach	Emphasizes higher cortical assessment and is flexible.	Standardization and validation are incomplete.
	Attention is focused on the patient's successes and failures.	Testing requires a high level of training and experience.
	Emphasizes process and strategy; similar deficits may reflect very different underlying processes.	
	Comprehensive in the areas of memory and language.	
	Useful and sensitive in rehabilitation planning.	
Muriel D. Lezac Approach	An individualized approach that emphasizes patient's successes and failures.	Test selection is critical.
	Contains the most comprehensive list of individual tests.	May require 6–9 hours of total administration time.

(continued)

TABLE 7–4. **Advantages and disadvantages of the most commonly used neuropsychological batteries and individualized approaches** *(continued)*

Batteries	Advantages	Disadvantages
Individualized approaches *(continued)*		
Arthur L. Benton Approach	An individualized and patient-oriented approach. Sequential process leads to a diagnostic decision. In 80% of cases, experienced neuropsychologists may complete testing in 60–90 minutes.	Tester requires a high level of training and experience.

Source. Based on Pendleton Jones and Butters 1991 (15, pp. 413–420).

TABLE 7–5.   **Misconceptions about neuropsychological testing**

A detailed clinical history and interviews of collateral sources are not necessary because such information may bias test interpretation. The neuropsychologist can simply rely on the patient's medical records to arrive at an understanding of the type of brain injury the patient sustained.

Defective performances on neuropsychological testing indicate cognitive dysfunction and/or brain damage, and defective performances on particular tests indicate dysfunction or damage to specific areas of the brain.

The neuropsychologist does not need to test or interview a particular patient if he or she has access to the patient's raw test data.

Collecting reliable test data is the neuropsychologist's primary goal. Careful interpretation of test data, using appropriate norms, is essential in arriving at accurate opinions about the patient's cognitive impairments or the localization of brain dysfunctions.

Changes in cognitive functioning are best determined by careful examination of serial neuropsychological test data.

It is unwise to continue testing a brain-injured patient if the patient becomes fatigued because the test data will become unreliable.

Brain-damaged patients should be tested in relatively quiet settings that are free from distractions or extraneous stimuli.

The neuropsychologist's primary responsibility is to record the patient's specific responses to specific test stimuli during testing. It is not necessary to record the amount and type of practice, cues, prompts, or various strategies given to or used by the patient during testing, because the raw test data are sufficient to determine the patient's cognitive impairments.

Test data can be interpreted accurately in the absence of information from other sources (e.g., historical information, medical records, academic records). Interpretations based on test data alone can predict the patient's ability to function at work, school, or home or in other real-world settings. It is not essential to observe the patient functioning outside the testing (laboratory) environment because careful interpretation of the test data will provide a sufficient basis for predicting how the patient is likely to respond in real-world settings.

(continued)

TABLE 7–5. **Misconceptions about neuropsychological testing** *(continued)*

Patients who sustain traumatic brain damage will make most of their recovery during the first 6 months and continue to recover for up to 2 years after the injury.

Intact performance on a standardized neuropsychological battery (e.g., WAIS-R, HRNB, LNNB) rules out the likelihood that the patient has cognitive deficits or sustained a brain insult.

Neuropsychological test reports need contain only a brief description of the reasons for referral, identifying information about the patient, the names of the test administered, the raw test data, and interpretation of the test data.

Neuropsychological tests can reliably identify brain damage if it is present. Intact performance on a variety of neuropsychological tests (e.g., the Category Test, the Wisconsin Card Sorting Test, the Trail Making Test) known to be sensitive to frontal lobe damage rules out the likelihood of frontal lobe pathology.

The results of neuropsychological testing should be consistent with the patient's complaints.

Source. Based on Sbordone 1997 (17, pp. 372–374).

■ SPECIFIC NEUROPSYCHIATRIC SYMPTOMS

Attention and Concentration Deficits

Attention processes are fundamental executive and neurocognitive functions that entail a variety of capacities, including sustained attention, selective attention, intensity of attention, and inhibitory control (18). Alertness, target detection, and vigilance are major components of the attention processes. *Alertness* refers to the readiness to process information and depends on the intactness of the right hemisphere. *Target detection,* or selection, depends on parietal lobe functioning and involves selective attention of a specific stimulus. The disengagement of attention from a given stimulus seems to be even more specific for intact parietal functions. *Vigi-*

lance refers to the mental effort needed to maintain attention. This "higher" aspect of attention involves effortless problem solving, motivation, and commitment to memory. Vigilance depends primarily on frontal lobe function (19, pp. 315–316). Subcortical structures (e.g., hypoactivity of the striatum) have been implicated in attention-deficit/hyperactivity disorder (ADHD) (19, p. 316).

Attention disturbances are implicated in a variety of psychopathologies: "Disorders of higher cognition may be related to attentive deficits. These include attention deficit/hyperactivity disorder, schizophrenia, traumatic brain injury and neglect syndromes" (20, p. 119). Disorders of attention are not unitary disturbances but "rather a loose association of symptoms affecting alertness or arousal, selective or focused attention, distractibility, sustained attention, and span of apprehension" (10, p. 365). Up to 20% of children with ADHD may also have a severe *social disability,* that is, profound deficits in interpersonal and social functioning.

ADHD is a primary disorder that can occur without other psychopathology; however, the disorder may accompany many neurological, psychiatric, and psychosocial conditions. Although distractibility and hyperactivity are the predominant features of ADHD, these symptoms are also found in many medical and neurological conditions. Garfinkel and Amrami consider the following conditions in the differential diagnosis of ADHD (19, p. 315):

- Organic disorders (e.g., lead intoxication; sensory disorders, especially deafness; frontal lobe lesions, such as abscesses and neoplasms; medication-induced attention deficit; antihistaminic, beta-agonists; substance abuse; mental retardation; seizure disorder; learning disabilities; pervasive developmental disorder)
- Functional disorders (e.g., conduct disorder, oppositional defiant disorder, affective disorder with manic characteristics, Tourette's syndrome and multiple tic disorder, adjustment disorder with disturbance of behavior, personality disorder, anxiety disorder, obsessive-compulsive disorder)

- Developmental disorders (e.g., age-appropriate hyperactivity) and situational, environmental, and family problems (e.g., inappropriate school placement involving gifted, learning disabled, or developmentally delayed children being placed in regular classrooms; a chaotic family setting; abuse or neglect)

Ferropenia; high doses of theophylline, cold medicines, decongestants; and conditions such as cerebral palsy or congenital and acquired brain disorders (e.g., brain injury sequelae) must be considered in the differential diagnosis of ADHD. Psychotropic medications may produce hyperactivity as a side effect: the stimulant medications used to treat ADHD, barbiturates, neuroleptics, antidepressants, and other medications may produce ADHD-related symptoms.

Delirium

Delirium occurs in children, but unfortunately it is seldom identified. Delirium is potentially life threatening and requires immediate medical attention. It usually has an acute or subacute presentation. Patients are inattentive and disoriented and display incoherent or rambling speech. They may appear to be in a stupor or a state of restless agitation. Perceptual disturbances (e.g., illusions and visual, auditory, or haptic hallucinations) are common. In addition, disturbances in the sleep-wake cycle or memory impairments may occur. Characteristically, the patient's level of alertness waxes and wanes: the patient may by oriented and alert at one moment and become disoriented and confused the next. This is the so-called sundowning effect. Autonomic instability (e.g., changes in heart rate, blood pressure, sweating, and pupillary changes) and mood and emotional alterations are common in delirium. Delirium should be suspected in patients who are taking psychotropic medications. Neuroleptic malignant syndrome and serotonin syndrome are life-threatening complications of psychotropic use.

The most common causes of delirium in children are physical

trauma, CNS infections, and intoxication. In adolescents, the most common culprits are CNS injuries caused by serious suicidal attempts (e.g., from hanging, carbon monoxide poisoning, or psychotropic drug overdoses), and side effects associated with abuse of hallucinogenic drugs and medication (including psychotropic medication side effects).

Seizure Disorders

The psychopathology related to seizure disorders has multiple causes: "Psychiatric morbidity related to seizure disorders is determined by several factors including underlying neuropathology, neural effects of ictal and interictal states, psychological effect of loss of consciousness or altered consciousness, family reaction to epilepsy, and psychotropic effects of anticonvulsant treatment" (6, p. 652). Commenting on Lindsay's studies, Cook and Leventhal say, "[A]s many as 85% of children with temporal lobe epilepsy had psychiatric disorders including mental retardation (25%) and disruptive behaviors (including 'hyperkinetic syndrome' and catastrophic rage), but only 30% had psychiatric disorders when followed to adulthood" (6, p. 652). Memory and attention are especially disturbed in patients with complex partial seizures, even in those with subclinical epileptiform discharges. This is particularly true if the left hemisphere is affected (10, pp. 324–325).

Aggressive behavior, mood disturbances, intolerance of frustration, poor integration into social groups, and marked dependency are common in children with seizures. Psychoses are more prevalent in children with left-hemispheric seizure foci. The following case example illustrates psychiatric consequences (i.e., aggressive behaviors and psychosis) in a child with poorly controlled seizures (see also Ralph's case example in Chapter 3):

> Ricardo, a 6-year-old Hispanic boy, was evaluated for oppositional and aggressive behaviors occurring at home and at school. His mixed seizure disorder (grand mal and complex partial) was poorly controlled primarily because of poor compliance with the

neurologist's recommendations. Ricardo was in the care of his maternal grandmother, who was frail, forgetful, and psychiatrically ill. The school had reported Ricardo's grandmother to the department of social services because Ricardo had come to school overmedicated on several occasions. When the school nurse checked on how much medication the grandmother had given Ricardo, it did not match the doctor's prescription.

The grandmother reported that Ricardo often stared into space and appeared confused. He would become unresponsive, his mouth would foam, and he would become cyanotic. The grandmother was more alarmed that the child often expressed fears that somebody was going to harm him. He had plucked out his teddy bear's eyes because, he reported, the teddy was "staring at me funny." Ricardo's sleep-deprived EEG confirmed the diagnosis of partial seizure symptomatology. Appropriate anticonvulsant medications and close monitoring ensured seizure control and produced marked improvement in Ricardo's aggressive behavior, paranoid symptoms, and overall symptomatology.

Cognitive Impairments

Cognitive impairments are either congenital or acquired. Congenital impairments constitute mental retardation. Children with mental retardation exhibit delays in neuromuscular and postural milestones and disturbances in attachment and social-relational behaviors, in language acquisition, and in communication competence. Several developmental assessment protocols aid in the assessment of cognitive impairments in infants and early preschoolers (e.g., Bailey Scales of Infant Development, Brazelton Neonatal Behavioral Assessment Scale, Denver Developmental Screening Test, Stanford-Binet, Vineland Adaptive Behavior Scales, Yale Revised Developmental Schedule). Ainsworth's Strange Situation aids in the determination and categorization of the infant's attachment competence. Children with mental retardation demonstrate academic difficulties and problems in the rate of acquisition of new skills. Because a number of mental retardation syndromes are potentially treatable (e.g., phenylketonuria), early identification is essential.

Ninety-five percent of genetic mental retardations are associated with the X chromosome. The most common causes of mental retardation are Down syndrome, fragile X syndrome, and fetal alcohol syndrome. These causes account for as many as 30% of the identified cases of mental retardation (21).

Because of diagnostic overshadowing, many psychiatric disorders are unrecognized in mentally retarded children. Such is the case with psychotic, mood, and anxiety disorders. ADHD and stereotyped habit disorders are common in these children.

Motor Coordination Deficits

Some children have a history of neurodevelopmental delays. For example, they sat and walked late or had late speech development. Other children display significant problems with fine and gross motor coordination. These children may not be able to walk straight, hop, skip, or jump; they have difficulty grasping and holding a pencil. Other children have problems learning to button their clothing and tie their shoelaces (this complex function requires efficient communication between the brain hemispheres). Some children have problems with balance, and others are delayed in learning to ride a tricycle or bicycle. Many of these children have difficulties in sports-related activities, which further contributes to their social isolation and problems with self-esteem.

Impulse-Control Difficulties

Many children with neuropsychological deficits demonstrate impulsive behaviors and a low tolerance for frustration. They become readily aggressive when things do not go their way, they demand immediate gratification, and they are intolerant of postponement of any of their wants. When not gratified, they throw temper tantrums or otherwise lose control. The extent and duration of the tantrums or the length of the dyscontrol depends on the child's capacity to modulate dysphoric states. Because of their aggressive behavior and lack of other social-interpersonal skills (e.g., sharing, empathy, reciprocity), these children have problems making and maintaining long-term friendships.

Impulsive behaviors reflect deficits in executive functions, and they may be a consequence of disinhibition, secondary to brain impairment. In these cases, children with a prior sense of propriety and solid judgment regarding sexual, aggressive, or appropriate social behaviors may display lapses in judgment in these areas. Impulsive behavior is common in children who have ADHD, conduct disorder, or psychotic disorders. Impulsiveness is a prominent feature of bipolar disorders and, in particular, mania.

Affect Dysregulation

Impairments in the expression, stability, and appropriateness of affect are common disturbances in neuropsychiatric patients. The neurological concepts of moria (an abnormal tendency to joke), apathy, brain-stem emotional lability, and others are examples of well-known adult emotional disturbances that are associated with specific neurophysiological or neuroanatomical impairments.

Depression and mania could be secondary to brain disorders. Explosive or blind rage in great disproportion to the eliciting situation are common after lesions of the frontal or temporal lobes. Otnow Lewis reviewed the neuroanatomical areas implicated in the regulation of aggressive behaviors: hypothalamus, amygdala, and orbital prefrontal cortex (22, p. 568). Functional impairment of these areas is implicated in behavioral dyscontrol.

Damage to the medial aspects of the frontal lobes renders the person incapable of initiating even primitive behaviors, such as getting out of bed or eating; the person also becomes devoid of affect or emotional responsivity. Even mild damage to this region produces a loss of spontaneity and creativity accompanied by flattening of affect; these symptoms may be misinterpreted as depression by well-meaning but uninformed psychotherapists (23, p. 145).

Aggressive behavior may have a neurological cause when

- The patient shows personality change and dyscontrol not shown previously
- The aggressive behavior is extreme in intensity and frequency
- The rage, violence, or destructive behaviors are unprovoked
- The patient has a history of or indications of brain injury (e.g., children who have been physically abused may have sustained a brain injury)
- The patient is remorseful and expresses disbelief about his or her loss of control

Although complex partial seizures are frequently implicated in intermittent aggressive dyscontrol, there is limited evidence to support this connection.

The following brain regions have been implicated in pathological aggressive behavior in adults: the medial hypothalamus (involved in rage, amnesia, and hyperphagia), the orbitofrontal cortex (involved in disinhibited, impulsive behavior and emotional lability), the temporal lobe (involved in interictal aggression; ictal aggression is uncommon), and the caudate nucleus (involved in irritability, impulsiveness, and emotional lability) (24, p. 123). Impaired functioning of analogous structures needs to be substantiated for corresponding disorders in children.

Regarding mood disorders in adults, depression is most common in disorders that produce dysfunction of the left frontal lobe, the temporal lobes, and the left caudate nucleus (24, p. 125). Most of the focal lesions that produce mania involve the right hemisphere: the inferior frontal lobe, temporo-basal region, or thalamic-perithalamic areas. Degenerative and infectious illnesses that affect the frontal lobes or frontal-subcortical systems have also caused mania (24, p. 126). Analogous lesions and symptom expression in children awaits substantiation.

The neuroanatomy of anxiety in adults is uncertain: "The focal lesions associated with increased anxiety have undergone relatively little investigation. Left frontal cortical lesions, temporal lobe disorders, and basal ganglia diseases have been associated with anxiety symptoms" (24, p. 126). Even less is known about the neuroanatomy of anxiety in children.

Neuropsychiatric Aspects of Social and Interpersonal Difficulties

Some children have selective deficits in social behavior secondary to an inability to process and understand affective cues or interpersonal nonverbal behavior. These deficits are the so-called social and emotional learning disabilities (25). Children with these disabilities cannot "read" affect or other nonverbal cues in social contexts and thus do not respond appropriately in social exchanges. As such, they have problems expressing affect appropriate to a given social situation and cannot understand the subtleties of complex social interactions. These children may also have difficulties understanding jokes and metaphoric language.

These children may have problems with the motor programming of face and limb affective gestures and affective prosody and, as a result, exhibit an emotional flatness, robotic speech, and an array of atypical social behaviors (25). They may be inappropriately affectionate and "sticky." Their lack of normal affective expression, their gaze disturbances, their tendency to violate social space, and their "stickiness" all contribute to their oddness. These children likely do not understand the perspective of others and as a result are apt to make disastrous social faux pas (25, p. 796). In adults these deficits frequently represent nondominant hemispheric dysfunction. The situation in the developing brain may not be as straightforward. These deficits may be dissociated from other academic and neuropsychological deficits associated with right-hemisphere impairments.

Psychosis

Psychotic symptoms are commonly observed in child and adolescent psychiatric practice. A variety of hallucinatory and delusional symptoms are caused by neurological dysfunctions. Temporal lobe epilepsy (complex partial symptomatology), although elusive in its detection, always must be considered in the differential diagnosis of psychotic disorders. Taylor et al. stress this issue in adult psychiatry: "[E]ven in the absence of a classic epileptic picture and course, temporal lobe disease should be considered in the differential diagnosis of psychosis" (3, p. 10). This is equally true in the differential diagnosis of psychosis in children and adolescents (see Ralph's case example in Chapter 3, Samuel's case example in Chapter 4, and Ricardo's case example earlier in this chapter). Rick's and Troy's case examples in Chapter 4 involve a variety of other neuropsychological deficits. See also Abe's case example later in this chapter for a connection between temporal lobe injury and psychosis.

When performing the perception portion of the AMSIT (see Chapter 3), the examiner should go beyond the customary questions regarding the presence of auditory and visual hallucinations and inquire about the presence of olfactory, gustatory, haptic, sensory, somatic, and other perceptual disturbances (e.g., out-of-body experiences, derealization, premonitions, déjà vu, jamais vu) and delusional symptoms.

Cummings implicated the limbic system and the temporal lobes in some delusional disorders in adults: "Although lesions associated with delusions occur in diverse brain locations, they commonly involve the limbic system. Lesions of the temporal lobes have the highest frequency of associated delusional disorders, and bilateral lesions are more likely to produce delusions than unilateral disorders" (24, p. 124). Analogous neuroanatomical attribution in children awaits pertinent substantiation.

Autistic Behavior

Autistic disorder, or autism, is one of the most severe psychiatric disturbances and the most dehumanizing neuropsychiatric condition. Autism is characterized by 1) a lack of communication language, 2) a lack of interpersonal relatedness, 3) an unusual preoccupation with inanimate objects, and 4) a need for sameness.

Cook and Leventhal asserted that the abnormal development of social reciprocity is one of the most striking features of autism and that the social, communicative, imaginative, and cognitive elements of the disorder are inextricably linked (6, p. 645). Autism is usually accompanied by a variety of profound neurodevelopmental problems. Brain anomalies and brain dysfunction(s) are considered the main cause of this perplexing syndrome (26, p. 773). Mental retardation is present in about 80% of patients with autism, and neurological findings are present in about 60%–70% of autistic children. By adolescence, up to 30% of autistic children develop a seizure disorder. Autism is associated with conditions such as phenylketonuria, fragile X syndrome, *Varicella* infection in utero, toxoplasmosis, cytomegalovirus infection, and other identifiable illnesses.

The Autism Diagnostic Interview, the Autism Diagnostic Observation Scale, and the Childhood Autism Rating Scale are standardized instruments for the diagnosis of autistic disorder. Chapter 4 (see section on very early onset schizophrenia) suggests exploratory questions pertinent to the interview of children with early severe developmental disturbances.

Obsessive-Compulsive Disorder

Obsessive-compulsive disorder (OCD) occurs in conjunction with diseases of the basal ganglia. The caudate nucleus or the globus pallidus may be involved. In adults, most disorders that produce OCD symptoms affect the basal ganglia bilaterally (24, p. 127). In OCD patients, an increase of bilateral prefrontal and anterior cingulate gyri activity has been reported. These observations have been interpreted as consistent with a "frontal lobe–limbic–basal ganglia loop" mechanism (27, p. 687). OCD is frequently associated with Tourette's syndrome: OCD is described in 10%–40% of children with Tourette's syndrome. See Chapter 4 for the differential diagnosis of OCD. The following case example illustrates the development of OCD in a child:

Donald, a 12-year-old Caucasian boy, was evaluated for possible ADHD and for behaviors that included stealing, lying, and cross-dressing. He had also voiced suicidal thoughts but had made no suicidal attempts. Learning disorders and expressive language difficulties were suspected.

Donald was an adopted child; his oldest brother was $4\frac{1}{2}$ years his senior and his parents' only natural child. Donald's parents had been divorced for 7 years prior to the evaluation; they maintained a very active, hostile relationship. Each parent spoke badly about the other in front of the children. Donald's mother had been sexually abused as a child and had a mood disorder. She was in poor health and, at the time of the evaluation, was receiving medical, psychiatric, and psychotherapeutic treatment. She was frustrated with the uncertainties of Donald's diagnosis.

Donald had been mainstreamed at school. There were no serious complaints about his behavior in the classroom. At home, however, Donald created a great deal of distress for his mother: he procrastinated about his homework and chores and frustrated his brother and mother on an ongoing basis. Donald irritated his brother by getting into his "things" and his mother by his persistent argumentative, oppositional, and defiant behavior. Donald also had a history of fascination with fires.

The mental status examination revealed the presence of a small, somewhat meek male who was not spontaneous. There was an air of immaturity about him. He displayed frequent tics in the upper left side of his face. His speech disclosed significant hesitation and a considerable degree of stuttering. The examiner observed occasional grunting and throat clearing. Donald's mood appeared mildly depressed. His affect was appropriate but constricted. There was no evidence of thought disorder or of any perceptual disorder. Donald denied suicidal or homicidal ideation. He indicated no concerns about his cross-dressing problem. His sensorium was intact, and he was of average intelligence. He displayed no insight into his problems, and in general, he demonstrated marked passivity about what was going on with him and around him.

One year after the initial evaluation, Donald's mother reported that he was becoming progressively more preoccupied with sex. She suspected that he masturbated frequently using stuffed animals. There were indications that he used the dolls for his sexual practices because his mother frequently found the dolls with openings that corresponded to the genital areas. On more than one occasion, Donald's brother and mother had seen him wearing feminine undergarments. Donald's mother often could not find some of her pantyhose, panties, brassieres, or shoes. Furthermore, when trying on her shoes, she would sometimes notice that they seemed stretched out. She suspected that Donald wore some of her shoes when he cross-dressed.

When Donald's mother received her latest telephone and credit card bills, she realized that Donald had charged thousands of dollars in calls to various sex lines. Donald seemed obsessed with sex. It was at this time that OCD was suspected. Donald was experiencing powerful sexual compulsions. He started taking fluoxetine with very positive results. On fluoxetine, Donald's sexual preoccupation lessened, and his compulsion to call the sex lines decreased.

Paraphilia and Hypersexuality

Regarding abnormal sexual behavior in adults, Cummings indicated that paraphilias have been associated with frontal lobe disorders (e.g., frontal degeneration, multiple sclerosis), basal ganglia diseases [e.g., Huntington's disease, Tourette's syndrome (see Donald's case example in the preceding section), or Parkinson's disease following treatment with dopaminergic agents), and epilepsy (24). Hypersexuality may be attributed to secondary mania, Klüver-Bucy syndrome, and septal lesions (24, p. 127) (see Ruben's case example later in this chapter). Similar neuroanatomical attributions in childhood await substantiation.

Memory Impairments (Amnesias)

Harris has commented that the various forms of memory are mediated by separate brain systems (20). Conscious memory (i.e., declarative or explicit memory) and nonconscious memory (i.e., nondeclarative or implicit memory—involved in acquisition of skills, habits, and other procedures) use different neuroanatomical systems. The hippocampus and its related structures are essential for declarative or explicit memory. Other structures are necessary for nondeclarative or implicit memory. The hippocampus and related structures are needed for the establishment of enduring memory, but long-term memory storage is believed to involve the neocortex. Nondeclarative memory appears to be stored in specific sensory and motor pathways. The cerebellum seems to be an important site for classical conditioning of skeletal musculature (20, p. 142). The role of the hippocampal region (medial temporal lobe) in amnesia is defined by Zola: "[T]he findings show that circumscribed bilateral lesions limited to the hippocampal region are sufficient to produce amnesia. Additional findings indicate that the cortical regions adjacent to and anatomically linked to the hippocampal region—i.e., the perirhinal, entorhinal, and parahippocampal cortices—are also important for memory function" (28, p. 458).

Heindel and Salloway (29) expand on the above concepts: "[S]tudies have convincingly demonstrated that memory should not be thought of as a single, homogeneous entity, but rather as being composed of several distinct yet mutually interacting memory systems that are mediated by specific neuroanatomical substrates" (p. 19). The authors integrate four memory systems: 1) *working memory,* composed of storing and manipulating information for a very short period of time (20–30 seconds), under central executive control, neuroanatomically based in the prefrontal cortex; 2) *episodic memory,* information that is remembered within a temporal or spatial context, mediated by the medial temporal lobe and the diencephalon; 3) *semantic memory,* the fund of general knowledge not dependent on contextual clues for retrieval, mediated by the temporoparietal association cortex; and 4) *procedural memory,* an unconscious way of remembering that is expressed through the performance of specific operations comprising a particular task, mediated by the basal ganglia (29, pp. 19–20).

Children with static encephalopathies or with anomalies in brain embryogenesis may experience serious memory dysfunction. Learning or language disorders in some children may be the result of memory difficulties. These deficits can be demonstrated with careful testing and must be confirmed with pertinent neuro-psychological testing. Memory difficulties are caused by encoding difficulties or by retrieval problems. The following case example illustrates a predominant encoding memory disturbance in a child who has multiple neuropsychiatric and neuropsychological problems:

Ruben, a 12-year-old Hispanic boy, was evaluated after his teacher overheard him saying that he had a person inside him who talked to him and told him to harm himself and others. During the evaluation, Ruben claimed he had this person inside him since he was 4 years old. He claimed that the person had asked him not to tell anyone and had even threatened to throw him in front of cars or trains if he were to do so. Ruben's mother learned about the "person" 2 days before the psychiatric evaluation when Ruben had been intercepted running toward railroad tracks, intending to kill himself. Apparently he was responding to commanding voices that were telling him to get run over by the train.

Ruben had a history of self-abusive behavior and had also displayed suicidal behavior. During the summer, 2 or 3 months earlier, Ruben's self-abusive behavior took a turn for the worse. Ruben had a number of unexplained accidents over the previous months. These incidents included cutting his finger, burning his left forearm, and falling frequently.

Ruben revealed that he had hurt a baby and another boy and that he had sexually abused a 7-year-old boy. He also disclosed episodes in which he had sexually molested his 9-year-old brother and had displayed sexual behavior toward his babysitter.

Ruben had been retained in school for 4 years in a row because "he didn't seem to be able to learn anything," according to his mother. He attended a special education program for second grade.

When Ruben was born, doctors discovered that he had a heart murmur and operated on him, after which time he remained in an incubator for 3 months. He also had three eye surgeries. He had no history of seizures. Ruben had a history of significant neurodevelopmental delays: he sat at 12–14 months, walked at 3 years, and talked between ages 3 and 4 years. He had been toilet trained by age 3 years. He had no history of enuresis. When Ruben was asked to do a chore, such as taking out the trash, he repeatedly came back to ask what he was supposed to do. Any expectation of him had to be repeated many times.

Ruben's mother had attempted suicide previously and had a history of psychiatric hospitalizations. She had a stroke 2 months before this examination and had ongoing problems with alcohol. Ruben's father had never cared for nor provided for Ruben or his brother.

During the family interview Ruben and his mother related positively. The mental status examination revealed a Hispanic male who appeared his chronological age. Ruben wore glasses, and at the beginning of the interview he displayed a serious countenance. Ruben endorsed auditory and visual hallucinations, saying that he heard and saw Robert, or Robbie, the person inside him. He also acknowledged hearing voices telling him to do bad things to himself and to others. He said that 2 days earlier, he had seen Robbie: he was all red and had horns. Ruben said that Robbie had always been like that. Ruben also heard people other than Robbie; these people were with Robbie. Robbie was real to Ruben, but he acknowledged that at times his actions were the result of his own thoughts. He claimed that he was able to put Robbie away from his mind for a little while. Ruben disclosed sexual excitement and preoccupation. He was oriented to time, place, and person. As Ruben began to relax, he became more pleasant. Ruben also exhibited expressive and receptive language problems and a limited vocabulary. The examiner had to repeat many of the questions more than once before Ruben could attempt to answer them. Ruben's intelligence, insight, and judgment were considered impaired.

Summary of positive findings (see Note 2 for other findings):

Physical examination.   Ruben exhibited synophrys (eyebrows meeting in the middle) and hyperthelorism (eyes appreciably more separated than normal. A periscapular surgical scar, related to the neonatal heart surgery, was present. Heart auscultation was unremarkable.

Neurological consultation. Ruben exhibited dysmorphic features (e.g., hyperthelorism, prominent ears, fragmented and abnormal palm creases). He had global difficulties with reading, writing, and mathematics, and multiple perceptual deficits, including sequential memory deficits (auditory and visual) and right-left disorientation. His human drawing showed a lack of detail, consistent with important body-schema deficits. Cranial nerves, muscle power, tone, deep tendon reflexes, gait, and stance all were normal. Multiple scars were noted, as was a birthmark on the left side of the neck. The diagnostic impression was of static encephalopathy, r/o chromosomal abnormalities (to rule out a genetic disease), and possible fragile X syndrome. Chromosomal studies, a sleep-deprived EEG, and an MRI were recommended. The chromosomal analysis showed a normal chromosomal count (46XY) and no fragile X abnormality. The EEG showed no focal or paroxysmal abnormalities. The MRI showed striking cell migration deficits, a fissure in the right temporo-parietal-occipital area, another milder cleft toward the central fissure, and evidence of pachygyria (abnormal clustering of gyri) and microgyria (gyri smaller than normal). Diagnosis: schizencephaly.

Cognitive testing. Scores on the WISC-III were as follows: full-scale IQ was 73, VIQ was 58 (intellectually deficient range), and PIQ was 93 (average range).

Projective testing. Ruben's performance was consistent with an affective psychosis with depressive features; significant organic impairment was present. He exhibited no psychosis at the time of testing, but on reality testing he showed a propensity to deteriorate under minor stresses. Schizotypal personality features were suggested.

Neuropsychological testing. The neuropsychologist elicited a history of head trauma at age 6 years when Ruben fell from the monkey bars at school. There was no loss of consciousness. Ruben's speech and language were remarkable for problems of syntax, grammar, word usage, and content organization. He used the word "thing" when he did not know the correct name for something or substituted a less accurate term (e.g., he called light bulb filaments "needles"). Ruben's expressive language suggested occasional loosening of the thought processes secondary to tangential thinking. His receptive language also appeared impaired. Ruben frequently did not understand instructions and questions. For example, when asked how many things make a dozen, he replied "eggs." Ruben appeared to have difficulty remembering previously attempted combinations when using a trial-and-error approach. He lost points on timed tasks because of task behavior (e.g., stopping to rub his forehead), and he appeared overly concerned with noncritical aspects of his performance (e.g., perfectly lining up cards on a timed sequencing task)

Language.   Ruben's language skills were generally impaired. His sentence construction was below average. His overall verbal abstraction and expressive skills were within the intellectually deficient range, and his receptive vocabulary was below expectations based on age.

Attention and memory.   Significant auditory and visuo-perceptual deficits interfered with concentration and encoding into memory. Ruben persisted at tasks; however, his distractibility score on the WISC-III was in the intellectually deficient range, reflecting his perceptual processing problems.

Ruben's immediate recall of digits was substantially below average, and his immediate recall of sentences was in the second percentile. His delayed recall for a story was below the first percentile; however, the difference between Ruben's immediate and delayed memory for the story was minimal, indicating a problem with encoding rather than with retrieval. Ruben's learning and recall for a word list was also below expectations; he did not appear to use organizational strategies to enhance learning. This pattern of performance further indicated encoding problems. Ruben's short-term memory for spatial coordinates was impaired. His visual reproduction memory, as assessed by drawing geometric designs, was in the ninth percentile for immediate reproduction.

Executive functions.   Ruben's executive functions were mildly impaired. He had some difficulty maintaining a cognitive set and generating new strategies when needed. His cognitive flexibility was mildly impaired.

Diagnostic impression.   In summary, Ruben's memory difficulties were more related to encoding difficulties secondary to attention-concentration deficits. Ruben also had broad language and cognitive impairments. These neuropsychological disorders are probably related to impairment of cell migration during cortical embryogenesis.

Although problems of retrieval are a common cause of memory difficulties, deficits of encoding need to be ruled out in children who demonstrate memory impairments: Ruben is a case in point (see also the case of Frances later in this chapter).

Soft Neurological Signs

Soft neurological signs have nonspecific neuropsychiatric significance. They are not localizing and are not invariably associated with specific structural lesions. Their clinical significance has been variably interpreted by different clinicians, and arbitrary hierarchical attributions have been assigned. They are closely related to the child's developmental status, because many of these signs are present at an early age. Soft neurological signs are often considered as evidence of developmental immaturity or of a developmental lag as they persist in older children. Soft signs are slightly more common in children who have several different types of psychiatric disorders. It is impossible to attach a well-defined clinical significance to soft signs. Within a specific diagnostic group, soft signs may have some predictive value (8, p. 455). The Physical and Neurological Examination for Soft Signs (PANESS) is the preferred assessment instrument for soft neurological signs.

Regressive Behavior

The loss of cognitive abilities or of acquired personal, social, or behavioral skills should call into question the integrity of the child's CNS. Clinicians should be cautious in making diagnostic closures in the assessment of regressive behavior. The following case example is illustrative:

Roger, a 7-year-old Caucasian boy, was referred for a psychiatric evaluation for regressive behavior. He had stopped talking and had problems eating. At school, he seemed listless and had limited academic progress. Roger also had problems with enuresis and encopresis. When Roger's mother was asked about a history of similar problems in the family, she casually commented that many boys in her family had died at a very early age. Because the neurological examination was positive for equivocal Babinski's signs bilaterally, and because Roger displayed feeding difficulties, he was referred to a pediatric neurologist. At first, the pediatric neurologist did not find reason to consider a neurological disorder; she suspected a functional disorder. A pediatric psychiatric consultation established that Roger had a psychotic disorder. Serendipitously, the neurologist later noticed hyperpigmented creases in Roger's hands, after which adrenal gland involvement (Addison's disease) was confirmed. A brain CT scan showed extensive demyelination in the frontal and temporoparietal areas. A diagnosis of adrenoleukodystrophy was made. The dementing and deteriorating course of the illness continued unremittingly until Roger became bedridden a few years later.

What was initially interpreted as a lack of academic progress was early evidence of a progressive loss of cognitive faculties, and what was initially called enuresis and encopresis was a loss of voluntary sphincter control, a sign of frontal lobe dysfunction.

Child psychiatrists have a key role in identifying dementing disorders with onset in childhood. Some of these disorders (e.g., Wilson's disease) are potentially treatable. Prompt identification is important for appropriate clinical management, including timely genetic counseling. Goodman recommends initiation of investigations to detect organicity and appropriate referrals 1) if the child loses well-established linguistic, academic, or self-help skills and performs below previous levels, 2) if features emerge that are suggestive of brain disorder, or 3) if risk factors for genetic or infectious disease (e.g., a father with Huntington's disease or a mother with AIDS) are present (1, pp. 179–180). According to Goodman, the most common disorders presenting with dementing symptoms in child psychiatric practice are as follows: Batten disease, Wilson's disease, Huntington's disease, adrenoleukodystrophy, juvenile-onset metachromatic leukodystrophy, subacute sclerosing panencephalitis, HIV encephalopathy, Rett syndrome, pervasive developmental disorders (e.g., disintegrative disorders, autism), convulsive disorders (e.g., Lennox-Gastaut syndrome, Landau-Kleffner syndrome), cerebral palsy, and head injury (1, pp. 180–186).

Some severely regressive patients may exhibit complex and confusing clinical pictures that mimic neurodegenerative disorders. For example, an 11-year-old preadolescent developed progressive speech difficulties and stopped eating. He was referred to a university hospital. The neurological workup (including neuroimaging) was negative. Under Amytal Sodium, he began to talk about his history of severe physical abuse. Acute regressive pictures with complex psychiatric symptomatology have been observed in children with complex partial seizures who did not have a history of seizures.

Traumatic Brain Injury

Birmaher and Williams have highlighted risk-taking behavior as one of the causes of traumatic brain injury:

> Implicitly, the issue of risk-taking behavior as an etiologic contributor to traumatic brain injury among children and adolescents is an important consideration. . . . [A] number of studies . . . point to the elevated incidence of documented alcohol use, preexisting cognitive deficits, preexistent deviant behavior, and diminished parental emotional stability among youngsters suffering traumatic brain injury. . . . Children with head injuries have tended to be impulsive, aggressive, attention-seeking, and behaviorally disturbed, engendering a greater probability of being in dangerous situations likely to result in accidents. The families of children experiencing accidents also show more parental illness and mental disorder, more social disadvantages of various kinds, and less adequate supervision of children's play activities than is found in the general population. (30, pp. 370–371)

It is not a simple matter to disentangle the sequelae of traumatic brain injury from antecedent deficits. Bennet et al. (23) classified the sequelae of traumatic brain injury into four categories (Table 7–6).

Many of the complications and sequelae of brain injury are illustrated in the following case example:

> Abe, a 13-year-old Caucasian adolescent, the son of two physicians, was evaluated for depression, suicidal behavior, and increasingly aggressive dyscontrol. He had hit a child with a rock, and on another occasion he had to be separated from the same child. Eighteen months earlier, on the first day of a vacation, he

---

TABLE 7–6. Sequelae of traumatic brain injury

Major cognitive sequelae

    Decrease in speed and efficiency of information processing

    Difficulties with attention and concentration

    Learning and memory problems

    Perception difficulties

    Language and communication problems

    Problems with executive functions

    Decrease in level of intelligence

Major affective and personality sequelae

    Organic personality changes

    Reactive personality changes

Noncognitive sequelae

    Sensory complaints

    Posttraumatic headaches

    Posttraumatic epilepsy

    Sleep disturbances

Psychological reaction to the brain injury

    Adjustment to adaptive impairments

    Changes in self-concept and body image

Source. Based on Bennet et al. 1997 (23, pp. 138–154).

was "accidentally hit" with a golf club in the left frontotemporal area. X rays demonstrated a depressed frontotemporoparietal skull fracture. Abe was comatose for 10 days. He sustained an intraparenchymatous hematoma (bleeding within the brain) and lacerations of the frontal and temporal lobes. After neurosurgical intervention, Abe experienced expressive aphasia and right-side hemiplegia (paralysis). He also had difficulties swallowing and controlling his bowel functions. By the time of the psychiatric evaluation, Abe had achieved a "wonderful recovery": most of the overt aphasia and hemiplegia had resolved. However, subtle impairments remained: he had difficulties writing because of a loss of a fine-motor coordination of the right hand, and he had episodic difficulties in word finding. Problems with concentration had also been observed.

Abe, who had been an honor student, was struggling to catch up at school and complained that the school's demands were harder to meet than before. Abe's parents noticed that he was painfully aware of his limitations and functional loss. They also noticed significant personality changes. Abe had become more irritable, and he was prone to angry outbursts and to frequent confrontations with his father. He had pushed his father and hit him in the chest on one occasion. He also had become destructive and self-abusive (e.g., he engaged in head banging). Abe became progressively more demoralized and began to show evidence of withdrawal and loss of motivation and interest.

The mental status examination showed a handsome teenager who was small for his age and was uncooperative and unfriendly during the interview. When Abe talked, he seemed to be making a deliberate effort to communicate. His difficulties with word finding and his loss of fluency of speech were observed intermittently. His sensorium was intact, and his intellectual function was assessed as above average. No disturbance in the thought processes was detected. Abe endorsed auditory hallucinations in the form of voices that talked to him and put him down; he denied other hallucinatory experiences. Abe denied paranoid ideation and denied suicidal thinking at the time of the evaluation. His judgment and insight were considered fair. Abe tended to argue and disagree with most of his parents' concerns.

A neuropsychological assessment before the psychiatric assessment, 18 months after the trauma, showed a dramatic recovery from most of the cognitive, language, and motor deficits seen 15 months earlier. Abe demonstrated some speech hesitancies but none of the dysfluencies and paraphasias observed earlier. He had motor-related problems in writing, but his problems with spelling and reading (i.e., pronunciation) had resolved. Motor coordination in his right hand had improved to the point that he could write slowly and perform many fine motor tasks, although he still needed to use the support of his left hand from time to time. His measured intelligence had increased to the superior range on IQ scores that did not require fine motor responses. The tactile response in Abe's right hand was mildly reduced. Abe was cooperative and easy to manage during a full day of testing, in contrast to problems seen earlier. Rapport with the tester was appropriate even though Abe had reported auditory hallucinations. The neuropsychologist suggested that the hallucinations could be related to the lesion of the temporal lobe and that the lack of motivation for reading could be related to residual language impairments.

Abe received the diagnosis of a mood disorder with psychotic features associated with a medical (i.e., neurological) condition. He was referred to a residential therapeutic program to help him to handle frustration and anger with more appropriate and adaptive behaviors and to help him to deal with issues of chronic demoralization and ongoing problems with his parents.

It is not true that the recovery from brain injury stops after the first year of the injury. Patients have shown significant improvements in cognitive functioning 2–5 years and 5–10 years after the injury. Patients who sustained severe traumatic brain injuries have demonstrated significant improvement in social, physical, and emotional functioning 2 years after the injury (17, p. 380).

In this book, we have presented some case examples in which postnatal brain injuries, involving neurocognitive and linguistic sequelae, had a prominent role in the patient's dysfunction (e.g., see Frances's case example later in this chapter and Johnny's case example in Chapter 10). In general, the prognosis after traumatic brain injury depends on the degree of intactness of the CNS (or on the degree of structural damage) as demonstrated by neuroimaging studies.

Learning Difficulties

Learning difficulties are rarely the primary reason for initial consultation with the child psychiatrist; however, they are common comorbid conditions for a number of psychiatric disorders (e.g., ADHD, Tourette's syndrome, conduct disorder, mood disorders). Language disorders are commonly associated with learning problems, and some experts believe that language deficits are the underlying cause of most learning disabilities.

Positron-emission tomography (PET) studies in men with persistent developmental dyslexia demonstrated a failure to activate "the left temporo-parietal cortex during a phonological and rhyme-detection task and the right temporal cortex during a nonlanguage task" (31, p. 12). These abnormalities are in contrast to "robust activation of the left inferior frontal regions during a syntax task involving sentence comprehension" (31, p. 12). The posterior portion of the large-scale language networks may be affected in dyslexia. Convergent findings indicate that the posterior temporal and nearby occipital and parietal regions are involved in dyslexia and in phonological deficits (31).

Language Disorders

The diagnosis of aphasia needs special consideration. Speech apraxias, dysnomias, and other production or expressive disorders need proper and timely identification. Among receptive language disorders, a congenital word deafness (verbal auditory agnosia) has been described. It entails an inability to differentiate speech sounds from other environmental sounds (so-called auditory imperception). Neologisms and idioglossia (unintelligible verbal utterances) are common in receptive disorders (10, p. 430). Among the expressive disorders, the examiner must distinguish dysfunctions secondary to neuromuscular control and coordination (i.e., dysarthria), defects at the motor level of speech production (i.e., apraxias), and defects in the production of language at the semantic level (i.e., lexical and syntax deficits) (10, p. 432).

The consequences of childhood-acquired aphasia appear to be long lasting and extend in time far beyond the disappearance of aphasic symptoms. Even when clinical signs of aphasia abate, full and functional pragmatic language will not necessarily be acquired or restored. Academic achievement continues to be poor, and failure to accrue new knowledge may be more pronounced over time, perhaps because of the increasing demands in the higher grades (12, p. 738; see also Frances's case example later in this chapter). Language disorders have far-reaching implications for children's cognitive, social, and learning competencies. Early identification and treatment are of the utmost importance (32).

A close association exists between language disorders and psychopathology. At least 50% of children with language disorders have associated psychopathology. When children with unsuspected language impairments (USLI) were compared with children with previously identified language impairments (PILI) and with children with normal language development, the USLI children were considered to have more ADHD symptoms and the most severe problems with aggression and delinquency when rated by teachers and parents. Parents of USLI children rated them as more delinquent than did the parents of children with PILI across all ages. The parents of children with PILI appeared to make accommodations for their children's communication difficulties, which protects these children from being blamed unnecessarily for some of their behavior (33). Early identification is so important because it seems to improve the parents' level of empathy toward the child and may decrease the frequency of negative interactions between the child and the parents.

Receptive language disorders have the worst prognosis among the language disorders. Disorders of pronunciation and stuttering are fairly common in childhood. See Chapter 3 for a discussion of issues related to the developmental language and communication components of the AMSIT.

■ INTERVIEWING CHILDREN WHO HAVE LEARNING DISABILITIES OR OTHER NEUROPSYCHIATRIC DEFICITS

An inner language is necessary for the formation of self-concept and for the understanding of the self in relation to others. Inner language also facilitates self-awareness and conceptualization of problem solving. It permits transmission of mental contents such as thoughts, memories, and emotions in ways that can be understood in interpersonal communication.

Inner language allows trial action and planning and is a prerequisite for understanding psychological and interpersonal problems. Verbalization or the capacity to communicate inner experience is necessary for the process of change. Children with learning disabilities have problems processing information and difficulties in encoding or decoding affects. As a consequence, mood disorders in this population may have a different clinical outlook, in particular, in their nonverbal display. This difference may mislead examiners.

Children with language disorders or learning disabilities lack the capacity to use language as an efficient and reliable information-processing tool; they also cannot use language for verbal, conceptual planning prior to action. These problems contribute to the child's sense of isolation, personal inhibition, diminished sense of competence, and poor self-concept. Rarely are these children able to convey their inner lives satisfactorily. For children with language disorders, communicating (or attempting to communicate) with others demands great effort, generates anxiety, and brings disappointing results. For these children, putting thoughts together and organizing thinking—in a relevant and meaningful manner—is usually a difficult, laborious, and frustrating task.

The challenge in the diagnostic assessment of these children lies in the timely identification of their communication difficulties. The examiner must open communication channels that compensate for the child's language limitations. By creating such pathways, the examiner facilitates the child's expression of his or her psychological and interpersonal problems.

Although verbalization is the most efficient modality for self-revelation, the diagnostic assessment of children with language impairments must be aided by a variety of expressive, nonverbal techniques (e.g., drawing, playing, puppetry, kinetic or mimetic enactments). In cases of receptive language deficits, the examiner has the added challenge of ensuring that the child understands what the examiner says or wants to convey. The examiner must use simple, deliberate, and redundant language. The examiner also needs to verify on an ongoing basis that he or she is being understood.

Many children with language difficulties acquired in the maturational-developmental process use so-called pragmatic behaviors (e.g., nodding to imply assent) to please others and to secure acceptance. The naive interviewer may misunderstand this adaptive nonverbal body language. For example, when the examiner is talking, the child may be nodding as if conveying that he or she follows the examiner's verbalizations. The nodding misleads the examiner because it is a learned behavior the child incorporated to fit into the social milieu; nodding does not guarantee that the child understands. The examiner needs to break through this adaptive facade by repeatedly asking for feedback until he or she is certain that the child is processing or understanding what is being communicated. We have evaluated children who have been referred because of apparent psychotic features. These children were said to "talk to themselves" and so on. Careful observations revealed that these children were thinking aloud or trying out the ideas they wanted to convey or were about to express. This self-talk was trial speech.

The following case example involves a child with aphasia, profound neuropsychological problems, and global cognitive deficits whose interpersonal behavior baffled his teachers.

Frances, an 11-year-old Caucasian girl, was referred by the school district for assessment of "psychotic behavior," specifically because "the child talks to herself frequently, she talks to imaginary friends, she laughs inappropriately." Frances had been diagnosed with global aphasia and was known to have global cognitive deficits. She attended a special education program in fifth grade because of demonstrated serious learning difficulties.

Frances's mother alleged that she had developed satisfactorily until age $2\frac{1}{2}$ years, at which time she sustained a severe head injury when her father, who had been holding Frances on his back, lost his grip and Frances fell on her head. Frances forgot how to speak after the accident. Her mother spent a great deal of time and effort teaching her to speak again and later to read.

Frances was born at full term and the delivery was uncomplicated; however, she was delivered by forceps and may have been oxygen deprived at birth. Frances's mother described her as an easy-tempered baby. She indicated that early developmental milestones had emerged at the expected times. She reported that developmental delays began after the fall. She had no history of seizures or of any other medical problems, and she had no psychiatric history.

At the time of the evaluation, Frances's parents were separated. Frances's father had abandoned the family some time earlier, and her parents' marital relationship was poor before her father left. Frances's mother alleged that her husband was mentally ill and that there was significant mental illness on his side of the family. The family was experiencing significant economic stress and received assistance from charity organizations.

The mental status examination revealed the presence of an attractive and engaging preadolescent female who appeared her chronological age. Frances was appropriately dressed and well groomed. She exhibited a significant degree of anxiety, and although she appeared euthymic, she demonstrated some social-adaptive but inappropriate smiling. Her affect was increased in range and in intensity.

As Frances began to talk, her dysprosody became apparent. Her voice was hoarse and rasping, like that of a very old woman. She had difficulties initiating speech and frequently showed hesitancy and significant problems in the expressive area. Frances tended to perseverate and the examiner frequently needed to repeat questions, because Frances seemed to have problems understanding speech. Frances's sentences were short and simple, and she had frequent problems with grammar and syntax, including improper use of prepositions and conjunctions. The examiner noted that Frances had recent and remote memory problems. She also displayed dysnomia and some illogical thoughts; however, she seemed coherent. There was no evidence of a mood disorder, suicidal or homicidal ideation, or psychosis.

Summary of positive findings (see Note 3 for other findings):

Physical examination. Findings were unremarkable.

Neurological screening. Frances showed evidence of receptive and expressive language disorders; she also exhibited some ataxia and frontal release signs.

Neurological consultation. Frances's left ear was mildly malformed, and mild facial asymmetry was observed. There was no evidence of dysarthria, but word usage and syntax problems were noted. Frances couldn't read at her grade level, and her reading comprehension was poor. Visual perceptual deficits were also observed. When challenged with medium complexity commands, Frances's speech comprehension was below the expected level. The diagnostic impression was of dysphasia (expressive-receptive speech deficits). A tic disorder was also suspected. The examiner recommended a speech evaluation and a sleep-deprived EEG.

Cognitive testing. Full-scale IQ of 75, with a VIQ of 66 and a PIQ of 87. Frances's scores on tasks requiring elaborate explanations were quite impaired, reflecting her significant aphasic deficits. Scores on subtests associated with perceptual organization also showed a scatter (i.e., a large spread in subtest score values), including borderline arrangement of pictures to tell a story and reproduction of designs using patterned blocks. She exhibited an average ability to scan for visual incongruities and a high average ability to assemble puzzles. Scores associated with attention and freedom from distractibility were average in repetition of digit strings and borderline in mental arithmetic. Processing speed scores were average in visual target detection and borderline in copying of symbols from a key. The pattern was consistent with a significant language deficit in the presence of better-developed visuoperceptual abilities.

Projective testing. Findings were consistent with the diagnosis of schizotypal personality disorder. Frances exhibited significant evidence of deficits in perceptual accuracy; however, there was no evidence of a thought disorder. Frances's behavior during the evaluation aptly depicted her internal confusion: she had difficulties interpreting the actions of others in a positive and caring way, and she was uneasy in interpersonal relationships, expecting that she would be misunderstood or that she would misunderstand others. Although she said that she was unwilling to participate in the evaluation, Frances's behavior was generally cooperative and pleasant, but she had a tendency to become disorganized under stress.

Neuropsychological testing. Findings were significant. The neuropsychologist reported that Frances was an attractive, slim girl, who was somewhat small for her age. She was adequately groomed and appropriately dressed. Her speech and language were unusual in several regards. Frances's word usage was quite concrete; she frequently used the word "thing" to refer to objects or made paraphasia errors (e.g., "eyelashes" for eyebrows). Frances talked almost continuously and at a rapid rate. Her spontaneous comments and questions appeared to reflect her personal concerns and anxiety (e.g., she frequently expressed fear of punishment) and were frequently off the topic. Frances tended to ask repetitive questions, such as asking what time it was every few minutes. Her receptive language appeared impaired; she often had difficulty understanding spoken instructions and needed more explanation and demonstration than would be expected based on her age.

Frances's motor activity and energy level were significantly increased. She fidgeted, squirmed, and attempted to get out of her chair and explore the room. Her motor activity increased every time she was faced with a task she found difficult. She had significant problems maintaining attention. Frances got off task frequently and required a great deal of redirection. Her approach to various tasks was less efficient; for example, she often indicated that she was finished with a task without checking it for accuracy. Her mood was anxious and her affect incongruent. For example, even when obviously frustrated and having protested that a task was too difficult, Frances continued smiling. Her cooperation fluctuated. She was most cooperative on tasks she enjoyed, and she appeared quite responsive to praise and encouragement. On tasks she found difficult, she protested verbally or responded in a random or silly manner until redirected. On one task, she simply refused to continue.

Visuospatial skills.   Right-left confusion and poor visuospatial construction skills were revealed.

Language.   Frances exhibited mild impairment in all aspects of language. Her receptive vocabulary was in the first percentile: Frances had problems understanding spoken questions and directions. Her expressive vocabulary was in the impaired range, and her abstraction skills were in the borderline range. Findings were consistent with a significant aphasic disorder.

Memory.   Frances exhibited impairments in immediate memory recall and learning. Her pattern of performance indicated poor initial encoding. On a task of learning and recall for a set of spatial coordinates, Frances became extremely frustrated, responded randomly, and refused to complete the task. The pattern of errors suggested inconsistent attention.

Executive functions.   Frances exhibited severe deficits.

Diagnostic impression.   Tests were consistent with multiple neurological deficits, most notably in Frances's receptive and expressive language, psychomotor coordination, and executive functions. These deficits significantly impeded Frances's ability to verbally problem solve or organize novel information, leading to a reliance on repetitive and often inappropriate behavior. Frances's neurocognitive problems were exacerbated by anxiety. Frances was not considered mentally retarded. Her symptoms were consistent with pervasive developmental disorder and appeared to be secondary to her neurocognitive deficits.

Regarding localizing principles of aphasia in children, Cummings says, "Children often exhibit non fluent aphasia regardless of the lesion localization in the left hemisphere" (2, p. 181). Severe linguistic deficits are rarely isolated. Frequently these deficits are associated with other neurocognitive and neuropsychological deficits. Understandably, depression, anxiety, and psychotic disorders are frequent comorbid conditions in children with language disorders and neuropsychological deficits. Receptive language disorders are frequently misdiagnosed as oppositional defiant disorders. In reality, children with these disorders do not understand the oral commands they are given. Impulse-control difficulties are common in these children. Consider the case examples of Ruben and Frances; these children were impulsive and demonstrated problems with executive functions.

Children with severe expressive language disorders display thought disorders that are similar to the thought disorders of schizophrenia (e.g., looseness of associations, incoherence, circumstantiality, neologisms). The main differences are in the areas of relatedness and affective expression. In general, children with language disorders are likable, have a strong interest in people, and frequently display broad and congruent affect. Schizophrenic children are usually schizoid and display blunt or inappropriate affect. Elaborate delusions and multisensory hallucinations are characteristic of schizophrenia.

Both Ruben and Frances demonstrated significant mixed language impairment and moderate-to-severe memory deficits, reflecting the close connection between language and memory functions. Surprisingly, parents and even teachers failed to recognize these communication problems. Even though Ruben had been retained 4 years in a row, no one had tried to find out why he could not advance at school or why he could not learn.

Patients with severe neuropsychiatric problems often grow up with deep-seated doubts about their competence and intellectual capacity. Because of their communication difficulties, they develop a sense of defectiveness and a poor self-concept. They may be demoralized or chronically depressed. Language limitations also interfere with their social relationships. These children have problems making friends and gaining acceptance from their peer groups; usually they are very isolated and insecure. Obviously neuropsychiatric impairments interfere with school and vocational achievement; this lack of achievement further interferes with these children's overall adaptation (i.e., sense of competence, self-esteem, and attitude toward life problems). Serious behavioral and attitudinal difficulties develop in children in whom these disorders are not properly diagnosed and treated. In general, learning disabilities and related neuropsychological impairments represent cortical association disconnections or cortical-subcortical disconnections caused by a variety of noxae. Finally, there is an interesting receptive language disorder associated with EEG abnormalities, and, in some cases with seizures: the Landau-Kleffner syndrome (32).

■ NOTES

1. According to Harris, "Neuro-imaging technology attempts to correlate specific aspects of information processing with specific brain regions. Structural imaging methods are used to link damage in particular brain regions with behavioral deficits; functional brain imaging investigates physiological changes associated with brain activity. Links to brain structure or physiology may validate neuropsychological assumptions for the developmental disorders" (14, p. 24).

2. Other findings in Ruben:

   Physical examination. Multiple self-inflicted bruises on the right arm and right foot, plus an old irregular scar in the lateral aspect of the right arm, corresponding to a self-inflicted burn.

   Neurological screening. Ruben was left handed; he exhibited marked right-left disorientation and dysnomia (e.g., he called a cross "two lines," a triangle "a rectangle," and didn't know the name of the diamond). This naming difficulty also reflected problems with abstract perception and thinking.

   Psychological testing. *Verbal tests scores* were very poor; all were below 4 (10 is average). *Performance test scores* were below average, except for object assembly, which was 11. *Academic test scores* were below third grade level in reading, spelling, and arithmetic. Ruben's reading performance met criteria for a diagnosis of a learning disability. His spelling and arithmetic performance was substantially below expectations based on age and grade placement.

Neuropsychological testing. Ruben wore glasses throughout the testing. His fingernails showed signs of severe nail biting; otherwise, he was well groomed and appropriately dressed. When approached initially, Ruben was concerned he would receive an injection and said, "She is gonna kill me," but he didn't appear nervous or frightened. He willingly accompanied the examiner and was polite and cooperative throughout the test session. Ruben related to the examiner in a friendly and outgoing manner.

Ruben's sentence organization was somewhat poor, although he managed to communicate his meaning. For example, he defined a thief by saying, "A thief is he's stealing stuff." Word usage problems contributed to his difficulty organizing his verbalizations. For instance, when attempting to communicate that a boy in the story wanted to be a violinist, Ruben said, "He just wants to be a violin, he wants to be a musical instrument thing. He wants to learn, I guess." Through such attempts to restate his thoughts, Ruben demonstrated an awareness that his verbal communications were ineffective.

Although Ruben fidgeted and occasionally got out of his seat, he was able to sit and attend for long periods of time. His mood was cheerful and his affect congruent. Ruben's approach to the testing was varied but generally systematic and efficient. He appeared to use analysis when solving visuoperceptual problems and worked systematically back and forth across rows when doing a target detection task.

Visuospatial skills. Evaluation of visuospatial skills revealed impairment of orientation judgment, spatial target detection, and visuomotor integration. Speed and accuracy for detecting spatial targets was below normal limits for all symbols except for complex embedded figure. Performance on constructional tasks using paper and pencil revealed very poor preservation of the spatial elements of the designs; Ruben's approach to this task was hurried and notably impulsive. Construction using puzzles and patterned blocks was within average range.

3. Other findings in Frances:

Cognitive testing. *Verbal test scores* were below average; the highest was 8. *Performance test scores* were higher than the verbal scores. One subtest score was 9, another was 13 (object assembly). These scores indicated that Frances's abilities based on visuoperception and some forms of motor response were substantially better than were her language-based abilities. Because of the large discrepancy between Frances's VIQ and PIQ scores, the full-scale IQ was not considered a meaningful descriptor of her cognitive abilities. Frances had below-average (borderline) scores on tasks requiring verbal comprehension, reasoning, and expression.

Sensory-perceptual functions.   Mild difficulty maintaining fixation during visual-field tests was revealed.

Motor functions.   Moderate-to-severe bilateral impairments were noted.

■ REFERENCES

1. Goodman R: Brain disorders, in Child and Adolescent Psychiatry; Modern Approaches. Edited by Rutter M, Taylor E, Hersov L. Oxford, England, Blackwell Scientific, 1994, pp 172–190

2. Cummings J: Neuropsychiatry: clinical assessment and approach to diagnosis, in Comprehensive Textbook of Psychiatry/VI, 6th Edition, Vol 1. Edited by Kaplan HI, Sadock BJ. Baltimore, MD, Williams & Wilkins, 1995, pp 167–187

3. Taylor MA, Sierles FS, Abrams R: The neuropsychiatric evaluation, in Textbook of Neuropsychiatry. Edited by Hales RE, Yudofsky SC. Washington, DC, American Psychiatric Press, 1987, pp 3–16

4. Gold AP: Evaluation and diagnosis by inspection, in Child and Adolescent Neurology for Psychiatrists. Edited by Kaufman DM, Solomon GE, Pfeffer CR. Baltimore, MD, Williams & Wilkins, 1992, pp 1–12

5. Menkes JH: Heredodegenerative diseases, in Textbook of Child Neurology, 4th Edition. Edited by Menkes JH. Philadelphia, PA, Lea & Febiger, 1990, pp 139–187

6. Cook EH, Leventhal BL: Neuropsychiatric disorders of childhood and adolescence, in Textbook of Neuropsychiatry, 2nd Edition. Edited by Yudofsky SC, Hales RE. Washington, DC, American Psychiatric Press, 1992, pp 639–661

7. Williams DT, Pleak R, Hanesian H: Neuropsychiatric disorders of childhood and adolescence, in Textbook of Neuropsychiatry. Edited

by Hales RE, Yudofsky SC. Washington, DC, American Psychiatric Press, 1987, pp 365–383

8. Young JG, Leven L, Ludman W, et al: Interviewing children and adolescents, in Psychiatric Disorders in Children and Adolescents. Edited by Garfinkel BD, Carlson GA, Weller E. Philadelphia, PA, WB Saunders, 1990, pp 443–468

9. Denckla MB: The neurobehavioral examination in children, in Behavioral Neurology and Neuropsychology. Edited by Feinberg TE, Farah MJ. New York, McGraw-Hill, 1997, pp 721–728

10. Spreen O, Risser AH, Edgell D: Developmental Neuropsychology. Oxford, England, Oxford University Press, 1995

11. Lewis M: Psychiatric assessment of infants, children and adolescents, in Child and Adolescent Psychiatry; A Comprehensive Textbook, 2nd Edition. Edited by Lewis M. Baltimore, MD, Williams & Wilkins, 1996, pp 440–453

12. Dennis M: Acquired disorders of language in children, in Behavioral Neurology and Neuropsychology. Edited by Feinberg TE, Farah MJ. New York, McGraw-Hill, 1997, pp 737–754

13. Grafman J, Rickard T: Acalculia, in Behavioral Neurology and Neuropsychology. Edited by Feinberg TE, Farah MJ. New York, McGraw-Hill, 1997, pp 219–225

14. Harris JC: Developmental Neuropsychiatry; Assessment, Diagnosis, and Treatment of Developmental Disorders, Vol 2. Oxford, England, Oxford University Press, 1995

15. Pendleton Jones B, Butters N: Neuropsychological assessment, in The Clinical Psychology Handbook, 2nd Edition. Edited by Hersen M, Kazdin AE, Bellack AS. New York, Pergamon, 1991, pp 406–429

16. Hartlage LC, Williams BL: Pediatric neuropsychology, in The Neuropsychology Handbook, 2nd Edition, Vol 2. Edited by Horton AM, Wedding D, Webster J. New York, Spring Publishing, 1997, pp 211–235

17. Sbordone RJ: The ecological validity of neuropsychological testing, in The Neuropsychology Handbook, 2nd Edition, Vol 1. Edited by Horton AM, Wedding D, Webster J. New York, Spring Publishing, 1997, pp 365–392

18. Taylor E: Development and psychopathology of attention, in Development Through Life; A Handbook for Clinicians. Edited by Rutter M, Hay DF. Oxford, England, Blackwell Scientific, 1994, pp 185–211

19. Garfinkel BD, Amrami KK: Assessment and differential diagnosis of attention-deficit hyperactivity disorder. Child Adolesc Psychiatr Clin

North Am 1:311–324, 1992

20. Harris JC: Memory, in Developmental Neuropsychiatry Fundamentals, Vol 1. Oxford, England, Oxford University Press, 1995, pp 138–153

21. King BH, State MW, Shah B, et al: Mental retardation: a review of the past 10 years; part 1. J Am Acad Child Adolesc Psychiatry 36:1656–1663, 1997

22. Otnow Lewis D: Conduct disorder, in Child and Adolescent Psychiatry; A Comprehensive Textbook, 2nd Edition. Edited by Lewis M. Baltimore, MD, Williams & Wilkins, 1996, pp 564–577

23. Bennet TL, Dittmar C, Ho MR: The neuropsychology of traumatic brain injury, in The Neuropsychology Handbook, 2nd Edition, Vol 2. Edited by Horton AM, Wedding D, Webster J. New York, Spring Publishing, 1997, pp 123–172

24. Cummings J: Neuropsychiatry, in Manual of Psychiatric Disorders. Edited by Simpson GM. New York, Impact Communications, 1995, pp 109–136

25. Voeller KKS: Social and emotional learning disabilities, in Behavioral Neurology and Neuropsychology. Edited by Feinberg TE, Farah MJ. New York, McGraw-Hill, 1997, pp 795–801

26. Kinsbourne M: Disorders of mental development, in Textbook of Child Neurology, 4th Edition. Edited by Menkes JH. Philadelphia, PA, Lea & Febiger, 1990, pp 763–796

27. Towbin KE, Riddle MA: Obsessive-compulsive disorder, in Child and Adolescent Psychiatry; A Comprehensive Textbook. Edited by Lewis M. Baltimore, MD, Williams & Wilkins, 1996, pp 684–693

28. Zola S: Amnesia: neuroanatomic and clinical aspects, in Behavioral Neurology and Neuropsychology. Edited by Feinberg TE, Farah MJ. New York, McGraw-Hill, 1997, pp 447–461

29. Heindel WC, Salloway S: Memory systems in the human brain. Psychiatric Times, June 1999, pp 19–21

30. Birmaher B, Williams DT: Acquired brain disorders, in Child and Adolescent Psychiatry; A Comprehensive Textbook, 2nd Edition. Edited by Lewis M. Baltimore, MD, Williams & Wilkins, 1996, pp 363–374

31. Rumsey JM: Brain imaging of reading disorders (letter). J Am Acad Child Adolesc Psychiatry 37:12, 1998

32. Bishop DVM: Developmental disorders of speech and language, in Child and Adolescent Psychiatry; Modern Approaches, 3rd Edition. Edited by Rutter M, Taylor E, Hersov L. Oxford, England, Blackwell Scientific, 1994, pp 546–568

33. Cohen NJ, Horodezky NB: Language impairment and psycho-pathology (letter). J Am Acad Child Adolesc Psychiatry 37:461–462, 1998

8

COMPREHENSIVE PSYCHIATRIC FORMULATION

Development of a comprehensive psychiatric formulation and creation of a relevant treatment plan are the ultimate objectives of the diagnostic interview. The formulation process is an indispensable conceptual aid in the overall understanding of and treatment planning for psychiatric conditions in children and adolescents. Skills in comprehensive psychiatric formulation are fundamental in clinical practice.

The formulation process is a baffling exercise for beginners in the field of child and adolescent psychiatry. This is due in part to a progressively widening schism between 1) the expectation—as espoused by sound and ethical practice—that clinicians should have a comprehensive understanding of the child and his or her family and 2) the pragmatics of contemporary practice, which deals mostly with DSM-IV descriptive psychiatric pathology. Even though the child psychiatrist may not be involved directly in administering individual or family therapies or other psychosocial interventions, he or she should have an overarching understanding of the patient's case and should offer appropriate input when the clinical course requires it.

Some biologically oriented child psychiatrists pay lip service to individual dynamic and systemic issues involved in child psychopathology; likewise, many psychodynamically oriented child psychiatrists disregard hereditary, constitutional, and organic factors that contribute to the child's dysfunction. A conceptual polarity also exists between individual- and family-oriented theorists. The former emphasize individual psychopathology with some disregard for family and other systemic factors; the latter overlook individual characteristics (i.e., temperamental, hereditary, constitutional, and developmental factors) and focus exclusively on family-systems points of view. Fortunately, the family field has begun to incorporate developmental thinking in its theoretical concepts.

The guidelines we introduce in this chapter attempt to bridge the gap between descriptive psychiatry and the practice of psychosocial interventions. More specifically, we consider developmental, psychodynamic, and systemic conceptualizations to be important components of overall diagnostic assessment and treatment planning.

■ REVIEW OF CHILD AND ADOLESCENT PSYCHIATRIC LITERATURE

The child and adolescent psychiatric literature contains limited references to the topic of formulation. Anna Freud contributed greatly to the process of child and adolescent assessment. She developed the *metapsychological profile,* an exhaustive inventory of mind functioning from drive, structural, and ego perspectives. The recommendations based on such an evaluation focus specifically on child analysis and psychoanalytic psychotherapy. Of particular importance, in the area of developmental assessment, is Anna Freud's concept of developmental lines (1, 2). We discuss the relevance of these concepts in more detail later in this chapter (see also Rick's case example in Chapter 4).

According to Cohen, "Case formulation and treatment planning are a ritualistic sham if one does not begin from a poly-therapeutic position" (3, p. 633) and "[W]hen that 'special moment' arrives which leads the clinician(s) to conclude that there are now enough objective data with which to formulate diagnostic judgments and make recommendations, then a careful and deliberate cognitive exercise must ensue" (3, pp. 633–634). Cohen adds, "In order to formulate and to make recommendations, obviously, one does not need to know everything. Indeed a good part of the information collected may not necessarily be relevant to decision making and recommendation" (3, p. 634).

Cox defends the need for the formulation process and describes its conceptual and therapeutic roles as follows: "A further process of diagnostic formulation is required to bring *the qualities which are different and distinctive* about the individual child and family. The formulation puts forward ideas and suggestions about *which psychological mechanism might be operating,* about *underlying causes and precipitants of the disorder of this child,* about factors leading to a continuation of the disorder and the potential strengths and ameliorating factors that could be used in formulating a treatment plan" (4, p. 26; emphasis not in the original). Cox stresses what the formulation should or should not be: "It's quite inadequate merely to collect a lot of facts in the hope that some sense will come of them when they're put together. *Rather the clinician must be formulating hypotheses to be tested from the very first moment he [or she] meets the family.* These hypotheses may concern family interactions or the nature of the child's problems." He also recommends that the interviewing and observation be specifically tailored to the relevant issues in each child's problems. He further advises that the interview should systematically cover a range of situations and difficulties (4, p. 26; emphasis not in the original).

Shapiro's contribution is a valuable one because he attempts to integrate developmental psychoanalytic thinking with descriptive psychiatry (5). He reviews the misconceptions applied to adult and child formulations. Some of his comments regarding reservations about formulation agreed with the views of Perry et al. (see Note 1): "1. That . . . formulation is only for a long-term treatment. 2. That it is primarily a training device. 3. That it requires an elaborate format and too much time. 4. That it need not be written. 5. That the clinician will become too invested in the formulation to permit change" (5, p. 675). To these misconceptions, Shapiro adds a sixth one: "a formulation is only useful for those who are planning to do a dynamic therapy with a child" (5, p. 675). He asserts that "dynamic understanding may guide the clinician towards other therapies as well . . . [A] dynamic formulation underlines the necessity for understanding the significance of symptoms to children and their families and permits anticipation of what the risk is in presenting a diagnosis, alleviating pain and symptoms, and changing the dynamic equilibrium of the person treated and of the family" (5, p. 675). Shapiro stresses the importance of psychoanalytic developmental psychology, particularly the three subsystems of ego psychology, developmental lines, and separation-individuation as the frames of reference to formulate. These points of view are of immense value in the developmental assessment component of a comprehensive formulation. Shapiro considers symptoms mostly from classical and ego-psychological points of view.

Harris offers a brief discussion of the importance of the formulation process: "[T]he clinical case formulation is not a list of difficulties but is a synthesis that describes the interplay and relative importance of various issues. It should be a clearly written dynamic explanation that leads to a plan of treatment and suggested prognosis" (6, p. 15). Harris includes biological and psychosocial considerations (e.g., psychodynamic, social, and phenomenological issues, and commentary on the protective factors) and connects them with the "developmental life tasks important for a child at this particular age" (6, p. 14). For a summary of other relevant contributions regarding the formulation process in adults, see Note 1.

■ THEORY OF THE COMPREHENSIVE PSYCHIATRIC FORMULATION PROCESS

The comprehensive psychiatric formulation deals with the integrative part of the child or adolescent psychiatric evaluation. The goal is to synthesize the collected information (e.g., referral information, patient and family interviews, testing) and to reach an integrated understanding of the data. The formulation needs to consider endogenous factors (e.g., hereditary, constitutional, biological, developmental, intrapsychic) and exogenous factors (e.g., familial, interpersonal) related to the chief complaint of the disorder under consideration.

The comprehensive formulation attempts to explain the problems or issues of the child as an individual and as a member of the family and other systems. A complex dynamic interaction occurs among the factors that contribute to the expression of an illness. All factors need not be addressed in the formulation of every case; each factor plays a role to a greater or lesser degree. In some cases, certain factors are more relevant than others; factors combine in unique ways to express or maintain a disorder in a given patient. Factors cannot be understood in isolation, and for most disorders, research does not support granting central etiological status to any single risk or causal factor (7, p. 4).

A good formulation stresses both protective and risk factors. *Protective factors* are those that promote normative development and satisfactory adaptation; *risk factors* create developmental deviations and contribute to psychopathology. The consideration and assessment of each factor is essential in the diagnostic formulation; this is relevant for the delineation of a rational and comprehensive treatment program. Rarely is an illness or disorder produced by one factor alone. Maladaptation and illness are frequently the result of an interaction of forces.

The diagnostic formulation has two objectives: one is diagnostic and the other therapeutic. A comprehensive descriptive (syndromic) diagnosis is essential for a comprehensive psychiatric formulation (in Chapters 4, 5, and 6, we focused on DSM-IV–guided diagnoses) and a valid treatment plan. The evaluator should consider how the identified syndromes (e.g., mood disorders, psychosis) organize and distort the patient's perceptions about his or her internal and external worlds. Table 8–1 summarizes the objectives of the diagnostic formulation.

■ ASSESSMENT OF INTERNAL (INTRINSIC) FACTORS

Developmental Assessment

Psychoanalytic developmental psychology concepts are relevant in this section. The *developmental assessment* addresses the de-

TABLE 8–1.	Objectives of the comprehensive diagnostic formulation

I. Descriptive (syndromic) diagnosis

II. Assessment of intrinsic and extrinsic factors (psychosocial assessment)

    A. Assessment of intrinsic factors

        1. Developmental assessment

        2. Psychodynamic assessment

        3. Assessment of other internal or intrinsic factors

    B. Assessment of extrinsic factors

        1. Assessment of parental and family dynamics

        2. Assessment of developmental interferences

        3. Assessment of other external or extrinsic factors

gree to which the child is at the developmental phase commensurate with his or her chronological-maturational age. This assessment identifies whether the child is mastering the developmental tasks associated with his or her developmental phase. For instance, in assessing a preadolescent, the examiner should note the child's adaptation to the extrafamilial environment (e.g., school, neighborhood), the child's progressive immersion in same-sex peership, the child's involvement in fantasy-oriented play, and the child's progressive internalization of rules, among others. When evaluating an adolescent, the examiner should explore how the adolescent is coping with adolescent developmental tasks such as separation-individuation, sexual exploration, identity consolidation, career orientation, formation of supportive groups in the extrafamilial social milieu, and so on.

    The concept of *developmental phases* is broad and nonspecific; more relevant and specific is the concept of *developmental lines,* which addresses the developmental vicissitudes of important ego-psychological and object relations functions. The assessment of developmental lines gives clinical focus and assists in the identification of areas of disturbance. Anna Freud added to Sigmund Freud's implicit developmental lines (i.e., psychosexual developmental, maturation and development of ego defense mechanisms, and anxiety transformation) the following developmental lines: from individual dependency to self-reliance, from egocentricity to peer relationships, from inability to manage the body and its functions to the child's control of them, and from play to work. She also suggested a developmental line from anaclitic (i.e., need-satisfying) relationships to object constancy. The number of developmental lines is not complete, and the lines are not independent of one another. Future progress in developmental psychology and child psychoanalysis may bring forward new developmental lines and conceptual refinement of the ones already described.

Anna Freud suggested that the examiner pay attention to the harmony or disharmony of the progression of the developmental lines (1, 2). The following case example illustrates disharmony in the developmental lines:

> Steve, a handsome 14-year-old Caucasian adolescent who weighed 250 pounds and was over 6 feet tall, was evaluated for suicidal behavior. He was in conflict with both of his divorced parents but had received a great deal of nurturing from his maternal grandfather, who died less than 1 month before the psychiatric examination. Steve felt that there was no point in living after his grandfather died. He appeared older than his stated age, was intelligent, and was a very good student; he had also been successful on his school's football team. Steve's mother had limited emotional sources of support and attempted to lean on him for emotional support.
>
> Steve's physical development contributed to a major disharmony in the developmental lines: because he looked older than his chronological age, his mother and other people had expectations of him that were not congruent with his emotional or psychological development. This promoted pseudo-maturity and precocious ego development. Steve had strong, ungratified dependency needs. There were ongoing power-control fights with his mother; he opposed her rules, saying that he was too big to depend on her. Because both parents were insensitive to his dependency needs, Steve found a group of troubled adolescents to

gratify his unmet narcissistic needs and to provide guidance, protection, support, and a sense of belonging. Behind Steve's robust adolescent body was a big "needy baby." His body size made him feel that experiencing dependency needs was proper only of a smaller or younger child. In contrast, because of his large size, his parents overlooked that he was still in need of tender and loving care.

Circumstances in which developmental disharmony is present (e.g., in precocious puberty, delayed sexual development, precocious cognitive development) bring about psychopathological risks (see Rick's case example in Chapter 4). If the child is at variance with developmental expectations, this variance needs to be explained. The developmental assessment will determine areas of developmental progression, regression, or arrest.

The diagnostic formulation distinguishes between normative developmental conflicts of a transitory nature (i.e., those commonly found at a given developmental stage) and internalized conflicts or character (personality) traits of an enduring nature. The latter indicate problems in the mastery of previous developmental tasks.

Psychodynamic Assessment

The *psychodynamic assessment* evaluates the child's internal mental operations and corresponding dysfunctions. It also evaluates the psychological forces that motivate the child's behavior. This assessment aids in the understanding of the quality and strength of the child's personality traits.

We discuss in the next several sections the most dominant psychodynamic points of view: ego psychology, object relations theory, separation-individuation theory, self psychology, attachment theory, and interpersonal theory.

Ego Psychology

As its name implies, ego psychology emphasizes the ego. According to Sigmund Freud's tripartite conception of the mind, commonly known as structural theory, the ego perceives the physical and psychic needs of the self and the qualities and attitudes of the environment (including objects), and it evaluates, coordinates, and integrates these perceptions so that internal demands can be adjusted to external requirements. The ego accomplishes these goals by utilizing the so-called conflict-free ego functions of perception, motor capacity, intention, anticipation, purpose, planning, intelligence, thinking, speech, and language.

The ego also deploys defensive mechanisms to protect the individual against the conscious awareness of the conflictive demands of the id (e.g., primitive urges, impulses, biological needs) and the superego insofar as these may arouse intolerable anxiety (8, p. 59).

Examiners who use ego psychology as the basis for the dynamic formulation should pay attention to the following ego functions:

- Ego boundaries
- Reality testing and preponderant ego defenses
- Impulse control and superego functioning
- Capacity for sublimation, insight, and verbalizing
- Intelligence and other adaptive ego strengths
- Motivation and long-term planning
- Capacity to develop a therapeutic alliance

Object Relations Theory

Object relations theory bases its psychological explanations on the premise that the mind is concerned with elements (issues) taken from the outside, primarily aspects of the functioning of other persons (objects). The processes of internalization are emphasized. This mind model explains mental functions in terms of relations between the various internalized elements (8, p. 131).

Examiners who use object relations theory as the basis for the dynamic formulation should pay attention to the following functions:

- Quality of object relations
- Integration and stability of self and object representations

- Degree of envy, projective identification, and splitting in psychological functioning

Separation-Individuation Theory

Separation-individuation concepts apply to a developmental theory, to a process, and to a complex stage of development. In the development of the individual, Mahler proposed normal, autistic, and symbiotic phases and the separation-individuation process, which comprises differentiation, practicing, rapprochement, and object constancy subphases (8, pp. 180–181).

Examiners who use separation-individuation theory as the basis for the dynamic formulation should pay attention to the following functions:

- Evidence of progress throughout the separation-individuation process
- Evidence of a rapprochement crisis
- Evidence of object constancy

Self Psychology

Self psychology emphasizes the vicissitudes of the structure of the self, and the associated subjective, conscious, preconscious, and unconscious experiences of selfhood. This point of view recognizes as the most fundamental essence of human psychology the individual's needs to organize his or her psyche into a cohesive configuration, the self, and to establish self-sustaining relationships between the self and its surroundings; these relationships evoke, maintain, and strengthen the coherence, energy, vigor, and harmony among the constituents of the self (8, pp. 174–175).

Examiners who use self psychology as the basis for the dynamic formulation should pay attention to the following functions:

- Self-concept and self-esteem regulation
- Self-esteem stability

- Self-cohesion versus self-fragmentation
- Nature of narcissistic injuries
- Nature of grandiose and exhibitionist needs

Attachment Theory

Attachment theory is gaining a great deal of support because it has a strong empirical foundation and its principles can be subjected to research, characteristics that set apart this model from its counterparts. Bowlby proposed that children have an innate (evolutionary) predisposition to become attached to a primary figure, usually the biological mother. The concept of attachment and attachment behavior describes both the underlying psychological constructs and the selective patterns of proximity seeking that a young child strives to maintain at times of stress. Although the process of attachment is clearly reciprocal, the term *attachment* usually refers to the behavior of the child in relation to the primary figure. Although patterns of selective attachment develop during the first year of life, the notion of attachment is applicable throughout the life cycle (9, p. 2354).

Examiners who use attachment theory as the basis for the psychodynamic formulation should pay attention to the following functions:

- Quality of the experience provided to the infant
- Attachment-exploration balance
- Hierarchy of attachment to major caregivers
- Presence of a secure base
- Nature of internal working models
- Presence of a secure or insecure attachment (10, pp. 385–388; 11).

Interpersonal Theory

Interpersonal theory, originated by Sullivan, postulates that a person's impulses, strivings, and personality patterns need to be understood in the context of interpersonal relationships. Interpersonal relationships are a human concern from the very beginning of existence. The primary striving of the mind is the satisfaction of physical and emotional needs, especially the need for human contact and the achievement of a sense of security. Anxiety is aroused when these needs are threatened. Anxiety is an interpersonal experience and the primary motivator of human behavior (12). Specific therapeutic interventions based on Sullivan's concepts have been effective in the treatment of depression (13) and other disorders.

Examiners who use interpersonal theory as the basis for the dynamic formulation should pay attention to the following functions:

- Sense of security, or evidence of anxiety and loneliness
- Predominance of modes of experience
- Nature of the security operations
- Presence of consensual validation

Pertinent questions in assessing internal factors or developmental areas include the following: Is the child mastering the tasks appropriate to his or her developmental state? Is the child progressing in the different developmental lines? Does the child show evidence of internalized conflicts? Does the child demonstrate lags in development from previous phases?

Other Internal or Intrinsic Factors

The examiner also must consider 1) other factors that influence the way the personality becomes organized and 2) the manner in which the primary caregivers respond to the developing child (e.g., temperamental traits, other individual qualities) (see Note 2). He or she also must explore other developmental acquisitions (e.g., psychosexual development, social and interpersonal functioning) and, when pertinent, other levels of functioning (e.g., physical functioning, motor coordination, cognitive and moral development). Other skills and abilities that affect the child's sense of competence, adaptive capacity, and self-concept should also be surveyed.

Competence in developing peer relations requires special attention. This capacity is a good measure of a number of intrapersonal and interpersonal skills such as self-concept, level of self-esteem, problem-solving skills, and capacity for reciprocity and empathy. Children's peer relations serve vital functions, have important short-term and long-term consequences, are linked to children's competence in coping with major social tasks, and can be facilitated by systematic interventions aimed at increasing social competence (14, p. 457). Poor peer relations predict school dropout, whereas aggressive behavior predicts criminality (14, p. 469). When intellectual impairment, learning disabilities, or other handicaps are present, the examiner must evaluate how these impairments affect the child's self-concept and self-esteem regulation. For example, how do the child and the family cope with the limitation and what adaptive compensatory mechanisms are called into play? Denial of a handicap is a common phenomenon; often the denial in the parent is far greater than that in the child.

Adolescents with behavioral and academic difficulties require careful assessment. A number of psychiatric syndromes—including developmental language and learning disorders and other neuropsychological deficits—need to be identified. Frequently, emotional and behavioral difficulties at school are merely surface behaviors caused by those unidentified problems.

■ ASSESSMENT OF EXTERNAL (EXTRINSIC) FACTORS

Parental and Family Dynamics Assessment

Parental and family dynamics assessment relates to the degree to which the parents or family as a whole promote normative development (e.g., provision of basic care, nurturing, love, consistent limit setting, gratification of healthy narcissistic needs, support for autonomy, identity formation) and to the degree with which the parents or family provide a warm and supportive environment with reliable and consistent boundaries. Issues related to social learning, modeling, conditioning, and other behavioral aspects within the family are relevant in this area (15). (See Note 3.)

When assessing difficulties in this area, the following issues could be addressed: Where is the preponderance of the dysfunction? Is it in the parenting function, in the marital subsystem, or in the family system as a whole? Are the parents allied in the provision of discipline? How cohesive are the marital system and the sibling subsystems? Do any of the parents (including stepparents) have any identifiable problems? Do any of the parents exhibit overt psychiatric pathology? Is alcohol or drug abuse a problem in the family? What are the family's strengths?

A number of functions, or dimensions, are critical in parenting behavior. The following areas are considered to be key dimensions of parenting behavior: emotional availability (degree of emotional warmth), control (degree of flexibility and permission), psychiatric disturbance (presence, type, and severity of overt disorder), knowledge base (understanding of emotional and physical development and basic childcare principles), and commitment (adequate prioritization of childcare responsibility) (16, p. 274). When assessing parenting behavior, the examiner must scrutinize each of these areas.

Assessment of Developmental Interferences

The concept of *developmental interference* relates to factors within the rearing environment that are outside of the child's control and have a negative influence on the child's psychological development. Such interference commonly includes marital or family dysfunction but also includes other adverse events such as illness, trauma, or loss. This area also pertains to persistent stresses in the physical, psychological, educational, or cultural environment. If the adversity is too intense or if it is too prolonged, it may be internalized and transformed into an internalized conflict, bringing about a negative developmental result. The new conflict then becomes part of the child's psychopathological organization (17, pp. 28–40).

A developmental interference occurs when the child does not receive the care needed at a given developmental phase or when the gratification goes beyond what a particular phase requires. Each developmental stage, or each developmental line, may be interfered with as a result of deprivation or overgratification.

Parents create developmental interference by omission or by commission. Interference due to omission is associated with situations of neglect or abandonment at one extreme or with the inability to set consistent limits (i.e., enforce boundaries through appropriate discipline) at the other extreme. Interference due to commission is secondary to physical or sexual abuse or to reversals of the child and parent roles. Physical and sexual abuse, overindulgence, and lack of appropriate discipline are common developmental interferences.

Other External or Extrinsic Factors

Chronic illness in children has a major effect on the boundaries between children and their parents, and it interferes profoundly with the process of separation-individuation. Compensatory overdependency may develop because of frequent separations (because of hospitalizations) or fear of death (see Rick's case example in Chapter 4 and Cory's case example later in this chapter). Parents may overindulge or overprotect the child, thus impinging on the child's self-concept and autonomy. This behavior has a negative effect on the child's sense of competence and on other adaptive functions. Parents of handicapped children often feel guilty and responsible for their children's limitations. These parents have problems with "letting go" and with setting consistent limits (see Chapter 7).

School refusal problems have multiple causes, including separation anxiety. Many children are afraid to attend school nowadays because they fear intimidation by older children, pressure to join gangs or use drugs, and so on. For example, an intelligent 12-year-old boy began to skip school, and after an intense exploration of the reasons for his behavior, he confided that he had been beaten up regularly by a group of children belonging to a gang.

Pertinent questions in assessing external factors include the following: Is the school milieu favorable for the child's learning and development? Is the school system meeting the child's psychoeducational needs? What kind of influence does the peer group have on the child's behavior? Is the neighborhood safe, or is it infested with drugs and crime? Are the child's and the family's behaviors culturally syntonic?

When a psychiatric syndrome is present, the formulation should postulate what developmental factors and environmental circumstances are facilitating the expression of the disorder in question. Issues related to precipitating and perpetuating factors are of relevance here.

No assessment is complete without an examination of areas of strength both in the individual and in the family. The assessment also needs to include observations on the regulatory functions within the child and within the family. For example, when the child or family members are involved in a crisis, how do they attempt to solve it? What do they do? Whom do they call for help? Is there any organized way of solving the problem? What soothing mechanisms help the child or family to get back on track? What mechanisms does the child activate to stop escalation of the problem and to initiate its resolution?

■ PRAGMATICS OF A COMPREHENSIVE PSYCHIATRIC FORMULATION

There is no definitive way to complete a comprehensive psychiatric formulation. Adherence to a particular explanatory model will influence the way the formulation is done by different practitioners. The model used (e.g., psychodynamic, cognitive, behavioral, or family theories) will influence the emphasis of the formulation. Details or emphasis of some aspects of the formulation vary depending on the circumstances at the time the formulation is done.

Coherence and comprehensiveness are two important elements in the formulation. The formulation needs to be relevant to the presenting problem(s) and to the most important developmental aspects of the case.

In this section, we suggest a format for a comprehensive psychiatric formulation. We suggest six sections, or components, each of which is illustrated with case examples.

1. *A succinct explanatory statement that indicates the major psychopathological issues. This statement answers the question "What is this case about?"*

   John is an 8-year-old Caucasian boy with a history of suicidal behavior, aggressiveness, and disorganized thinking.

   Andrew is a 13-year-old African-American adolescent with a long history of impulse-control difficulties and a recent history of violence, depressive affect, and suicidal behavior.

   Maria is a 17-year-old Mexican-American adolescent with a long history of major depressive disorder and borderline personality traits.

2. *A succinct explanatory statement that indicates the perceived main problem (i.e., core issue or conflict). This statement answers the question "What are the main issues of the case?"*

   John's main conflicts are related to his perception of rejection and abandonment by his adoptive mother. He perceived this event as a psychological death; because of this, in his own words, "There is no reason for me to live any more."

   Andrew's main conflict was confusion over his primary maternal object.

   Maria struggled with developmental issues of autonomy and individuation in a very pathological nonsupportive environment: her father was psychotic, and her mother was controlling and lacked empathy for Maria.

3. *A succinct explanatory statement indicating the hereditary, constitutional, or organic factors related to the main problem. Any medical or neurological difficulties may be included here.*

This statement answers the question "What are the contributory biological factors of the case?"

John's natural mother was a drug abuser. He was exposed to drugs in utero. Previous psychological assessments had shown a disparity between his verbal and performance abilities. He also exhibited language deficits and electroencephalogram (EEG) abnormalities, and there were concerns about his nutritional state. John had asthma and inconsistent bladder control.

Andrew's mother had a background of alcohol and polysubstance abuse, and she probably abused drugs during pregnancy. Genetic factors were probably involved because Andrew's mother had a chronic psychiatric disorder and his maternal grandmother had an affective disorder.

Maria had a severe depressive disorder and strong anxiety disorder features. Management of the depressive syndrome with antidepressants was difficult because of cardiovascular complications.

4. *A succinct explanatory statement of the dominant intrinsic or internal factors that contribute to the problem(s). This statement answers the question "What are the predominant developmental and psychodynamic factors of the case?"*

For John, the threat of parental loss had precipitated significant regression, including impairment of thought organization and reality testing. He also displayed prominent somatization, which represented an affective regression and an identification with his very sick adoptive mother (she had severe diabetes with multiorgan complications). Recurrent somatic symptoms ensured gratification of John's unmet narcissistic needs. John sometimes expressed intense ambivalence toward his mother and family as a whole. His self-concept was very negative. He felt hopeless and showed marked desperation and torment. He attempted to take responsibility for the perceived rejection by psychotic guilt, the latter secondary to his intense aggression. Anger against his rejecting objects taxed his ego capacities and stimulated regression and serious compromise of his adaptive capacity. There were also concerns about John's capacity to bond emotionally to other people.

Andrew's loyalty conflicts were strong. His mother and grandmother competed for his love and affection. Andrew displayed impairment in the development of object constancy and lacked a stable object and self-representations. Competition for Andrew's love had blocked the resolution of infantile omnipotence and facilitated the creation of manipulative interpersonal traits. Lack of object constancy rendered him vulnerable to separations and impaired the separation-individuation process; these difficulties also contributed to an unstable self-concept and to a faulty superego development. Parent-child role reversal was a prominent feature in Andrew; he worried continuously about his mother.

Maria struggled with identity consolidation issues; she had a rigid system of defenses and had very high expectations for herself. Her strong defenses against sexuality appeared to be eroding. Control was a major coping defense for Maria. Anger and hostility were pervasive maladaptive features and highly valued coping mechanisms.

5. *A succinct explanatory statement of the relevant external or extrinsic factors (e.g., developmental interferences and other risk factors). This statement answers the question "What are the detrimental factors in the child or in the rearing environment that have a bearing on the case?"*

John had a history of multiple placements and ongoing rejection by his adoptive mother (she had made explicit threats to reverse the adoption). There were ongoing questions regarding abuse and neglect. His adoptive mother was very sick, and his adoptive father had been given the diagnosis of organic affective disorder, secondary to a stroke. Other siblings also had emotional problems: a younger sister had a history of psychiatric problems and had been hospitalized previously.

Andrew's family situation was extremely chaotic and confusing. His mother was dysfunctional and had alcohol and drug abuse problems. He had never had a male parental figure as a source of masculine identification and as an appropriate model for aggressive expression.

Maria's family was highly dysfunctional: violence, scapegoating, and rejection were common.

6. *A succinct explanatory statement of the protective factors—in the child, within the family, or in the rearing environment—that promote normative development and adaptive resolution of the problem(s) or conflict(s). Issues related to resilience and self-regulatory functions for the child or the family may be mentioned here. This statement answers the question "What are the strengths of the child or the family?"*

John was likable and engaging; he was verbal and intelligent. He did well in supportive and structured environments. He was attached, though ambivalently, to his adoptive sister. Finally, John had a strong bond with his natural sister, who had been adopted along with him.

Andrew was handsome and very intelligent and had some degree of insight. His grandmother was genuinely involved with him. Appropriate placement of Andrew and stabilization of his rearing environment was considered essential to regulate his inner world and to ameliorate his pervasive psychological turmoil.

Maria was a likable, honest individual who displayed integrity. She was tenacious and determined. She was intelligent, insightful, and very committed to helping herself and her family. Although her father was prone to intermittent psychotic functioning, he was the main source of affection for the children.

As the clinician advances in the formulation process from sections 1 to 6, he or she should gain progressively more understanding of the child and his or her circumstances. Note that sections 2, 3, 4, 5, and 6 address areas or factors that could become the target of specific therapeutic interventions. These sections could be considered to represent circumscribed or specific formulations themselves.

It is not enough to identify the factors that contribute to the creation and maintenance of symptoms or a disorder. The formulation should go one step further: it should make conceptual or explanatory bridges among the different factors. As the examiner advances from sections 1 to 6, he or she should attempt to make relevant connections among the components of the formulation. According to the clinical evidence and the examiner's theoretical bias, any of these sections could receive particular emphasis or amplification; this format is flexible.

Brevity in the presentation of the formulation is stressed. A very long and elaborate write-up renders this exercise impractical and clinically cumbersome. Because the formulation is offered as a conceptual guide to clinicians who have different levels of sophistication and expertise, it should be written without technical language.

Consider the following neuropsychiatric case example:

1. Cory was a 15-year-old African American adolescent who had significant difficulties with anger control (she pulled a knife on her brother twice and had done the same to her father 2 years earlier). She had poor interpersonal relationships and was oppositional and unruly toward her mother.
2. The main issues in Cory's case were 1) lack of stabilization of a partial seizure disorder, secondary to a lack of compliance with anticonvulsant medications; and 2) frequent power-control struggles with her mother.
3. Hereditary and constitutional factors were involved. Cory's mother made a suicidal attempt in her youth, and Cory's brothers had problems with aggression and impulsiveness. At birth, Cory almost died and underwent major abdominal surgery. More fundamental was the presence of complex seizure symptomatology (there was a positive EEG with right-side spiking). Furthermore, features of a receptive aphasia were present. Other symptoms, such as paranoia and perceptual distortions, were compatible with psychomotor seizures. Cory would become disoriented in space, and on a number of times, she lost her way home and became helpless. She wandered around and would start crying.

4. Salient issues regarding internal developmental factors centered around massive denials and pervasive externalization of blame for her persistent and recurring problems. She did not take any responsibility for her aggressive and impulsive behaviors and was prone to blame others when she lost control. Cory defended against strong dependency needs toward her mother with hostility and was very ambivalent about her. Her feelings toward her mother vacillated from open rebellion to regressive behavior characterized by baby talk and the need for frequent body contact with her mother. Somewhat aware of her perceptual inaccuracies, she relied on her mother a great deal for consensual validation. Seizure phenomena and twilight states contributed to her idiosyncratic experiences and her conviction that what she felt and experienced was real. Cory felt that everyone misunderstood her, and she was very suspicious of most people. Her lack of insight was remarkable.

5. Cory's mother had been overprotective of and lenient with Cory because she feared for Cory's life. Her mother was also inconsistent with discipline. Cory's mother was a single parent with a limited support network. Because of a strong denial, Cory didn't comply with her medications, which were essential to control her seizure disorder, the main cause of a great deal of her psychopathological functioning.

   Cory needed her mother's supervision and tighter controls because she was very impulsive, misjudged situations, and was prone to distort interpersonal events. She regularly broke her mother's rules and didn't meet her mother's expectations. Cory was sexually active and had sneaked some of her partners into her bedroom. She believed that people were out to get her.

6. Cory was a tall, attractive, and intelligent adolescent. In spite of her neuropsychological problems, which affected her learning, she liked school and was motivated to do her school work.

   Cory's developmental features and her conflicts with her mother were major factors in her dysfunction. No progress was possible with Cory until the therapist understood and validated Cory's idiosyncratic experiences.

The case examples provided in this section could have been written with a different emphasis or from other theoretical perspectives, or with a different systemic or ecological focus. The proposed model allows this variability. There is no perfect theory to support the psychodynamic aspects of the formulation. Each theory has an explanatory richness that needs to be exhausted before using alternative theories to fill the conceptual gaps. It is preferable to know one theory in depth than to know a variety of theories superficially. The clinician needs to know the explanatory power and the limits of a chosen theory, and the advantages of choosing one over the others. When the limits of a theory are reached, the clinician can appeal to other theories to satisfy explanatory gaps.

In the following case example, the examiner attempted to explain the patient's symptoms from a self psychology psychodynamic perspective:

> Rudolf, a 19-year-old Asian-American adolescent, exhibited poor self-concept and chronic self-esteem difficulties. His compulsive sexualization reflected evidence of an ongoing narcissistic disturbance and a lack of affirming and supportive self-objects. His compulsive anal masturbation reflected the transformation of body functions into soothing self-objects when supportive self-objects were not available to him. This autoerotic involvement represented a substitutive restorative (reparative) self object. His fantasies during masturbation expressed exhibitionistic gratification of his arrested primitive grandiose self. His feeling that people were looking at him during his compulsive activities was another manifestation of his projected grandiose self.
>
> Rudolf's need for a heating pack on his back at night was again a restorative self object (it stood for the absent grandmother who used to warm his back as a child). A body sensation was transformed again into a soothing self object. Suicidal ideation emerged when his sense of self was at risk of fragmentation. Because he had not internalized his supporting self objects, he was hopelessly dependent on others for his self-esteem regulation. Rudolf's drug use was another method with which he

attempted to avert fragmentation of his enfeebled self.

This explanatory alternative is interesting; there is a sense of coherence in the systematic application of self psychology concepts even though other psychodynamic propositions could be equally useful.

■ COMMON PROBLEMS IN THE ELABORATION OF A COMPREHENSIVE FORMULATION

The following common problems may be encountered in reviewing formulations:

1. Some formulations recite or agglomerate the data without integration.
2. Some formulations lack an orderly presentation of the explanations. They mix concepts and lack clarity or internal consistency.
3. Some formulations do not "grasp" or represent the core problem.
4. Some formulations overlook the patient's subjective issues (i.e., internal factors). They overemphasize external factors at the expense of developmental, intrapsychic, and interpersonal conflicts.
5. Some formulations are psychodynamically incoherent. Clinicians new to the formulation process may use a confusing mixture of concepts or explanatory models to explain internal factors.
6. Some formulations fail to explain the presenting problem.

■ REFORMULATION

The formulation is a dynamic process. The psychiatrist needs to change the formulation when new clinical data emerge, when there is a negative development in the clinical course, or when there is no progress after the treatment plan has been implemented.

Piggot's approach to refractory OCD is relevant in cases that need reformulation as a result of lack of progress (18). She advises the following:

1. Review the accuracy of the diagnosis
2. Review the comorbid conditions
3. Review the adequacy of the treatment trials
4. Review the integration of the treatment modalities
5. Review compliance
6. Review whether expectations about the therapeutic objectives are unrealistic

To the preceding list, we add a seventh recommendation: consider the possibility of countertransference factors (see Chapter 11). At times a reinterview may provide data or observations that have previously been missed and allow reconceptualization of the formulation.

■ NOTES

1. Review of contributions to the formulation process in adults:
   Gelder et al.'s format for formulation consists of six components: 1) statement of the problem, 2) differential diagnosis, 3) etiology, 4) further investigations, 5) plan of treatment, and 6) prognosis (19). These authors include in the etiology section predisposing, precipitating, and maintaining factors. Elucidation of these factors is of particular importance in child and adolescent psychiatry.
   Perry et al. represent a significant advance in the integration of dynamic thinking and nondynamic considerations (20). These authors offer many valuable ideas: they regret that the "psycho-dynamic formulation is seldom offered and almost never incorporated with the written record" (20, p. 543). In comparing the clinical diagnosis with the dynamic formulation, they say, "[T]heir primary function is to provide a succinct conceptualization of the case and thereby guide the treatment plan" (p. 543). They also declare that the formulation is a "fundamental component of all treatments" (p. 544), and they assert that "the dynamic formulation is consistent with the bio-psycho-social model, is relevant to all forms of psychiatric treatment, and is not re-

served only for those psychiatric conditions in which biologic factors are less well referred (e.g., personality disorders) and only for those treatments that are insight-orientated (e.g., exploratory psychotherapy)" (p. 546). Their examples demonstrate the importance of addressing dynamic factors in obviously organic conditions.

Sperry et al. made a major contribution in the area of formulation (21). Theirs is one of the few texts extant on this subject. According to Sperry et al., "A psychiatric formulation can be defined as a prescribed method for the orderly combinations or arrangement of data and treatment recommendations about a psychiatric patient according to some rational principles . . . [I]t is the clinician's compass, guiding treatment . . . [I]t should include a wealth of information about a patient yet be clear, concise, and usable in clinical practice" (21, p. 1). These authors describe three components of an effective psychiatric formulation:

i) The *descriptive component* is a phenomenological statement about the nature, severity, and precipitant of an individual's psychiatric presentation. It is cross-sectional in nature and answers the question "What happened?"

ii) The *explanatory component* attempts to offer a rationale for the development and maintenance of symptoms and dysfunctional life patterns. It is more etiological and longitudinal and answers the question "Why?"

iii) The *treatment prognostic component* serves as an explicit blueprint that governs treatment interventions and prognosis. It answers the question "What can be done about it and how?"

Crayton and Offenkrantz's contribution warrants special discussion (22). Their presentation of the subject is clear and didactic. According to these authors,

> The 'formulation' has long been considered an essential feature of the psychiatric work up. As a synthesis of what is known about the patient, it becomes the key exercise in the development of a rational treatment plan. . . . Despite this perceived centrality of the formulation in both teaching students and treating patients, the formulation is also one of the most puzzling exercises for psychiatry trainees and, in particular, for psychiatric board candidates. (22, p. 2)

Crayton and Offenkrantz continue, "Knowledge of the content and form of the formulation, then, greatly enhances the candidate's [examiner's] awareness of which questions to ask, what issues require elaboration, and how the data of the interview may begin to take a coherent form" (22, p. 3). The authors present "a model of the formulation which we believe addresses the current need in psychiatry for a comprehensive formulation" (22, p. 3). Crayton and Offenkrantz distinguish circumscribed from comprehensive formulations: "'The formulation' has frequently meant 'the psychodynamic formulation' which focuses just on one set of causal factors and explanatory systems. We wish to encourage the adaptation of a more comprehensive formulation that accommodates a wide variety of social, psychological, and biological data" (22, p. 4). This integration of descriptive psychiatry with psychodynamic thinking and other etiologic factors is meritorious. There are significant parallels between these authors' model and the one we present in this chapter.

According to Gabbard, "Although the formulation is intended to explain the patient's condition, it is not intended to explain everything. It should succinctly highlight the major issues, especially their relevance to treatment planning." Commenting on the dominant psychodynamic points of view (ego psychology, object relations, and self psychology), Gabbard says, "With some patients, one theoretical model will appear to have more explanatory value than the other two. With other patients, however, all three theoretical perspectives may seem useful in conceptualizing various aspects of the patient's psychopathology . . . [C]linicians should be open minded to all three theoretical frameworks and should embrace a 'both-and' rather than an 'either-or' attitude" (23, p. 84).

2. Cloninger et al. defined temperament as "the dynamic organization of the psychobiological systems that regulate automatic responses to emotional stimuli. Individual differences in temperament are known to be moderately heritable and stable throughout life regardless of culture or ethnicity" (24, p. 3). Cloninger proposed "three dimensions of personality that are genetically independent and that have predictable patterns of interaction in their adaptive responses to specific classes of environmental stimuli. The three underlying genetic dimensions of personality are called *novelty seeking, harm avoidance* and *reward dependence*" (25, p. 574). The novelty seeking, a dopaminergic pathway, is a behavioral activation system; the harm avoidance is a serotonergic, behavioral inhibition system; and the reward dependence is a

norepinephrine-mediated behavioral maintenance system that facilitates the acquisition of conditioned signals of reward or relief from punishment. Each system has discrete neuroanatomical areas of influence. Cloninger developed a personality typology based on these dimensions. For instance, antisocial personalities are high in novelty seeking and low in harm avoidance and reward dependence, obsessive individuals are high in harm avoidance and low in novelty seeking and reward dependence, and so on (25, p. 581). According to Cloninger, advances in gene mapping promise to elucidate the genetic architecture of a variety of temperamental traits.

3. Concepts such as "the average expectable environment" or "good enough mother" do not do justice to the role of the rearing environment. They imply that the developmental environment plays a passive, unimportant, and often detrimental role. Rarely is there an explicit articulation or recognition of the positive contributions of the environment in the developmental process; it is as if the whole issue of the nature of the developmental environment (the role of the mother or caregiver, in particular) is taken for granted. Neuroscience and developmental research are beginning to elucidate the specificity of factors that promote optimal development. Schore presented the following summary of evolving views on this subject:

> [W]e now know that the early environment is fundamentally a social environment, and that the primary social object who mediates the physical environment to the infant is the mother. Through her intermediary action environmental stimulation is modulated, and this transformed input impinges upon the infant in the context of socioaffective stimulation. The mother's modulatory function is essential not only to every aspect of the infant's current functioning, but also to the child's continuing development. She thus is the major source of the environmental stimulation that facilitates (or inhibits) the experience-dependent maturation of the child's developing biological (especially neurobiological) structures. Her essential role as the psycho-biological regulator of the child's immature psychophysiological systems directly influences the child's biochemical growth processes which supports the genesis of new structure. (26, p. 7)

■ REFERENCES

1. Freud A: The concept of developmental lines, in An Anthology of the Psychoanalytic Study of the Child. Edited by Eissler RS, Freud A, Kris M, et al. New Haven, CT, Yale University Press, 1977, pp 11–30

2. Freud A: Child analysis as the study of mental growth (normal and abnormal), in The Course of Life: Psychoanalytic Contributions Towards Understanding Personality Development; Vol 1: Infancy and Early Childhood. Edited by Greenspan SI, Pollock GH. Mental Heath Study Center, National Institute of Mental Health, 1980, pp 1–10

3. Cohen R: Case formulation and treatment planning, in Basic Handbook of Child Psychiatry, Vol 1. Edited by Noshpitz JD, Berlin IN. New York, Basic Books, 1979, pp 633–640

4. Cox AD: Diagnostic appraisal, in Child and Adolescent Psychiatry; Modern Approaches. Edited by Rutter M, Taylor E, Hersov L. Oxford, England, Blackwell Scientific, 1994, pp 22–33

5. Shapiro T: The psychodynamic formulation in child and adolescent psychiatry. J Am Acad Child Adolesc Psychiatry 5:675–680, 1989

6. Harris JC: Developmental Neuropsychiatry; Assessment, Diagnosis, and Treatment of Developmental Disorders, Vol 2. Oxford, England, Oxford University Press, 1995

7. Mash EJ, Dozois DJA: Child psychopathology; a developmental systems perspective, in Child Psychopathology. Edited by Mash EJ, Barkley RA. New York, Guilford, 1996, pp 3–60

8. Moore BE, Fine BD: Psychoanalytic Terms and Concepts. New Haven, CT, Yale University Press, 1990

9. Volkmar F: Reactive attachment disorders of infancy or early childhood, in Comprehensive Textbook of Psychiatry/VI, 6th Edition. Edited by Kaplan HI, Sadock BJ. Baltimore, MD, Williams & Wilkins, 1995, pp 2354–2359

10. Belsky J, Cassidy J: Attachment theory and evidence, in Development Through Life; a Handbook for Clinicians. Edited by Rutter M, Hay DF. Oxford, England, Blackwell Scientific, 1994, pp 373–402

11. Bacciagaluppi M: The relevance of attachment research to psychoanalysis and analytical social psychology. J Am Acad Psychoanal 22:465–479, 1994

12. Weiner MF, Mohl P: Theories of personality and psychopathology: other dynamic schools, in Comprehensive Textbook of Psychiatry/VI, 6th Edition. Edited by Kaplan HI, Sadock BJ. Baltimore, MD, Williams & Wilkins, 1995, pp 500–502

13. Mohl P: Brief psychotherapy, in Comprehensive Textbook of Psychiatry/VI, 6th Edition. Edited by Kaplan HI, Sadock BJ. Baltimore, MD, Williams & Wilkins, 1995, pp 1879–1880

14. Asher SR, Erdley C, Gabriel SW: Peer relations, in Development Through Life; a Handbook for Clinicians. Edited by Rutter M, Hay DF. Oxford, England, Blackwell Scientific, 1994, pp 456–487

15. Mash EJ: Treatment of child and family disturbance: a behavioral-systems perspective, in Treatment of Childhood Disorders. Edited by Mash EJ, Barkley RA. New York, Guilford, 1989, pp 3–36

16. Mrazek DA, Mrazek P, Klinnert M: Clinical assessment of parenting. J Am Acad Child Adolesc Psychiatry 34:272–282, 1995

17. Nagera H: Early Childhood Disturbances, the Infantile Neuroses, and the Adulthood Disturbances. New York, International Universities Press, 1966

18. Piggot TA: Personal communication, 1996

19. Gelder M, Gath D, Mayou R: The Concise Textbook of Psychiatry. Oxford, England, Oxford University Press, 1994

20. Perry S, Cooper A, Michaels R: The psychodynamic formulation: its purpose, structure and clinical application. Am J Psychiatry 144:543–550, 1987

21. Sperry L, Guddeman JE, Blackwell B, et al: Psychiatric Case Formulations. Washington, DC, American Psychiatric Press, 1992

22. Crayton JW, Offenkrantz W: The Psychiatric Formulation; A Handbook for Board Candidates, 4th Edition. Chicago, IL, University of Chicago Press, 1994

23. Gabbard GO: Psychodynamic Psychiatry in Clinical Practice. Washington, DC, American Psychiatric Press, 1994

24. Cloninger CR, Adolfsson R, Svrakic NM: Mapping genes for human personality. Nat Genet 12:3–4, 1996

25. Cloninger CR: A systematic method for clinical description and classification of personality variants. Arch Gen Psychiatry 44:573–588, 1987

26. Schore AN: Affect Regulation and the Origin of the Self; The Neurobiology of Emotional Development. Hillsdale, NY, Lawrence Erlbaum, 1994

9

SYMPTOM FORMATION AND COMORBIDITY

Certain clinical syndromes are commonly associated with particular psychodynamics. For example, patients who have panic attacks display traits of helplessness, dependency, passivity, and behavioral avoidance; similarly, patients who are depressed feel unmotivated, devalued, and hopeless. When these syndromes are clinically active, certain dynamic traits are expected to be present. These traits are considered *state dependent,* meaning that the traits are present when the patient becomes panicky, depressed, or the like. Those personality traits vanish or are less salient when the syndromes are under control. The intimate relationship between certain syndromes and associated psychodynamics is such that clinicians are advised to defer making Axis II diagnoses when dealing with active syndromes.

Do psychodynamic constellations unleash clinical syndromes? This does occur, and there are a number of examples. The most common example is a person's response to a loss. People have different thresholds for, and different ways of responding to, loss. Many factors, including constitutional and temperamental factors, determine this variability. In the so-called psychosomatic disorders, an intimate connection is assumed between the somatic and mind realms. In these illnesses, people become ill in response to a variety of stresses. This vulnerability probably depends on response thresholds and on individual organ vulnerability to stress. The coping dysfunction, or breakdown, may be in the somatic realm or in the mental realm; either diathesis may have an underlying genetic predisposition. When children break down, they do it in different ways: one child may become depressed, another may become psychotic, a third may activate a psychosomatic illness, and a fourth may evolve a mysterious inhibition of the release of growth hormone.

What happens when a chronic syndrome, such as anxiety or depression, improves or remits? Common clinical observations show that control of chronic mood disorders may produce only partial improvement in personality functioning. Although the depression or anxiety may be controlled, many areas of the patient's personality dysfunction may remain. In chronically anxious patients, patterns of avoidance or inhibition, pervasive doubting, and strong dependency traits may remain. In chronically depressed patients, patterns of passivity, inhibition, low self-esteem, and fear of failure outlast the affective disorder symptoms. In either situation, these patients have a greater vulnerability to stress. The lasting dysfunctional traits are impervious to further psychopharmacological treatment. These observations have made mandatory the combination of treatment modalities.

What is the relationship between dysfunctional personality traits and affective dysregulation? It could be postulated that chronic mood disorders promote maladaptive patterns of coping that gain stability or even functional autonomy. It could also be argued that affective dysregulation and associated personality traits have different though parallel origins. Alternatively, the affective disorder could interfere with adaptive processes of learning and skill development in interpersonal relationships and in other areas; the unresolved symptoms could represent lags in learning adaptation (see Note 1).

The precise nature of the phenomenon of comorbidity is a challenge in the ongoing elucidation of the origin and expression of psychopathology. Puig-Antich and colleagues have made interesting observations concerning the association of major depressive disorder and the concomitant manifestation of anxiety and conduct disorder (1, 2). For the latter association, they noted that in a group of depressed preadolescents, the conduct disorder features waxed and waned, according to the reactivation or improvement of the affective disorder. When the depression was active the conduct disorder features were active, and when the depression was in remission the conduct features were also in remission. In the same vein, there is a strong association between conduct disorder and bipolar disorder: the conduct disorder may precede, be concurrent with, or follow the onset of bipolar illness. According to Kovacs and Pollock, conduct disorders are equally likely to antedate or postdate the onset of the first episode of bipolar disorder (3).

The factors that stabilize a syndrome or that are important in symptom expression or maintenance may not have anything to do with the origin of the disorder.

The complexity of interactions in the process of symptom formation and symptom maintenance can be observed in the following case example:

> Kirk, a 16-year-old Caucasian male, was evaluated for depression and suicidal ideation. Kirk's mother had a history of chronic depression: she was chronically suicidal and episodically self-abusive. The father, a scientist, qualified for the diagnosis of obsessive-compulsive disorder. He would repeatedly check his laboratory door to ensure that it was locked, and in the parking lot, he would walk around his car several times, checking all the door locks. On occasion he would go back to the laboratory at night to ensure that it had been locked securely.
>
> Kirk's parents were involved in an ongoing conflict over issues of power and control. Kirk's mother complained that her husband was tyrannical and very controlling. When tension in the marriage increased, Kirk's mother would become depressed, self-abusive, and suicidal. At these times, Kirk and his 13-year-old sister (who exhibited regression) would come to their mother's rescue and unite against their domineering father. Kirk's father found himself progressively isolated and felt rejected and undermined. At those times, the father's insomnia and symptoms of obsessive-compulsive disorder worsened.

Kirk's acting out also increased at those times.

Kirk's mother undermined his father's efforts to set limits on the children. Kirk, in spite of superior intelligence, was flunking most of his school classes. School authorities earmarked Kirk as a problem child; he was very unconventional in his manner of dress, he associated with troubled peers, and most likely he used drugs.

The preceding case example illustrates the additive influences of negative factors. For Kirk, some psychiatric features (such as depression) had biological-hereditary contributory factors (probably coming from both parents). These factors, added to prolonged exposure to parental psychopathology and marital discord, created significant developmental interferences, promoting negative social learning and ultimately negative internalization and defective self-concept formation.

A caregiver's affective disorder will have multiple effects on his or her parental functioning. Allen and Gross quoted Ferguson et al., who investigated the relationship between maternal depression and children's behavioral problems:

> These investigators found that correlations between family life events and maternal reports of child-rearing problems were largely attributable to the mediating effects of maternal depression. It was suggested that children of depressed mothers may respond to mothers' depressive style by developing increasingly more behavioral problems. A second explanation suggests that depressed mothers perceived their children's behavior differently from non-depressed mothers. Regardless of the specific mechanism, however, maternal depression is a very important diagnostic clue. (4, p. 317)

Keitner and Miller agree with this conceptualization:

> It is not certain whether problematic family relationships predispose to or facilitate the emergence of depressive illness or whether the depressive illness and its attendant impact on pa-

tients' interpersonal styles create family difficulties in coping. There is evidence to support both points of view. In addition, the combination of a number of different stressors can obviously have an additive effect in leading to family dysfunction. (5, p. 22)

Kirk's case example also demonstrates the formation and stabilization of psychopathology in a developing child through concomitant parallel systems. Although the adolescent's affective disorder improved, the developmental, internalized conflicts and the negative learning persisted. A protracted course of family therapy was required to disentangle Kirk from maternal enmeshment and to facilitate a closer relationship between Kirk and his father. The improved relationship was necessary for the consolidation of the child's masculine identity. The case example also showed mutual balancing, or stabilization, of the parent's individual pathologies: the mother's chronic affective disorder with periodic acute reactivations and the father's obsessive-compulsive disorder and unremitting insomnia.

We have followed a number of adolescent patients who exhibited chronic, stable, maladaptive regressions. Crucial in the stabilization of the psychopathology is the symbiotic link of these children to their mothers. Positive steps in the treatment have been achieved every time the symbiosis has been fractured. A positive sign in this respect is the development of depression in mothers when they begin to separate from the enmeshed adolescents.

Negative factors in the development of psychopathology, as in Kirk's case example, may act additively, by summation, or may potentiate themselves by synergism. An example of the latter is a recent outcome study that seems to predict a criminal outcome at age 18 years, when two conditions occur together in a male infant: 1) complications at birth and 2) maternal rejection by the first year of age. Neither condition in isolation produced the adverse development (6). The aggregate of negative factors may, unfortunately, have combined results far more negative than the mere addition of the individual factors.

Psychopathology in the child may be a reflection of the degree of stress in the caregiver. According to Keitner and Miller,

> Goodyer and colleagues, 1988, identified maternal factors that were related to increased frequency of anxiety and depression in children. . . . They examined the role that lack of emotional support in the mother's life played in the rates of pathology in their children. They identified three factors: recent stressful life events in the mother's life, the degree to which the mother was distressed (maternal distress), and the quality of the mother's supportive confiding relationships. . . . The risk of emotional disorder in the child was multiplied by the presence of these adverse factors. . . . In other words, the effects were independent and multiplicative rather than merely additive. (5, pp. 79–80)

Contemporary conceptualization of the nature-nurture relationship establishes a mutual influence between the factors. Pike and Plomin explain:

> [E]nvironmental factors, both shared and nonshared, were found to be important to varying degrees. . . . Parents who are negative cast a shadow over their families and put all children in these families at risk for depression in adolescence. . . . Nonetheless, nonshared family environment also appears to have some effect. Nonshared environment is a fresh way of thinking about the environment of the family. It suggests that important experiences lie within the families, not just between families. For example, . . . adolescents who are the object of more maternal negativity than their sibling are more likely to be depressed, independent from the effects of genetics or shared family environment. (7, p. 568; see also Note 2)

■ NOTES

1. Kandel has proposed that behaviors that characterize psychiatric disorders are disturbances of brain function, even in those cases where the causes are clearly environmental in origin (8). Genes and their protein products are important determinants of the patterns of intercon-

nection of the neurons and the details of their functioning. Learning, including learning that results in dysfunctional behavior, produces alteration in gene expression. Kandel discusses the gene's template and transcriptional (phenotype) functions. The template function can be altered only by mutation and is not regulated by social experience of any sort. The transcriptional function, in contrast, is highly regulated, and this regulation is responsive to environmental factors. This epigenetic regulation is influenced by internal and external factors including brain development, hormones, stress, learning, and social interaction. The regulation of gene expression by social factors makes all bodily functions including the brain susceptible to social influences. In humans the modifiability of gene expression through learning in a nontransmissible way is particularly effective and has led to a new kind of evolution: cultural evolution (8, pp. 460–461; see also Note 2).

2. Pike and Plomin summarize a number of concepts related to behavioral genetic research: Quantitative genetic theory postulates that variation observed among individuals in a population can be ascribed to genetic and environmental sources; this stems from individuals' genetic variability and the variability of the environments experienced by the individuals. Genetic effects can be either additive or nonadditive. *Additive genetic influence* refers to genetic effects that add up linearly in their effect on the phenotypic variance. *Nonadditive genetic influence* refers to effects caused by interactions among the genes. Environmental influences consist of two categories: those shared by siblings reared in the same family (i.e., *shared environment*) and those not shared by siblings in the same family (i.e., *nonshared environment*). *Environment* in behavioral genetics is defined more broadly than is typically the case. It includes all sources of variations not explained by heritable genetic effects. In addition to psychosocial experiences, the environment includes perinatal factors, accidents, illnesses, and even chromosomal events such as chromosomal anomalies that are not inherited (7, pp. 560–561).

■ REFERENCES

1. Puig-Antich J, Blau S, Marx N, et al: Prepubertal major depressive disorder; a pilot study. J Am Acad Child Adolesc Psychiatry 17:695–707, 1978

2. Puig-Antich J, Gittelman R: Depression in childhood and adoles-

cence, in Handbook of Affective Disorders. Edited by Paykel ES. New York, Guilford, 1982, pp 379–392

3. Kovacs M, Pollock M: Bipolar disorder and comorbid conduct disorder in childhood and adolescence. J Am Acad Child Adolesc Psychiatry 34:715–723, 1995

4. Allen JB, Gross AM: Children, in Diagnostic Interviewing, 2nd Edition. Edited by Hersen M, Turner SM. New York, Plenum, 1994, pp 305–326

5. Keitner GI, Miller IW: Family functioning and major depression, in The Transmission of Depression in Families and Children. Edited by Sholevar GP. New York, Jason Aronson, 1994, pp 79–80

6. Raine A, Brennan P, Mednick S: Birth complications with maternal rejection at age one year predispose to violent crime at age eighteen years. Arch Gen Psychiatry 51:984–988, 1994

7. Pike A, Plomin R: Importance of nonshared environmental factors for childhood and adolescent psychopathology. J Am Acad Child Adolesc Psychiatry 35:560–570, 1996

8. Kandel ER: A new intellectual framework for psychiatry. Am J Psychiatry 155:457–469, 1998

SPECIAL SITUATIONS DURING THE PSYCHIATRIC EXAMINATION: DIAGNOSTIC OBSTACLES OR RESISTANCES

It is hoped that when the examiner encounters difficult or complex situations during the psychiatric examination, he or she does not readily appeal to the concept of *resistance*. Only by making a dedicated effort to understand the patient's circumstances, no matter how complex, intractable, or hopeless they may appear, will the examiner learn to identify the issues surrounding difficult and complex diagnostic presentations. If the examiner appeals to the concept of resistance every time difficulties are encountered during the psychiatric examination, many opportunities for growth, both professionally and personally, will be lost. The statement "the child was resistant" could be easily transformed into "the examiner was unable to engage the child." In the same way that a good chess player knows different openings and knows how to respond to the opponent's moves, the child and adolescent psychiatrist should know different strategies to respond to diverse clinical situations.

> The child and adolescent psychiatrist needs to have a variety of engagement skills and other rapport-enhancing strategies readily available to meet difficult clinical challenges during the diagnostic examination.

Katz suggests a number of skills or qualities the therapist (examiner) needs to have at his or her disposal. These include knowledge, understanding, empathy, and a positive, warm approach toward patients (1, p. 81). To these we add equanimity and a solid awareness of the child's developmental level (see Chapter 1).

The child psychiatrist should remember that trying or difficult children (and their families) are not creating difficulties anew for the examiner; the pathology that children and their families display during the psychiatric examination represents enactments of long-standing patterns of maladaptive behaviors (e.g., internalized conflictive relationships). These patterns require clarification and understanding.

The concept of resistance relates to intrinsic protective factors that block an individual's awareness of internal conflicts. Because the concept of resistance puts the burden of the diagnostic difficulties on the patient (discounting the examiner's shortcomings in the interview process), and because this concept somehow conveys that the patient is deliberately opposing the psychiatrist's efforts, we prefer the terms *interviewing difficulties* or *interviewing obstacles*.

A child who is not verbally productive is not necessarily resistive. Conditions such as deafness, elective mutism, schizoid disorders, and developmental learning disorders interfere with optimal communication. Language and communication disorders, intellectual limitations, or other neuropsychological deficits also impair receptive or expressive communication processing.

If a child indicates that he or she doesn't want to participate in the interview, the examiner should review with the child what he or she knows about the reasons for the evaluation (i.e., the so-called contractual aspects of the examination) and should invite the child to explain what he or she thinks is the reason for the evaluation. Children often are cajoled or manipulated into a psychiatric evaluation by deceptive means. For example, a child's parents may say, "Let's go to see a doctor. We'd like you to see a counselor." Correspondingly, the child may come to the evaluation intending to "get mom and dad off my back." In circumstances of passive compliance, it is uncertain whether the child is aware of a problem or whether he or she acknowledges any feeling of internal distress.

In each diagnostic interview the examiner needs to ascertain how the child was prepared for the examination. If the examiner suspects deception, he or she should attempt to understand why the family needed to manipulate the child. If deception has been identified, the examiner should attempt to discover other patterns of manipulation or communication deviancy within the family; family deception may be secondary to the power and control the child has gained over the family.

The challenge with a defensive and uncooperative child is to transform the child's mistrust and defensiveness into a working alliance in order to conduct a productive diagnostic interview. If information may need to be released to the authorities (e.g., police, school officials, abuse investigators), the examiner needs to let the child or his or her family know that they will be informed of the need for such a disclosure. The examiner should also convey that he or she is working on their behalf and that no step in the process of the evaluation will be taken without their participation.

The examiner needs to continually safeguard the purpose of the interviewing process. If the patient is uncooperative or plainly resistive, the great temptation for the examiner is to plead for cooperation in one way or another. This is not recommended; the patient is likely to provide only partial or even deceptive information, which will leave the nature of the difficulty unclarified and unresolved and the obstacles of the communication unexplored. A better approach is to attempt to understand the obstacle every time it presents itself. Clarifications and interpretations are the optimal means to deal with any difficulties with communication or rapport or in the face of any obstacle in building an alliance. The following vignette illustrates a novice examiner's inadequate management of interviewing obstacles:

A 14-year-old Caucasian adolescent with a history of conduct problems, self-abuse, suicidal behavior, and polysubstance abuse entered the interviewing room and sat facing away from the examiner. The examiner asked the patient to "sit more appropriately"; she complied. The examiner then pleaded for cooperation and received passive compliance on many other occasions. The quality of the ensuing interaction was bland and detached; no rapport was established.

In the preceding vignette, the emotional tone of the evaluation could have been different if the examiner had addressed the resistance from the very beginning, for example, by saying, "It seems you do not want to talk to me," or "It doesn't seem that you want to participate in the interview." This approach also addresses negative affects that motivate the patient's lack of cooperation. The same approach should be taken when a patient acts out during the interview. Novice examiners take what seems to be the easiest (but by no means the optimum) approach when they simply ask the child to stop misbehaving.

Effective and therapeutic interventions connect the child's acting out with the presenting problem and appeal to the child's adaptive ego (the part of the ego struggling for optimal adaptation). This helps the child to improve his or her participation in the examination. In this manner, the patient's self-awareness of what he or she is doing is increased, and the patient's internal self-controls are stimulated. Rather than asking the child to stop misbehaving, a better intervention would be for the examiner to make the child aware of an overall pattern of maladaptation by saying, for example, "The way you are behaving during this examination makes me wonder if this is the way you behave in other situations. . . . I am beginning to understand why you get in trouble, or why people complain about you." Demanding passive acquiescence or taking over the patient's controls is an intervention of last resort. Occasionally, the interviewer has no other alternative but to take over the control of the situation for the sake of the patient's or the examiner's welfare.

■ CLASSIFICATION OF INTERVIEWING OBSTACLES

Interviewing obstacles may be classified as either pseudo-resistances or true resistances. The latter category may then be subdivided further into categories of superficial, moderate (approachable), or severe (insurmountable) interviewing obstacles.

Pseudo-Resistances

Pseudo-resistances are obstacles to the interview objectives that are not created directly by the child's defensiveness or unwillingness to participate. Pseudo-resistances can be considered from both the examiner's and the child's perspectives. There could be a failure in the interviewing process secondary to the examiner's inability to engage the child, because of a lack of skill, a lack of sensitivity to the child's problems, or a lack of attunement to the child's developmental level. For example, the examiner may not be attentive or sensitive to the presence of language disorders or neuropsychological deficits. In these cases, the obstacles are apparent only because the communication deficits interfere with the child's ability to participate in the diagnostic interview. An attentive examiner should notice the child's efforts or attempts to communicate.

When it becomes obvious that the child does not understand what he or she hears (and it is clear that the child does not have a hearing deficit), the examiner should attempt to ascertain the child's communication intent, by paying special attention to the child's nonverbal behavior (e.g., pointing, signaling, gesturing) or use of elementary vocabulary. If the examiner concludes that the child has communication difficulties, he or she should try to maximize the use of nonverbal media (e.g., play observation, drawing) to get access to the child's internal world.

Abused children often act "dumb" and learn not to say anything that may bring the family into contact with the law or other agencies. These children appear superficially resistant; they have learned that being silent prevents them from getting into further trouble.

Children who are very anxious frequently become inhibited and "freeze" in the presence of strangers. Elective mutism should also be considered in this category of resistances (see Pedro's case example in Chapter 1).

The examiner needs to be sensitive to the child's inner sense of internal disorganization and chaos. Children who are on the verge of a psychotic breakdown display strong denials and avoidance, with all the external appearances of resistance; this is the patient's attempt to cope with impending psychotic fragmentation.

Superficial Interviewing Obstacles

Interviewing difficulties that are readily amenable to cognitive, educational, or reassuring interventions are classified as superficial. They may be approached in the following ways:

1. The examiner should clarify the reasons for the evaluation (i.e., the contractual elements), if these reasons are unclear.
2. The examiner should stress the importance of the child's participation.
3. The examiner should deal with the deceptive issues and openly and honestly explain to the child what the evaluation entails, what may be gained by it, and how the examination may help the child.
4. The examiner should express concern and empathy for the child's plight.

Children and adolescents who display superficial obstacles commonly use a number of avoidant strategies. For instance, they commonly or repeatedly say, "I don't know," "I don't remember," "I forgot," and so on. In general, these responses indicate a deliberate decision not to participate in the interview or not to tell the truth. The examiner should not take these statements at face value. Suggested responses to these evasive and avoidant statements are

"Tell me what you know," "Tell me what you remember," or "Let's talk about what you've forgotten." Frequently, the child may give an "opening" after these simple interventions, and the interview may be elevated to a more productive level; the child may become more revealing or more straightforward, and the new material may improve the diagnostic alliance.

Children who respond to prompts or questions with repetitive or monotonous and unproductive answers such as "I forgot" and "I don't remember" are frequently lying and distorting the truth. The examiner should attempt to transform the lying into a problem for the child or into an issue that may cause problems for the child. For example, the examiner could ask the child, "What happens when you don't tell the truth?" or "What happens to you when you lie?"

Sometimes children become evasive and selective because they do not want to say anything that may jeopardize their significant others. They do not want to get anybody into trouble. Some children have been ordered not to disclose what is going on in their homes or in their lives. Abused children may have been threatened by the perpetrators not to tell anybody about the abuse. The examiner needs to be aware of this possibility.

Moderate Interviewing Obstacles

Moderate interviewing obstacles involve situations in which a great deal of externalization of blame and responsibility, overt oppositional stances, bullishness, scapegoatism, and intimidating and aggressive behaviors are present. In attempting to overcome these obstacles,

1. The examiner should follow steps 1 through 4, described in the preceding section.
2. The examiner should attempt to help the child gain insight into his or her current behavior. In a calm, nondefensive manner, the examiner may ask the child what happens at home, at school, or in other places when he or she behaves in the same manner as he or she is behaving in the office. The examiner

may also ask the child how he or she feels while behaving this way. What are the reactions of others? The child may gain some awareness of how much he or she enjoys upsetting people. The child may also state that he or she likes to be in control or that he or she protects himself or herself against the anticipation of being controlled by others. These new observations may provide an understanding of the child's problems and may provide new opportunities to establish or to further the diagnostic alliance.

3. If the previous approaches do not work, the examiner should use the oppositional behavior (or bullishness or so on) to make connections between the child's problems in the real world and what the examiner is observing during the interview. The examiner should attempt to connect the provocative enactment with the presenting problem. For example, if a provocative and oppositional child becomes defiant or evasive and keeps externalizing blame and responsibility onto others, the examiner should make the child aware of the similarities between the presenting problem that others complain about and the provocative enactment during the interview.

As the oppositional patterns of behavior unfold or begin to be enacted during the interview, the examiner must attempt to deal with such behavior by saying, for instance, "I'm having a hard time trying to understand you," or "You are giving me a very hard time." Comments like these usually elicit some affective response—a smile, a gesture of satisfaction, a sense of control, or verbalizations indicating that the child likes to be provocative or give people a hard time. When this issue is brought into the open, the examiner should interpret the child's characterological trait or transference enactment and then attempt to make the child aware of how acting out in that way can create problems for him or her. The examiner may also attempt to connect the enactment with the presenting problem, by saying, for example, "I imagine that when you act like this, you may bring problems upon yourself," or "What happens to you when you act like this?" The first intervention is more empathic, the second more confrontational. These reflective statements will place the examiner in the child's realm, in the sphere of the child's subjective state.

A similar approach could be taken in dealing with openly aggressive, provocative, or seductive children. For example: "I am beginning to see why you are here. If you behave like this at school [or at home], it's no wonder your teachers [or parents] are getting so upset or so mad at you!" This approach is the most risky because it is the most confrontational; however, if done with compassion, it may have a powerful effect. The following case example illustrates a moderate but approachable interviewing obstacle:

Carlos was a 14-year-old Hispanic adolescent with a history of severe neurodevelopmental problems, including Tourette's syndrome and developmental aphasia (with speech apraxia and fluency difficulties). Carlos also displayed psychotic features and had become aggressive at home. On several occasions he had threatened to kill his mother and her boyfriend(s). Carlos was interviewed because of complaints that he had molested a 5-year-old boy and had attempted to bite the boy's penis. In the past, there had been allegations of homosexuality and inappropriate sexual behaviors.

During the interview, Carlos displayed a great deal of shame: he tried to cover his face with either his T-shirt or his hands. Carlos was extremely self-conscious of his expressive language problems but had been able to respond to most of the questions until the examiner chose to explore the molestation.

The examiner started by saying, "Let's discuss what you did to the 5-year-old." Carlos exhibited signs of shame or embarrassment. The examiner proceeded, saying, "I understand you bit his penis." Carlos took a defensive stance and said, "I don't remember what happened." To this the examiner replied quickly, "I don't see any reason why you can't remember. You don't want to discuss this. There is no reason why you can't remember what happened." The examiner asked again, "What happened?" Carlos began to report what happened with the boy. He said that he had tried to molest a number of children before, adding, "I was going to do to other kids what was done to me."

Carlos then reported that when he was 7 years old, five or six men had raped him on a number of occasions. He said that no one knew; he had not told his mother, fearing that the disclosure could send her to the hospital. He showed significant relief after revealing this victimization. The examiner's confrontations and challenges to Carlos's defensive denials were effective and quite productive. Issues related to sexual abuse, posttraumatic stress disorder, and enactment of sexual abuse with other children had been missed previously.

The following case example illustrates the management of a moderate-to-severe interviewing obstacle through the use of confrontation, interpretation, and humor:

Jackie, a 12-year-old Caucasian girl with cerebral palsy, was evaluated for suicidal behavior. She had been living in a group home for a number of months prior to the assessment. During the 48 hours preceding the psychiatric evaluation, Jackie had put a knife, a screwdriver, and a fork to her neck. She had tried to kill herself many times before.

Jackie was not living at home because of her violent behavior toward her mother and younger sister. She also had attempted to fall from her wheelchair in an effort to harm herself. The staff at the group home felt they could no longer take care of Jackie because she was very disruptive to other children and to the program in general. Jackie claimed that she was hearing voices telling her to kill herself. She had a number of previous psychiatric hospitalizations for similar suicidal and aggressive behaviors. Jackie also had mild cognitive impairment and some degree of language disorder, in particular, expressive language difficulties related to cerebral palsy.

As soon as the examiner came into the evaluation room, he was aware of this small, spastic child in a big wheelchair. The examiner had many feelings and intuitions about Jackie's sad situation and about how much Jackie hated to be a handicapped person.

Jackie came to the evaluation accompanied by her mother and two female staff members from the group home. She had dictated a suicide note to one of the staff members the night before. When a child psychiatry fellow came into the room, just before the examiner arrived, Jackie gave the suicide note to her. She advised Jackie to give the note to the examiner, at which time Jackie crumpled up and destroyed the note.

After the examiner sat down and began the interview, Jackie kept making eye contact with one of the group home staff members, ignoring the examiner. When the examiner called her attention to this behavior, Jackie said that she was hearing voices and added that the voices were telling her not to listen to the examiner. She told one of the staff members that she could not understand the examiner because of his accent. To this, the examiner replied that he also had problems understanding Jackie (because of her expressive language difficulties), saying, "We are in the same boat." Jackie smiled and made direct eye contact with the examiner. The examiner realized that the child was very manipulative and that she could be deceptive or "tricky" throughout the interview.

As the examiner began to explore Jackie's suicidal behavior, Jackie said again that the voices were telling her not to pay attention. The examiner said, "The voices do not want you to get any help," and added, "I expect you to block the voices so we can go ahead with understanding what is the matter with you." The "voices" stopped interfering.

When Jackie was asked why she was not living with her family, she ignored the examiner again. The examiner said to Jackie in a humorous manner, "You are full of tricks," and "You are a tricky girl." Jackie smiled and began to talk about her violent behavior, emphasizing with emotion that this was why she was not living with her mother.

When the examiner asked Jackie why she was mad at her mother, Jackie became evasive and turned her head away. The examiner proposed that Jackie was mad at her mother for a number of reasons. The examiner suggested that Jackie blamed her mother for her being in the wheelchair. Jackie smiled and renewed eye contact. By this time, she had begun to use the word "trick" in a playful and insightful manner. For example, she said, "My mind plays tricks on me," to which the examiner replied, " Like when your mind tells you that the reason you aren't living with your mom is because she doesn't love you?" Jackie said that she wanted to go home. The examiner asked Jackie what was expected of her before she could go home, and Jackie said she didn't know. The examiner then advised Jackie that she could ask her mother what she was supposed to do. Jackie's mother said that they had already discussed this issue and that she expected Jackie to control her temper prior to returning home.

The examiner then focused on why Jackie wanted to kill herself. The group home staff members indicated that they had the distinct impression that Jackie believed that if she were to be expelled from the group home she would automatically be returned home. "That's not the right way to return home," the examiner told Jackie, adding, "You need to learn to control yourself first."

The examiner explored Jackie's problems with self-concept and her sense of hopelessness. He said, "You probably feel worthless and that you're not good for anything because you're in a wheelchair." He then asked Jackie, "What kinds of things are you good at?" Jackie immediately replied that she liked to take care of plants. The examiner praised her for that. The staff members added that Jackie liked listening to the radio and watching television, especially a couple of comedy programs. The examiner asserted that the reason Jackie felt worthless and suicidal was that she "blocked" the positive qualities she had and paid attention only to her limitations. The examiner added that in the same way that Jackie was able to block the voices, she would have to learn to block bad feelings about herself. The examiner continued, saying that Jackie seemed to focus mainly on her limitations and on bad aspects of herself, disregarding her strengths and that, instead, Jackie needed to pay more attention to her positive qualities and the things she could do.

Humor was used a number of times during the interview, especially when the examiner discussed how "tricky" Jackie could be and when he discussed Jackie's current use of blocking and the other kinds of blocking she needed to do. Although this interview started out with a negative, resistive, and aversive tone, it changed into a very productive exchange. Major gains were made in the therapeutic alliance. The examiner's active stance against a variety of resistances (e.g., avoidance, denial, oppositional, manipulation, dissociation, and activation of psychotic symptoms) was very productive.

After Jackie was admitted to an acute psychiatric program, her case was assigned to another psychiatrist. Jackie's mother complained about the change and asked that the examiner be in charge of the case. The examiner thought the mother was satisfied with the way he had conducted the evaluation, but he felt that Jackie should have a say in the matter. The examiner went to the unit to speak with Jackie and told her that her mother was upset because of the change of doctors. The examiner asked Jackie, "What do you have to say about this?" Jackie replied, "I kind of . . . want you to be my doctor." The examiner responded with humor, "But I gave you a hard time!" To this Jackie replied, "You helped me!" This response seemed to confirm that the interview had been effective and promoted insight.

Clinicians are very apprehensive about using confrontational techniques. Clinical observations are reassuring in this regard: Hopkinson et al. quoted Anderson as stating, "[C]onfrontations given by warm, empathic interviewers increased self-exploration, whereas this was not the effect with the interviewers who lacked these qualities" (2, p. 413). Turner and Hersen agree with the role of confrontation during the clinical interview: "Mild confrontation, when accomplished with skill and interviewer openness, will also prove to be beneficial in cutting through patient denial and defensiveness. However, the clinician will realize, with increasing experience, how far to push a given patient. Of course with aggressive patients, the issue may become one of safety for the interviewer and those others in the surroundings" (3, p. 16).

Confrontational techniques are usually contraindicated in children with severe oppositional traits and in those with very strong passive-aggressive features. In these cases, there is a risk of a hostile withdrawal or, worse, of unleashing overt aggressive behaviors. In either situation, the diagnostic alliance will be lost. Attempts to reengage these children after an episode of dyscontrol are usually unsuccessful. Confrontation should not be used in working with children who have psychosis or prominent organicity.

Children with a long-standing history of encopresis use marked denial, splitting, omnipotent control, isolation of affect, and dissociative defenses to deal with this humiliating symptom. Confrontation of these children should be avoided, as the following case example illustrates:

Billy, an intelligent 14-year-old Caucasian adolescent, presented for clinical consultation at the local state hospital. The consultation was requested because of Billy's lack of progress in the adolescent acute program and because of conflicts between the program staff and Billy's mother regarding discharge criteria. Billy had been admitted to the program for suicidal behavior and serious conflict with his siblings. Encopresis had been an important complaint, and both Billy's mother and his siblings were upset over the offensive smell and the associated behaviors. Billy had been in the hospital for almost 4 months, an unusually long stay for an acute admission. Two weeks before the consultation, Billy had been furloughed home; he was returned to the hospital 1 week later because of the encopresis. During the time that Billy stayed in the hospital, encopresis had not been active and he had denied having such a problem.

It was hard to engage Billy during the individual interview; he came across as passive and distant. Billy denied knowing why he had been in the hospital in the first place and denied knowing why he was back. The examiner's efforts to find out what was going on at home were unsuccessful. The only thing Billy was clear and explicit about was that he didn't like the hospital and wanted to go home. During the interview, Billy's only active behavior was frequent glancing at his watch. Sensing major resistance, the examiner promised that Billy would be allowed to leave in about 15 minutes. Billy responded by turning around his chair, to face away from the examiner. He slouched and stretched out in his chair, clearly conveying that he was going to sleep and that he did not want to be bothered. As Billy started to withdraw, he began to breathe deeply.

The examiner interpreted these behaviors as self-regulating mechanisms and acknowledged to Billy that he understood that he was trying to calm himself down. The examiner began to direct Billy's breathing, asking him to breathe deeply in and out. The examiner also periodically informed Billy how soon he could leave. Billy remained calmed. When the time was over, he stood up and left right away. The examiner stayed calm throughout the session and did not respond to nor confront Billy's passive-aggressive and provocative behaviors.

Encopretic patients are markedly oppositional and very passive-aggressive. In discussing the case with the staff, the examiner agreed that the best way to deal with Billy's encopresis and his denial was for Billy's mother to take him on leaves of absence, making it explicitly clear to Billy that he would be taken back to the hospital every time he became encopretic. It would thus be very hard for Billy to hold to his tenacious denial and blame the hospital for his separation from his family.

Severe Interviewing Obstacles

Children and adolescents with major behavioral and emotional problems display severe resistances. These children externalize blame and responsibility for their actions and defend themselves with very strong denials and projections. They are also mistrustful, if not overtly paranoid. The following is an example of a severe resistance:

Johnny was a 14-year-old Caucasian adolescent at the time of his diagnostic psychiatric evaluation. He had been in an unending conflict with his parents during the previous year, and the situation had deteriorated during the previous 4 months. In spite of ongoing outpatient therapy for Johnny and his family, no significant progress had been achieved. Johnny had been in a child psychiatric hospital twice when he was 8 years old. He had received antidepressants in the past, but had stopped taking medications 3 months earlier.

A couple of days before the evaluation, Johnny announced to his family that he was going to orchestrate his getting kicked out of school, and he accomplished this goal a day before the examination. Johnny had been extremely provocative at school; he had a history of multiple school suspensions for behavioral and aggressive problems. At home he was unruly: during the previous week, he had come and gone at his own will. He was defiant and had threatened to kill his mother and father many times. Two months earlier, he had taken his grandparents' van without permission and had stolen a gun from them.

During the previous 3 months, Johnny's parents had carried out the following routine before retiring at night: they unplugged the phones, collected their money and other valuables, and put a theft-deterrent device on the car to ensure that Johnny would not call gang members (with whom they suspected him of associating) or steal during the night. Johnny's parents suspected that he was associating with gang members. His mother had discovered aerosol cans in his room, and the day before the psychiatric examination, he was found with evidence of spray paint around his mouth and nostrils. When confronted, he cried and appeared remorseful, claiming that this had been the first time he had done something like this.

At age 10 years, Johnny had sustained a brain injury in a car accident. After the accident, Johnny forgot and had to relearn many things.

At the time of the evaluation, Johnny was very angry and contemptuous. He constantly externalized blame for his conspicuous acting out, not taking responsibility for his multiple transgressions. He pinned all the blame for his problems on his parents, accusing them of not loving him. He had felt unloved all his life and was quite jealous and hostile toward his younger sister; he was convinced that his parents favored her. His parents were at their "wit's end" and didn't know what to do about their son's behavior. They felt totally helpless in the face of Johnny's provocative and defiant behaviors. They also feared for their lives.

Johnny's father had been a peripheral figure in the family and in Johnny's life. He had delegated all forms of discipline to his wife, and to make matters worse, she had been incapacitated because of a fractured foot. Doctors were not optimistic about her prognosis for unassisted walking. Johnny believed that his father was his ally, and he manipulated him. Johnny's father undermined his wife's efforts to provide consistent discipline. Partly because of this perception, Johnny's hostility, antagonism, and vicious verbal attacks and intimidations of his mother had no limit.

The family's financial situation had worsened since Johnny's mother became ill. She had a highly paid, skilled job before becoming incapacitated. Johnny seemed oblivious to economic realities and continued making demands the family couldn't meet. Finally, Johnny's parents were concerned that he was turning into a delinquent and anticipated that he would end up in jail.

It may be believed that this child was anxious to leave home and that he would welcome any placement recommendations, but that was not the case. Johnny strongly rejected any suggestion of placement. Whenever placement was suggested, Johnny would blame his parents for wanting to get rid of him; obviously this baffled his parents. He threatened suicide when placement was discussed, because he wanted to continue living at home.

Johnny said that the examiner didn't like him either. From the start he didn't believe that the examiner was on his side. He doubted the examiner could help him. The examiner sensed that Johnny wanted to get into a conflict with him from the very beginning. Johnny's seemed angry; he was also depressed and labile. He denied suicidal ideation but acknowledged homicidal intentions against his parents. Johnny displayed a very rigid projective system, refused to acknowledge any responsibility for his behavior, and perseverated in blaming everything on his parents. The examiner was unable to engage Johnny and couldn't undermine his projective system.

This is a severe example of a child caught up in a very conflictive, deeply ambivalent relationship with his parents. Strong dependency and regressive tendencies opposed separation-individuation strivings. Jealousy of paranoid proportions was present. Furthermore, the previous brain trauma had left Johnny cognitively impaired, which was reflected in his rigid and narrow cognitive coping style and in his primitive defense mechanisms. Other stressors in the marriage and in the family contributed to Johnny's maladaptation. In spite of the examiner's efforts, the child rejected his suggestions of help.

The following case example illustrates a marked denial and a severe resistance with a different quality:

Robert, a 17-year-old Caucasian adolescent, was being evaluated after making a suicidal gesture. He had cut his right wrist, expressing a desire to kill himself. Six months before the evaluation, Robert had undergone an above-the-knee amputation of his left leg to prevent the spread of bone cancer. The cancer had been discovered when he was examined in the emergency room after his left foot was run over by an all-terrain vehicle. X rays taken at the time revealed the malignancy. Robert had received chemotherapy treatment, and he was using a prosthesis at the time of the psychiatric examination.

Robert had been very athletic and had participated in track and field at school. He dropped out of school after the surgery. According to Robert, the school objected to his presence because a boy on crutches "could pose liability risks." Robert had always been in special education classes for learning disabilities. When he was 10 years old, his brother (5 years his senior) "accidentally" shot him in the abdomen with a gun. The circumstances surrounding the accident were unclear. One year before the evaluation, Robert's father had left home. Robert explained that his father was gay.

Robert limped into the interviewing room, sat quietly, and displayed a polite, pleasant demeanor. When Robert was asked to explain the reasons for his being in the hospital, he said that he had tried to cut his wrist "to stop his mother from threatening suicide." He displayed an anxious and peculiar smile that had an inappropriate quality; this smile resurfaced frequently throughout the evaluation. He denied any previous suicide attempts. He added that his mother was "crazy," reporting that she yelled at herself in the mirror and had threatened suicide many times before. He made all of these statements while exhibiting bland affect and his peculiar smile.

Because the loss of his leg seemed to be such an important issue, the examiner asked Robert to describe what it was like for him to hear about the cancer. He responded in a nonchalant manner, "It was okay." When the examiner encouraged him to discuss the loss of his leg or the changes that it brought to his life, he blandly answered, while smiling, that he could no longer run or do a number of things he used to do. The examiner's multiple attempts to draw from Robert any emotional reaction regarding the loss of his leg and the impact that it had on his self-concept and self-image were met with strong denials. The examiner's use of countertransference (e.g., the sense of loss, of being handicapped, of being unattractive to the opposite sex) met with no success.

It was not surprising then that Robert's response to explorations regarding the accidental shooting by his brother, having a gay father, having a "crazy" mother, and other potentially emotion-laden experiences were met with the same blandness encountered when the examiner probed his emotional response to the loss of his leg. Robert displayed massive denials, marked isolation of affect, affect reversal or reaction formation, and repression (of aggression). He was also a very immature adolescent. Factors that may have contributed to Robert's affective disturbance were severe learning disabilities and cognitive impairments, plus major developmental problems associated with defective parenting (Robert's mother had alcoholism and abused alcohol throughout her pregnancy with him).

It is impossible to build a diagnostic and therapeutic alliance with patients who show intense mistrust (and are unable to believe in the goodness or at least in the neutrality of the examiner) as a result of strong psychopathology (e.g., severe trauma, fears of psychotic disintegration, or suspicious-paranoid behavior). When sensing panic of fragmentation in prepsychotic children, the examiner should respect the adaptive defenses and support reality testing and any efforts at self-control. Abused adolescents are very apprehensive about psychological evaluations; this makes any trustful engagement difficult. The examiner should empathize with the adolescent's feelings about previous betrayals of trust and should encourage verbalizations regarding misuse (or abuse) of prior psychological or psychiatric evaluations.

If an adolescent persists in being resistive and remains uncooperative, it is better "to lose a battle" and not "lose the war." When the accounts about the adolescent do not raise questions regarding safety to self or others, the examiner should concede that without the adolescent's participation it is impossible to reach any understanding or any conclusions. The examiner should indicate to the adolescent that without his or her participation there is no point in continuing the process. The examiner should tell the adolescent that as soon as he or she is willing, the examiner will be available for further contact and work. When the examiner deals with an uncooperative adolescent and suicidality, homicidality, or severe functional impairment secondary to mental illness is present, the examiner is obligated to pursue involuntary commitment.

■ OBSTACLES IN INTERVIEWING FAMILIES

The concept of interviewing obstacles applies equally to the family or to other complex systems. The next case example illustrates the phenomenon of defensiveness within the family system:

> Marta, a 15-year-old Mexican American adolescent, was referred to an acute psychiatric program after an almost successful suicidal attempt. She had decided to hang herself with a dog chain after a fight with her boyfriend. She was unconscious an undetermined amount of time before she was found. Marta had neither a history of suicide attempts nor a psychiatric history. She was admitted to a pediatric ward for a complete neurological assessment. A computed tomography scan of the brain was unremarkable, and a cervical spine series was normal. The extent of the neuronal damage caused by hypoxia was uncertain. A psychiatric consultation in the pediatric ward indicated severe thought disorganization and severe impairment of the sensorium, compatible with delirium.
>
> After Marta was stabilized, she was referred to the acute psychiatric unit. The referring physicians met a significant obstacle when they requested family permission for the transfer. The family insisted that there was nothing wrong with Marta, that this was an accident, that she didn't mean to kill herself, and so on. Only by using strong persuasion were the physicians able to convince the family to agree to the transfer.
>
> Marta spoke blandly about the events preceding the suicide attempt. She referred to the incident nondefensively and without any emotion. The most striking results of the mental status ex-

amination were abnormal findings in mood and affect: her affect was blunted markedly, and she was not dysphoric in any significant way. Her thought processes were unremarkable, but Marta was concrete. She denied suicidal ideation and denied that she would ever try to kill herself again. Marta did not endorse any feelings of sadness or any other depressive feelings. Her sensorium was intact at the time of the assessment.

When the family came to the acute unit, they demanded that Marta be released. They stressed, once again, that nothing was wrong with her. They said that if she were to need treatment, they would take her to the local mental heath center. Any attempt to diminish the family's resistance was unsuccessful. Marta was discharged from the acute program against medical advice.

Marta's family is by no means exceptional. In this case, denial within the family is as prevalent and as impervious as it is in the child. In severe family resistance, the identified or symptomatic child is likely a stabilizing figure in the dysfunctional family. In such cases, the family will interfere with any change in the child that may jeopardize the family's homeostasis. Gross denials are common in dysfunctional families in which the family's parental subsystem is impaired and the child is necessary to keep the family together. In severe cases of family resistance (see Johnny's and Robert's case examples earlier in this chapter), the examiner often encounters families that are chaotic and have multiple problems.

■ REFERENCES

1. Katz P: The first few minutes: the engagement of the difficult adolescent, in Adolescent Psychiatry, Vol 17. Edited by Feinstein SC. Chicago, IL, University of Chicago Press, 1990, pp 69–81
2. Hopkinson K, Cox A, Rutter M: Psychiatric interviewing techniques; III: naturalistic study: eliciting feelings. Br J Psychiatry 138:406–415, 1981
3. Turner SM, Hersen M: Interviewing process, in Diagnostic Interviewing, 2nd Edition. Edited by Hersen M, Turner SM. New York, Plenum, 1994, pp 3–24

SPECIAL SITUATIONS DURING THE PSYCHIATRIC EXAMINATION: COUNTERTRANSFERENCE

The topic of *countertransference* is discussed last because it is the most subjective and probably the most complex area of the psychiatric examination. The ideas presented here are tentative. It is hoped that these ideas will stimulate examiners to think about these difficult, intriguing, and interesting factors of the diagnostic interview. These suggestions may help evaluators to improve their interviewing skills.

The diagnostic interview is a transactional process between the child and family and the examiner. It is not surprising that during the interview process the examiner may be stimulated by a number of emotions or affective states. Sometimes patients can "infect" examiners with positive or negative emotions. Other times the examiner unexpectedly experiences unwelcome emotions during the diagnostic assessment.

Countertransference difficulties are at the root of many diagnostic and therapeutic mistakes. The experienced interviewer uses the understanding and articulation of his or her own personal affective responses during the interview to increase diagnostic information and to further the diagnostic and therapeutic alliance.

A professional attitude, the wish to help, and feelings of compassion, sensitivity, and other empathic emotions are positive affective states that aid or assist the interview process; technically, we would not call these positive emotions countertransference. In this book we define this term as the emotions or affective states that interfere with the goals of gathering diagnostic information, developing a treatment plan, and helping the patient. Any emotional state or thought process that diverts the examiner from helping the patient and his or her family in the diagnostic process will be designated as countertransference.

Countertransference occurs, for instance, when the examiner, out of frustration with the child or family, makes a hasty diagnostic closure, overlooking important diagnostic data, or when the examiner assigns a poor prognosis to a child because of an aggressive counterresponse to the child or family.

For the purposes of this chapter, we will consider the concept of countertransference in a broader sense, paralleling Khan's definition of the term, as a nonpathological capacity of the interviewer's affectivity, intelligence, and imagination to comprehend the total reality of the patient (and family) (1, p. 410). Khan's definition of the concept corresponds to contemporary meanings of the term.

Nersessian and Kopff's considerations regarding the analytic process are applicable to the psychiatric diagnostic examination. A broader definition of countertransference is considered advantageous. It is now assumed that the entire array of an examiner's emotional responses—those specifically induced by the child and the family and those brought by the examiner from his or her personal background—must be taken into account in studying the diagnostic and therapeutic process (2, p. 438).

Children with aggressive, provocative, and defiant behaviors tend to elicit primary responses in examiners; the same is true of callous and narcissistic children. Parents who are physically or sexually abusive and those who are overtly neglectful elicit strong affective responses in examiners.

Simplistic notions of the psychopathological process increase the risk of countertransference. The examiner may attribute the child's problem to the parents, thinking, for example, that the parents are bad. Alternatively the examiner might think that the child is constitutionally defective (i.e., "a bad seed"). Psychopathology is complex and multidetermined. Another conception that promotes primary responses is the attribution of linear causality. In examining interpersonal psychopathology, circular causality has a better heuristic value.

The emotions that most frequently interfere with the diagnostic interview are anger, frustration, boredom, and dislike toward the patient or family. These emotions are not difficult to identify and could be transformed and worked through productively for the benefit of the patient; however, they may interfere with the thoroughness of the diagnostic process and may contribute to diagnostic and therapeutic mistakes.

Other emotions (e.g., sexual feelings, desires to obtain gratification from the patient) are more insidious and subtler to detect; their negative influence may be more difficult to identify, understand, and transform. The examiner has more difficulties acknowledging and working through these emotions, which may be more ego-syntonic to the examiner.

Lewis discusses a number of issues that may elicit countertransference in clinicians working with children and adolescents; he also indicates common difficulties in these transactions. Aggressive children tend to mobilize strong defenses (or counter-responses) in clinicians. Mentally retarded children are often overlooked and inadequately served, and deformed children may repel some examiners (3, p. 443). Lewis lists a number of diagnostic circumstances in which the examiner's countertransference may become problematic (Table 11–1). The list by no means exhausts the range of complexities or potential complications of countertransference responses.

The management of countertransference responses is a complex area. Good self-awareness, equanimity, and extended supervision are fundamental requirements to master this problematic area. In this chapter, we will sketch only a few practical ideas for dealing with countertransference responses that may occur during the interview process.

Beginning interviewers tend to avoid or put aside any feelings or emotional reactions that patients evoke in them. These reactions are commonly disregarded; usually the interviewer finds these

TABLE 11–1.	Diagnostic circumstances in which countertransference may be problematic

Persistent difficulties in understanding the child's point of view

Failure to recognize the child's developmental level

Expectations are not commensurate to the child's developmental level

Regressive pull; identification with the child's acting out; wishes to encourage the adolescent to act out against the parents or other authority figures

Failure to understand the transference enactments of the child (i.e., misperceiving the child's relationship with the examiner or failing to detect the child's seductive behavior toward the examiner)

Reactivations of previous conflictive areas in the examiner's life (e.g., problems with aggression or sexuality) or prior problems with the parents

Reactivations of affective states in the examiner (e.g., depression or activation of affective states such as frustration, boredom, or anger)

Projection onto the child or the family of prior psychological or interpersonal problems

Need for approval from the child or the parents and repeated arguing or competing with the child or the parents

Negative response to children with certain personality traits (e.g., conduct problems, drug abuse, promiscuous behavior)

Negative reactions toward children with deficits or handicaps

Lack of understanding or dislike for parents who are neglectful or abusive

Lack of sensitivity to gender, racial, cultural, or religious differences

Source. With modifications from Lewis 1996 (3, p. 443).

feelings unacceptable to his or her professional or moral standards. The feelings thus evoked do not promote the diagnostic process. In contrast, experienced interviewers pay close attention to their subjective responses and attempt to use them to gain further information about the patient's problems. In this manner, the experienced examiner deepens his or her emotional understanding of the patient (or family) and increases his or her knowledge of the patient's pathology.

For the examiner to be able to accomplish this process in an effective and sensitive manner, he or she needs to have a good level of self-awareness and good emotional self-knowledge. The examiner needs to know his or her normal affective state and range or usual emotional tone, so that when this range or tone changes, the examiner has a sign that a particular emotional or affective state has been activated during the examination.

The examiner masters the countertransference by introspection. When the examiner's emotional tone changes in quality or intensity, the examiner needs to wonder whether he or she is taking part in a patient's emotional enactment. The examiner may suspect, then, that the patient is dramatizing or enacting an emotional transaction with the examiner. The patient may be unaware of this transaction or of his or her emotional intentions toward the examiner. In other words, the patient may be completely unaware that he or she is "reliving" an emotional script (a pattern of interaction) with the examiner. In these circumstances, the child or the family attempt to provoke particular emotional responses from the examiner. This occurs most frequently because the child or the family project certain emotional states onto the examiner (i.e., projective identification).

The examiner attempts to integrate the information gathered from his or her subjective-introspective awareness with the data obtained throughout the interview process; this is accomplished by bringing the elicited emotions into a contextual understanding. When the examiner takes into account the context in which these emotions have been activated, he or she may gain an understanding of the patient's conflictive emotions and may gain meaning from the intruding affective states.

Countertransference feelings are helpful in aiding the patient to verbalize and to understand certain emotional problems. Some patients are unable to verbalize their emotional problems for a variety of reasons; they enact or dramatize them instead. Technically, they act out the emotional conflict with the examiner rather than expressing it verbally.

By verbalizing the way the examiner feels when the patient

talks about a given problem, the examiner helps the patient become aware of affects or emotional states that he or she may be unaware of or is disconnected (i.e., dissociated) from. The interviewer may state openly that he or she feels a particular way when the patient talks about a given subject. Usually the patient responds productively to this intervention, abreacting an emotion that had been difficult to put into words, making connections with other aspects of his or her life, bringing forward new material, or reaching a new depth in understanding.

Whatever feeling is evoked during the interview (e.g., fear, anger, anxiety, sexual arousal), the examiner should attempt to make sense of it within the context of the interview. Frequently the examiner is able to feel or experience affects that the patient has difficulties acknowledging. Several situations present an opportune time for the examiner to use subjective responses to help the patient find meanings or connections that have eluded him or her: when the patient begins to display difficulties verbalizing the problem, when the examiner notices that the patient struggles to find the words to express what he or she feels, or when the patient does not make connections that are rather obvious to the examiner.

If the experienced interviewer becomes aware of a change in his or her normal affective tone, he or she begins to ask a number of private questions: "Why am I feeling angry or anxious now?" "What is it about what the patient is saying or attempting to say that makes me feel fearful or bored?" In trying to make sense of these questions, the examiner gains important information about the patient's inner conflicts.

How does the interviewer move from his or her subjective realm to the interaction and reality of the interview? When the examiner is contaminated or infected by the patient's prevailing affect, a simple sharing of the examiner's emotional state may be productive. Thus if the examiner begins to experience depression or hopelessness, he or she may disclose these feelings to the patient and may wonder aloud what they have to do with the patient's circumstances, with what the patient is talking about, or with the way the patient is feeling. The patient's response may help illuminate his or her conflicts or the source of his or her emotional problems. If the examiner feels drawn to the patient's emotional state, senses compassion for the patient's situation, or experiences a need to save or to rescue the patient, the examiner may wonder about the patient's sense of helplessness and dire need for help. If this protective feeling is activated by preschoolers or by children who have difficulties verbalizing their needs, the examiner needs to consider deprivation or neglect in the rearing environment.

Sometimes the understanding and handling of the countertransference responses is more complex, requiring careful introspection, discrimination of the examiner's affective state(s), assessment of the context of the examiner's responses, and choosing of an appropriate language to stimulate the patient's own introspective abilities.

Let's assume the interviewer begins to feel scared, and these feelings represent a change in the examiner's normal affective tone. We will discuss three approaches to deal with this emotional response. The first one is an indirect approach; the others are direct:

1. **Indirect approach.** The interviewer reflects on his fear, becoming aware that the patient has limited control over her aggressive impulses. The examiner proceeds with the interview, inquiring about the patient's sense of control when she gets angry, how close she feels to losing control when she gets upset, what things would help her to stay in control, and so on.

2. **Direct approach.** The interviewer becomes aware of her fear and tells the patient the feeling she is experiencing, by saying, for example, "As you talk about this, I am feeling scared," or "You are making me feel scared." Depending on the patient's response, the examiner may connect the interviewer's response with the presenting problem or with responses that people have when they feel scared or intimidated by the patient. For example, the examiner could say, "I wonder if this is the way some people feel about you," or, better, "I wonder if that is the way you make people feel." These two approaches are helpful when the patient is provocative or is acting out during the interview.

3. **Direct approach.** An even better alternative (applicable when the patient has difficulties connecting his feelings with his thoughts) is for the examiner to pay close attention to her own emotional reactions and attempt to link those responses to the patient's narrative. For example, if a patient begins to talk about problems with his father and the examiner senses fear, she may approach the awareness of her emotional response in the following manner: "As you begin to talk about the problems you have with your father, I began to feel fearful. Is that the way you feel about him?" Or "I am feeling fearful. Is that the way your father makes you feel?" Notice that both responses are very empathic; they connect with the patient's emotional responses. Interventions like these improve the patient's trust of the examiner and build the therapeutic alliance. This tentative exploration could be continued in many alternative ways.

When the intervention is correct and timely, the patient's response or the information that follows may validate the interviewer's assumptions through the emergence of new data. Such data may provide new diagnostic evidence, which, of course, enriches the interview process.

Sometimes the examiner is overcome by subjective responses whose meaning may be somewhat familiar. The following is an example of a drowsiness response to an overwhelming, probably hopeless, clinical situation.

> Martin, a 14-year-old Hispanic adolescent, was brought for a psychiatric reevaluation because of progressively worsening difficulties at school, including academic and behavioral problems. According to Martin's mother, school officials were fed up with Martin's lack of response to progressively harsher disciplinary measures. Martin was now scheduled to attend an alternative middle school, the most restrictive and structured form of special education programming. According to his mother, this was the last step the school would impose on him prior to expulsion. Martin's mother believed that her son was no longer wel-

come at school because he had been relentlessly provocative and didn't seem to care about the consequences of his behavior. He had earned such a poor reputation that whenever something bad happened at school, his name was at the top of the list of suspects. Martin also had a problem with stealing, and the school had pressed theft charges against him, for which he was on probation. Martin's mother had found a hiding place in one of the walls of her home, where Martin kept money he had taken from her. To complicate matters, Martin was dabbling in drugs, the extent of which his mother was unaware. He also was running around with troublesome peers and was failing most of his classes.

Martin continually argued with his mother about her rules. He told the examiner, "I would be better off if my mother stopped bothering me." His mother was concerned that he had become more isolated, that he stayed in his room a great deal, and that he appeared withdrawn and sad. He cried when he talked about his father's death. His father had died in a plane crash 3 years prior to the reexamination. Apparently his father was an experienced pilot and was giving flying instructions at the time of his death. The circumstances of the crash were unclear, and they were the subject of ongoing litigation. Martin had been a marginal student before his father's death, and he and his father reportedly had a close relationship. After his father's tragic death, Martin's life began a progressive decline: he was asked to leave a private school because of poor academic achievement, and he had been placed in the public school with the expectation that more psychoeducational resources would help him with his learning difficulties. Instead, he developed behavioral problems.

Understandably, Martin's father's death had been a shocking experience for the whole family. Martin's parents had marital difficulties and had been separated prior to the accident. Martin's mother had been devastated by the accident; she struggled with the loss and had attempted to reorganize her life by going to college. She also had started working on a law degree. Martin's only sibling was his 21-year-old sister, who was married and doing well.

Martin had a limited grief reaction after his father died. His mother had complained to the examiner that Martin had not cried during the funeral and that he was averse to talking about his father's death.

The examiner had evaluated Martin 6 months earlier for oppositional behaviors and limited interest in schoolwork. At that time, his symptoms were not as severe as they appeared during the reevaluation.

Martin's mother was very confused and was feeling overwhelmed by her son's problems and by his lack of response to the school and the family's efforts. She had some unrealistic academic expectations for him and was hoping that putting Martin back in a structured private school would get him on the right path. Martin had told his mother that he wanted to quit school. At some point during the interview, Martin's mother started crying; she confessed that she feared Martin could end up in jail.

At the time of this examination, Martin and his mother displayed behaviors that had been observed during the previous assessment: Martin sat impassively and quietly, offering no comments about any of his mother's concerns. His mother cried frequently, conveying a sense of helplessness and confusion. She was puzzled over Martin's lack of an effort to change. This small adolescent's passivity, his silent opposition, and his lack of introspective capacity had struck the examiner earlier. After hearing about the worsening of the overall symptomatology, the examiner asked Martin's mother to leave. The examiner then made an effort to engage Martin.

Soon after beginning the individual interview, the examiner began to feel so drowsy that it was very hard for him to stay awake. He was aware that he was prone to experience drowsiness when 1) the clinical situation was overwhelming (hopeless), or 2) the patient was actively opposing or resisting his efforts. After the examiner recognized his drowsiness, he attempted to understand and to mobilize the drowsiness to continue with the clinical reexamination. The examiner said to Martin, "You don't want to be here." Martin responded, "I'd rather be at home playing." The examiner asked, "What is your view? What is going on?" Martin said, "If only my mother were to leave me alone, everything would be okay." The examiner asked, "How come you are getting into so much trouble?" Martin said that he didn't know. There was a pause, after which Martin displayed a smile briefly. The examiner wondered what had made him smile, what had gone through his mind. He said, "It was funny the way you are looking at me." Martin responded, "Maybe I am running around in circles, maybe I'm confused." The examiner praised Martin for saying this. He told Martin, "This is the most honest and positive thing you have said today."

When the examiner recognized the emerging drowsiness and began to connect it to Martin's passive-resistive behavior, his drowsiness started to clear. He began to refocus his cognitive, diagnostic, and therapeutic functions on the case. In this manner, by dealing with the overt obstacle to the examination (i.e., Martin's resistance), he was able to resolve his drowsiness and regain his optimum level of awareness (see Chapter 10 for a discussion of obstacles). The examiner was able to proceed with this difficult examination.

Patients with obsessional personalities have difficulties communicating emotions and display marked isolation of affect during the psychiatric examination. They evoke a variety of countertransference responses from the examiner, as illustrated in the following case example:

Amy, a 15-year-old Caucasian adolescent, was evaluated for aggressive and destructive flare-ups. She had a history of suicidal behavior at age 11 years, and before the evaluation she had overdosed on fluoxetine. Amy was intelligent and had been in the gifted and talented program at school; however, her academic performance had deteriorated during the preceding year. When Amy was 3 years old, her 8-month-old brother drowned; he was comatose for 18 months, sustained permanent brain damage, and required intensive daily care. She was 8 years old when her parents divorced. She believed her father divorced her mother because he couldn't stand to see his "brain-damaged child." Apparently Amy's father complained that after the accident his wife focused so exclusively on the injured child that he and the other children were neglected. Amy had displayed some antisocial acting out during the previous year.

Amy was an attractive and articulate adolescent. She elaborated her thoughts with extreme ease, used sophisticated language, and described events with great detail. After interacting with her for a while, the examiner began to feel bored and became aware that he was not listening. The examiner realized that the patient was not expressing any emotions (the examiner considered that boredom was a sign that the patient was not communicating affectively). Her productions were filled with rationalizations, marked isolation of affect, displacements, intellectualizations, and strong denials. These are common defense mechanisms in obsessional character disturbances.

When the examiner became aware of his boredom difficulty, he began to pay closer attention to the process of Amy's communications and commented on it. He told Amy that she had problems expressing emotions. Amy responded positively to this simple intervention: the emotional tone of the interview changed. She began to place less emphasis on factual issues and began to verbalize more affect-laden communication. Her stiff posture, rapid speech, and dry tone changed; her demeanor softened, and she became more at ease and more animated. Also, the quality of her speech improved, becoming more melodious and lively.

Thereafter, questions with affective content were emphasized, and Amy rose to this task; however, she tended to revert to affect-less communication and to her circumstantial verbalizations. Amy displayed no emotion when narrating her brother's accident, her parents' divorce, or her problematic behavior. She displayed more affect when she was asked what kind of help she needed. She said with emotion that she needed individual therapy and therapy with her mother. She explained that she and her mother depended too much on each other. Amy struggled with her mother around issues of control and Amy's increased need for autonomy.

The preceding case example shows the constructive use of countertransference. The example also shows the importance of providing feedback on the patient's communication style, or communication process (see the "Process Interviews" section in Chapter 1). It was very helpful to indicate to the patient that she had problems dealing with her emotions.

In the next case example, the examiner experienced anger and transformed this dystonic feeling into a therapeutic understanding:

> Britt, a 13-year-old Asian American adolescent, was experiencing hallucinations and was talking about killing herself. Her school counselor had called the examiner to request an emergency evaluation. The examiner experienced anger, and instead of personally evaluating Britt, whom he had seen before, he delegated the examination to a fellow in child psychiatry. After the fellow examined Britt, she concluded that Britt needed to be in an acute psychiatric program. The fellow presented this recommendation to Britt and her mother. Upon hearing this, Britt began to cry and pleaded that she didn't need to be in the hospital. Her mother's demeanor was bland and passive, but she expressed concern about Britt's fear of hospitalization. Because Britt was so distressed about the possibility of hospitalization, the fellow presented alternatives to inpatient care. More specifically, partial hospitalization was recommended. Britt's mother remained impassive. Britt said that she wanted to see her classmates, hinting that she didn't like the partial hospitalization option either. The examiner asked the fellow to write an appropriate prescription and refer Britt for outpatient therapy. The examiner remained highly aroused with anger toward Britt's mother.
>
> The following night at 3:00 A.M. the examiner was awakened by a call not related to Britt. After answering the call, Britt's case came to the examiner's mind. He began to explore why he was so angry at Britt's mother.
>
> The examiner had evaluated Britt for the first time 6 months earlier for severe depression and a severe obsessive-compulsive disorder. At the time of the evaluation, Britt was experiencing auditory hallucinations commanding her to kill herself. Britt had severe school difficulties centered around profound immaturity and regressive behaviors; her classmates regularly teased and ridiculed her. Britt's mother was skeptical of her suicidal intentions and didn't give any credence to her hallucinations. Britt made allegations of physical abuse by her father and

claimed that her father abused alcohol. Her mother denied these complaints.

Britt was small, unattractive, inhibited, anxious, and immature. She displayed a regressed demeanor and a somewhat inappropriate affect. She endorsed a number of compulsive features, including nail biting and compulsive eating of the skin of the knuckles of both hands. The look of her hands was remarkable: the backs of both hands had large areas of denuded skin. Her mother rejected acute care or partial hospitalization options. The examiner prescribed an antidepressant and a neuroleptic. He asked Britt to report back a few weeks later. When the examiner saw Britt for the second time, Britt denied suicidal ideation, but she continued complaining of psychotic features and prominent obsessive-compulsive disorder and anxiety symptoms. There were no significant symptom changes partly because Britt had not taken the antidepressant on a consistent basis and because her mother had refused to give her the neuroleptic. The examiner experienced irritation about the lack of compliance.

Britt's school continued to express concerns about her inappropriate behaviors. School officials had also heard Britt's complaints about her father's alcohol abuse and physically abusive behaviors. When Britt's mother was presented with these allegations, she explained that these were a thing of the past, that her husband had stopped drinking a number of years earlier, and that he was not physically abusive. She also reported that her husband did not believe that Britt's condition was serious or that she needed psychiatric help. Britt was seen two times more before the latest crisis.

The examiner's introspection in the middle of the night threw light on the intense anger he had felt toward Britt's mother. He was aware that he tended to respond with anger in situations of passivity and helplessness. He came to understand his anger and frustration at the mother as a response to her passivity and helplessness regarding her husband's and daughter's difficulties. The examiner recognized that Britt's mother had been hoping her husband's alcohol abuse and physically abusive behaviors would go away. She was also hoping that Britt's symptoms were not serious and that they would go away. The examiner realized that Britt's mother had difficulties asserting herself, and this explained her passive and ineffectual behavior with her husband and her daughter.

This insight dissipated the examiner's anger. Armed with these understandings, he approached the mother in a constructive and positive manner. He made her aware of her passive and ineffectual behavior, of her wish that the problems with her husband and her daughter would go away, and of her fears of confronting her husband and her daughter. For some reason she was afraid of asserting herself with her husband and hesitated to fight for what she felt her daughter needed. She gained an understanding of her difficulties in dealing with her husband's and her daughter's problems, changed her attitude, and began to approach these difficulties in a more resolute manner.

The examiner did not direct his raw, unmetabolized anger at Britt's mother. Instead he used private, introspective work to transform the anger into a therapeutic tool. The transformation of a raw feeling (i.e., anger) into a therapeutic insight helped the examiner to help Britt's mother become a more competent parent and a more effective wife.

By using subjective feelings skillfully, the interviewer will learn something new and important about the patient's problems. A similar approach may be used when attempting to understand other feelings elicited during the interview (e.g., sadness, anger, sexual feelings). The examiner needs to integrate the subjective responses evoked during the psychiatric examination and make use of the understanding of these responses in configuring the patient's comprehensive diagnostic formulation.

■ REFERENCES

1. Khan MR: Vicissitudes of being, knowing and experiencing in the therapeutic situation, in Classics in Psychoanalytic Technique. Edited by Langs R. New York, Jason Aronson, 1981, pp 409–417
2. Nersessian E, Kopff RG: Textbook of Psychoanalysis. Washington, DC, American Psychiatric Press, 1996
3. Lewis M: Psychiatric assessment of infants, children and adolescents,

in Child and Adolescent Psychiatry; A Comprehensive Textbook, 2nd Edition. Edited by Lewis M. Baltimore, MD, Williams & Wilkins, 1996, pp 440–453

INDEX

Page numbers printed in **boldface** *type refer to tables or figures.*